Oral Implantology and Periodontology

Oral Implantology and Periodontology

Editor: Owen Richardson

MURPHY & MOORE
www.murphy-moorepublishing.com

www.murphy-moorepublishing.com

MURPHY & MOORE

Cataloging-in-Publication Data

Oral implantology and periodontology / edited by Owen Richardson.
p. cm.
Includes bibliographical references and index.
ISBN 978-1-63987-415-6
1. Dental implants. 2. Periodontics. 3. Implants, Artificial. 4. Dentistry. I. Richardson, Owen.
RK667.I45 O73 2022
617.693--dc23

Murphy & Moore Publishing,
1 Rockefeller Plaza,
New York City, NY 10020, USA

ISBN 978-1-63987-415-6 (Hardback)

Contents

Preface

In my initial years as a student, I used to run to the library at every possible instance to grab a book and learn something new. Books were my primary source of knowledge and I would not have come such a long way without all that I learnt from them. Thus, when I was approached to edit this book; I became understandably nostalgic. It was an absolute honor to be considered worthy of guiding the current generation as well as those to come. I put all my knowledge and hard work into making this book most beneficial for its readers.

Periodontology is a specialty of dentistry that is concerned with the study of the diseases and conditions affecting the supporting structures of the teeth. These supporting tissues are termed as periodontium. They include alveolar bone, gingiva, periodontal ligament and cementum. Periodontology involves the diagnosis, treatment and prevention of periodontal diseases and the placement of dental implants. Anatomically, the gingivae are broadly categorized into three categories. These are free gingiva, attached gingiva and interdental gingiva. Periodontal therapy is broadly classified into 4 phases. These are disease control phase, surgical phase, restorative phase and maintenance phase. Dental implants are surgical fixtures which are placed on the jawbone. Over a period of a few months, they are allowed to fuse with the bone. This book studies, analyses and upholds the pillars of periodontology and its utmost significance in modern times. It traces the progress of this field and highlights some of its key concepts. This book attempts to assist those with a goal of delving into the field of periodontology.

I wish to thank my publisher for supporting me at every step. I would also like to thank all the authors who have contributed their researches in this book. I hope this book will be a valuable contribution to the progress of the field.

Editor

1

Platelet-Rich Fibrin: Utilization in the Treatment of Periodontitis

Apoorv Goel, Lester Jack Windsor and Steven Blanchard

Abstract

Periodontitis is a chronic inflammatory disease affecting the supporting structures of the teeth and results in loss of supporting bone around the teeth leading to eventual tooth loss. It is a multifactorial disease that involves bacteria and host responses. Advanced options to treat periodontitis are aimed at regeneration procedures to restore lost periodontal structures. These include bone replacement grafts and the use of biological materials to enhance regeneration. Platelet-rich fibrin (PRF) is an autologous platelet-rich concentrate derived from a fibrin clot and is a natural source of growth factors derived from platelets, which are released over time and have been shown to have potential in periodontal procedures to enhance wound healing and regeneration. This chapter will focus on the past, current and future scope of PRF for treating periodontitis.

Keywords: platelet-rich fibrin, periodontitis, autologous, growth factors, regeneration, healing

1. Introduction

Blood is an integral part of the human body, which is responsible in delivering necessary nutrients and oxygen to different cells and also transports the metabolic waste products from those cells to be excreted out of the body. Blood includes four components: platelets, white blood cells (WBCs), red blood cells (RBCs) and plasma. Particularly, platelets play a major role in the release of growth factors at the site of injury to initiate wound healing [1]. Wound healing is an essential inflammatory process which requires cellular organization and remodeling, cellular migration and cellular proliferation. Platelets play a crucial role in all of these functions. Due to these properties, the concept of using platelet concentrates for therapeutic purposes was introduced. The main aim was to isolate large numbers of platelets from the whole blood and then use them to enhance the wound healing process. Initially, platelet-rich plasma (PRP) was developed for this purpose and can be considered as the first generation of the platelet concentrates. Whole blood was collected and anticoagulants (i.e., calcium chloride or bovine thrombin) were added to the blood prior to centrifugation to prevent clotting. The platelet-rich fraction was removed after the blood components were separated by centrifugation. Various studies showed that the final product after processing contained 95% platelets and played direct roles in influencing osteoblasts, periodontal ligament cells, connective tissue cells and epithelial cells [2]. Due to the lengthy centrifugation protocols, the need for specialized equipment, and the need to combine the liquid PRP with other biomaterials made it cumbersome to use in a clinical setting for outpatient oral and maxillofacial surgeries and periodontal surgical procedures. To overcome the limitations presented by PRP, the second generation of platelet concentrates (i.e., platelet-rich fibrin, PRF) was developed [3].

With the main objective of obtaining platelet concentrates without the addition of the anticoagulation agents, a new protocol was developed which included centrifuging the blood at high speed (3000 rpm) for 10 minutes to separate different components that included the heavier RBCs in the bottom of the centrifugation tube, clear serum at the top of the tube with an interposed fibrin clot layer consisting largely of platelets and WBCs [3, 4]. Because no anti-coagulation factors were used, a three-dimensional yellow fibrin clot was obtained between the two liquid layers and was termed as PRF (**Figure 1**). It was shown that approximately 97% of the platelets and >50% of the leucocytes in the blood sample were concentrated in the PRF clot and due to its additional

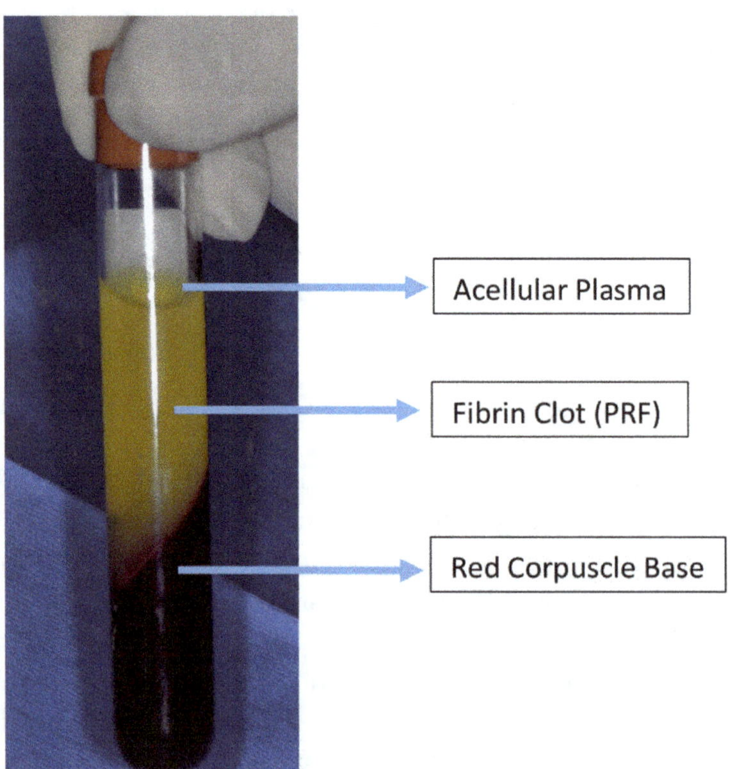

Figure 1. PRF clot after centrifugation.

leucocyte content, these platelet concentrates are also sometimes referred to as leucocyte-PRF (L-PRF) [4].

1.1. PRF processing

Intravenous blood is collected through venipuncture (superficial veins in arm: median cubital vein, cephalic vein, basilica vein or dorsal metacarpal veins) and collected in 10-ml sterile tubes without anticoagulants (**Figure 2a**). The volume of blood depends upon the application of the PRF. Immediately after collection of the venous blood, the tubes are centrifuged at specified speed and time as shown in **Figure 2b**. This centrifugation allows the formation of the fibrin-scaffold in the middle of the tube as shown in **Figures 1** and **2c**. This fibrin clot is separated from the red corpuscles base with the help of the sterile tweezers and scissors and is transferred to the sterile PRF box for compression (**Figure 2d**). The minimum compression period required is 4–5 minutes for uniform thickness. This converts the clot into PRF membrane (**Figure 2e**) which can be used for various applications in the field of periodontics as discussed later. The lower chamber of the box collects the exudate after the compression which may be used for hydration of other regenerative materials (**Figure 2f**).

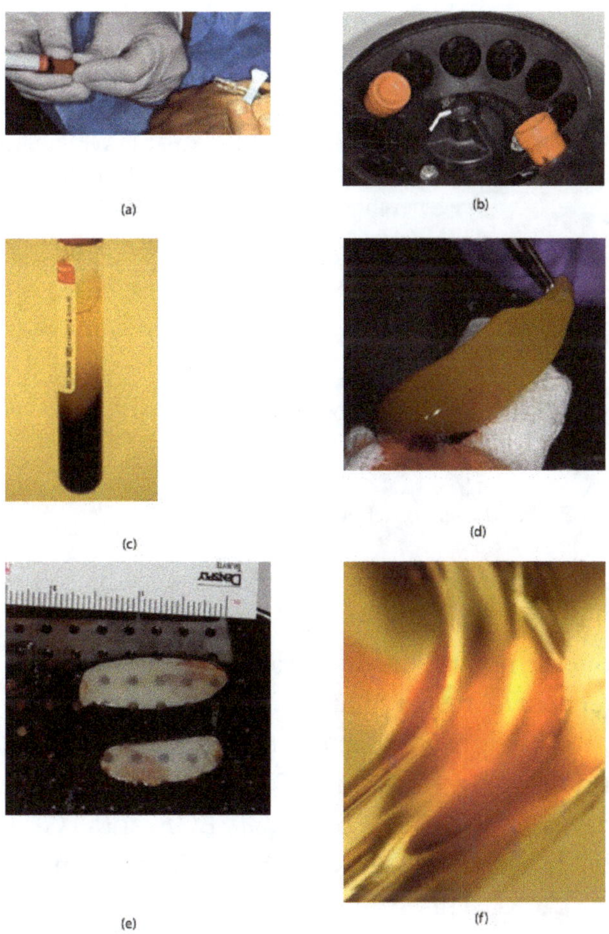

Figure 2. (a–f) PRF procedure. (a) Blood collection, (b) centrifugation, (c and d) fibrin clot, (e) PRF membrane after compression, (f) Exudate collected in lower chamber.

1.2. Properties of PRF

With the advancement and research to explore the properties of the PRF, various procedures have been established for the formulation of the PRF [5]. Studies have been carried out to evaluate the significance of different protocols which are based on different centrifugation speeds and times [5, 6]. The L-PRF procedure includes centrifugation at 2700 rpm for 12 minutes was the first well-documented procedure. It was followed by an advanced-PRF (A-PRF) procedure, which includes centrifugation at 1500 rpm for 14 minutes [5–7]. The differences in the properties due to different procedures will be discussed based on the available evidence. All three concentrates of platelets (PRP, L-PRF, and A-PRF) have been shown to release growth factors when processed as described above but each differs in its growth factor release kinetics [6]. PRFs, the most commonly studied platelet concentrate, have been shown to contain growth factors that are produced by and released from platelets including: platelet-derived growth factors (PDGFs), transforming growth factor β1 (TGF-β1), vascular endothelial growth factor (VEGF), endothelial growth factor (EGF) and insulin-like growth factors (IGFs). These are slowly released over a period of time, which may extend up to 28 days when PRF is used as the membrane to cover a periodontal defect [3, 6]. The primary functions of each growth factor are discussed in **Table 1**.

Growth factor	Functions
Platelet-derived growth factors (PDGFs)	Specific roles include proliferation of cells, cellular migration and collagen production for remodeling of extra-cellular matrix to repair the wound.
Transforming growth factor β1 (TGF-β1)	Tissue repair, extracellular matrix synthesis and immune modulation. Specific roles played by TGF-β1 includes angiogenesis, re-epithelization and regeneration of connective tissue. Due to bone morphogenetic proteins (BMPs) being part of TGF family. They also play role in bone formation.
Vascular endothelial growth factor (VEGF)	Primary function is angiogenesis. Also, plays a role in tissue remodeling.
Endothelial growth factor (EGF)	Proliferation and multiplication of endothelial and mesenchymal cells, which leads to epithelization.
Insulin-like growth factors (IGFs)	Cell-protective in nature and participates in proliferation and differentiation of a variety of cells.

Table 1. Growth factors found in PRF and their functions.

The most important aspect of PRF is growth factor release, which is why PRFs are being used as a material to promote healing and regeneration of tissues. Information about the number of growth factors released over time will aid in understanding the roles played by PRF in tissue repair. The most comprehensive research in this regard was done by Kobayashi and co-workers [6]. They evaluated the growth factor release from PRP, L-PRF, and A-PRF over a period of 10 days and found that L-PRFs and A-PRFs released significantly higher amounts of growth factors compared to PRPs. PDGF, VEGF, IGF, EGF, and TGF-β1 were evaluated in this study [6]. The same study showed that A-PRF had significantly more growth factor at 1, 3 or 10 days when compared to L-PRF. This study demonstrated that second-generation PRFs were superior over first-generation PRP with respect to the number of growth factors released and A-PRF (low centrifugation concept) can enhance the level of growth factors entrapped in the fibrin clot.

To understand the roles of PRFs in the wound healing process, it is important to understand the biological properties of PRFs. It is important to study how the fibrin network releases growth factors over time leading to enhanced cell migration and proliferation, and thus cell maturation. The periodontium is a unique complex structure of soft and hard tissues consisting of gingival connective tissue, periodontal ligament tissue, cementum and bone that tends to repair and heal by collagenous fibrous tissue reformation and maturation. One of the important factors responsible for regeneration of the periodontal structures involves periodontal ligament cells. Periodontal ligament cells primarily consist of periodontal ligament fibroblasts, which play a key role in the maintenance of periodontal health as they are responsible for formation and remodeling of alveolar bone in the development of periodontitis [8]. Also, studies have found that human periodontal ligament fibroblasts (HPLFs) form a heterogeneous population, whereas some cells exhibit phenotypic characteristics of osteoblast-like cells which might have the potential to further differentiate to osteoprogenitor cells leading to osteoblasts or cementoblasts [8]. Another important cell type which aids in the maintenance of the periodontal structures along with HPLFs is human gingival fibroblasts (HGFs), which are abundantly present in the gingival tissue and support the periodontal tissues. It is important to understand how PRF biologically affects both HPLF and HGF. Chang and co-workers [9] investigated the effects of PRF from healthy individuals on HPLF. They measured the expression of phosphorylated extracellular signal-regulated protein kinase (p-ERK), osteoprotegerin (OPG) and alkaline phosphatase (ALP) activity. This study showed that PRF significantly increased ERK phosphorylation and OPG in HPLF in a time-dependent manner, along with upregulated ALP activity. This demonstrated that PRF may provide benefits for periodontal tissue regeneration. Another study by Vahabi et al. [10] showed that PRF when cultured along with HGF for a period of 24, 48 or 72 hours and evaluated through a methyl thiazol tetrazolium assay led to statistically significant proliferation of HGF at 24 hours, but no proliferation of HGF was observed at 48 and 72 hours along with the viability of the cells also decreasing with time. The explanation for proliferation seen up to 24 hours could co-relate with the maximum number of HGF being reached per available area. More recently, Fujioka-Kobayashi et al. [11] compared L-PRF and A-PRF with regards to their effects on HGF proliferation and viability. They used the same assay as mentioned in the Vahabi study [10] to measure proliferation, but additionally, they performed real-time PCR analysis where RNA was harvested from HGF samples to assess RNA levels of PDGF, TGF-beta, and collagen type I. This study demonstrated a 200% increase in the proliferation of HGF when combined with PRF at 24 hours and increased cellular proliferation was noted with increased numbers of cells at 3 and 5 days. A significant increase in growth factor levels was seen in the culture when combined with PRF. All of this data supports that PRFs can play a significant role in the healing and regeneration of periodontal structures when used as biological modifier during periodontal and oral-maxillofacial surgeries.

2. Applications of PRF: an overview

A true regenerative procedure in periodontology includes regeneration of both soft tissues (periodontal ligament) and mineralized tissues (cementum and alveolar bone) [12, 13].

Guided tissue regeneration (GTR) procedures are advocated for regeneration of periodontal defects and involve the use of barrier membranes which prevents the downgrowth of the epithelium and excludes gingival connective from the healing wound to allow selective cell repopulation from the periodontal ligament in alveolar bone. The barrier membranes can be bioresorbable (made of collagen material) or non-bioresorbable (made of polytetrafluoroethylene material) and studies have shown that resorbable membranes show comparable results with fewer post-surgical complications for GTR procedures when compared to non-resorbable membranes [12, 14]. Some periodontal regenerative techniques include using bone replacement grafts like demineralized freeze-dried bone allograft or biological modifiers (i.e. enamel matrix derivative and recombinant human platelet-derived growth factor-BB) [15–17]. These commercially available growth modifiers have been shown to have significant roles in stimulating wound healing and tissue regeneration [12]. PRFs can be used as a potential barrier membrane with enhanced wound healing properties due to its rich growth factors content [7]. PRF membranes can be used as an adjunct in the future implant site preparation [18, 19]. Subepithelial connective tissue grafts (SCTGs) are considered to be the gold standard for root coverage procedures but involve a second surgical site in the oral cavity to harvest the graft [20, 21]. The use of PRF for root coverage procedures has been shown to be an alternative to the SCTG for root coverage procedures with reduced patient post-surgical discomfort [22, 23].

2.1. Management of extraction sockets with PRF

Following tooth extraction, alveolar bone dimensions are reduced both in vertical and horizontal dimensions as part of the normal healing process [24]. Various treatment interventions have been carried out to reduce changes in post-extraction alveolar ridge dimensions either for esthetic purposes or for future implant placement [25]. Treatment options which include use of allograft or xenograft bone graft materials with or without barrier membranes have shown positive results in preventing alveolar ridge collapse when compared to sites without any intervention [25]. Considering the beneficial properties of the PRF, it has been used as an adjunct in socket grafting procedures with or without bone graft material to improve the healing and maintenance of the alveolar ridge dimensions [18, 26]. Groups treated with the PRF showed better results when compared to the non-grafted control groups with respect to vertical and horizontal dimensions of the alveolar ridge with less discomfort and better clinical and histological healing pattern in the socket [18, 26, 27]. **Figure 3** shows a clinical case of a patient with a non-restorable molar seeking future implant placement. The tooth was extracted and the socket was filled with allograft bone particles and covered with a PRF membrane. Healing at 1 week (**Figure 3d**) demonstrated enhanced soft tissue healing over the socket with no reported patient discomfort.

2.2. Guided bone regeneration (GBR) with PRF

Edentulism for long periods or following trauma can cause ridge deficiencies that are not suitable for implant placement. GBR procedures using barrier membranes and bone grafts

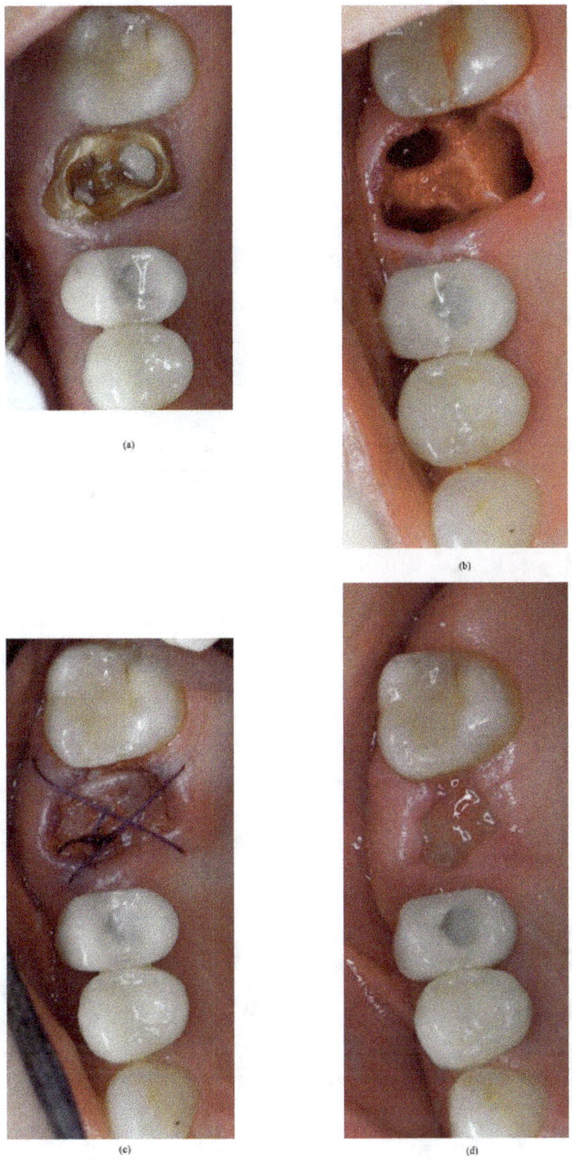

Figure 3. Management of extraction socket and site preparation for future implant placement. (a) Hopeless #30 to be replaced with dental implant, (b) Atraumatic surgical extraction, (c) allograft bone graft placed in the socket for space maintenance and covered with PRF membrane, (d) healing at 1 week with visible PRF membrane.

bone regeneration have shown good clinical outcomes [28, 29] and successful long-term results with implants placed in the regenerated bone [30]. Based on the defect size and the required amount of bone to be regenerated, a decision tree is available in the literature which helps the clinician to decide on the GBR technique [31]. Although GBR procedures for horizontal bone augmentation have shown predictable results, there are multiple reported complications associated with such procedures which can lead to poor or failed treatment outcomes [32]. The most common wound healing complication reported is membrane exposure which can eventually lead to treatment failure or infection [32]. The membrane exposures can happen either due to the insufficient blood supply to the flaps leading to necrosis or due to the inability of achieving and maintaining passive primary closure of the flaps [32]. PRF can be used as an adjunct in such procedures to enhance healing and regeneration [7, 19, 27]. The patient illustrated below (**Figure 4**) presented with insufficient bone dimensions for implant placement and underwent a GBR procedure with PRF as an adjunct with resultant good healing without any reported discomfort.

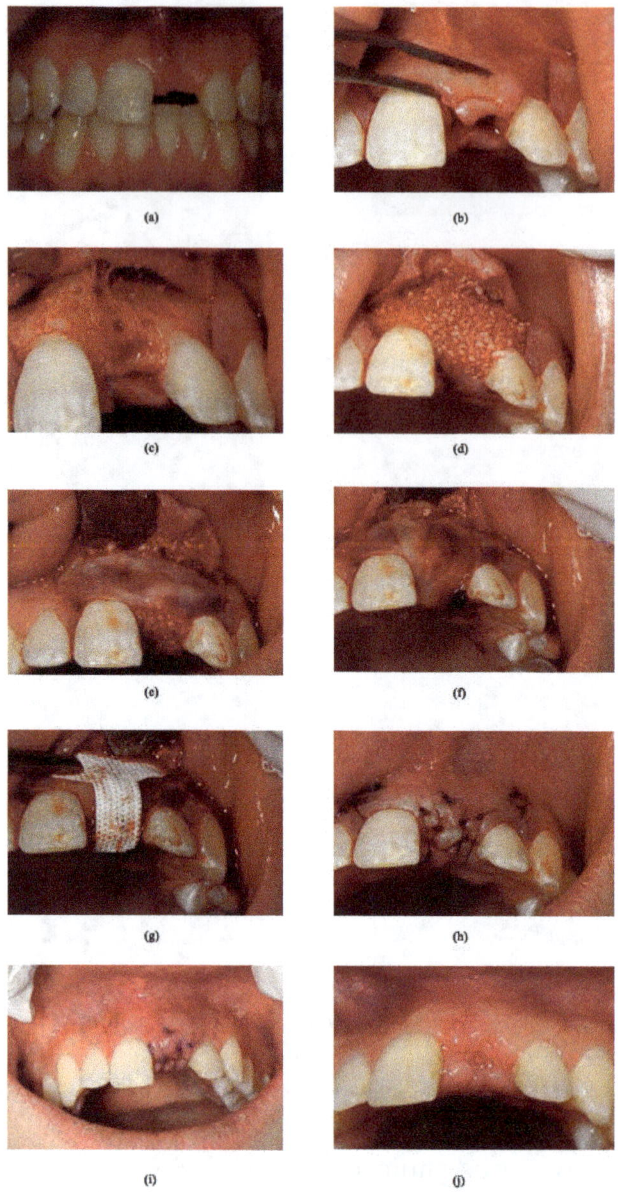

Figure 4. GBR at site #9 for future implant placement. (a) #9 Edentulous site with insufficient bone for implant placement, (b) incisions, (c) defect with decortications, (d) particulate bone allograft to fill the defect, (e) PRF membrane placed horizontally over the bone graft. (f) Second PRF membrane placed vertically, (g) titanium-reinforced d-PTFE membrane for space maintenance placed over the PRF membrane, (h) primary closure achieved, (i) healing at 1 week, (j) healing at 4-months after titanium-reinforced d-PTFE membrane removal.

2.3. PRF used in sinus procedures

The edentulous posterior maxilla can be a challenging site to restore with implants due to alveolar ridge resorption and the presence of maxillary sinus pneumatization which tends to increase over time. Sinus augmentation procedures are the treatment of choice to restore posterior maxilla with deficient bone height due to sinus pneumatization [33]. The two most common sinus augmentation procedures include the osteotome sinus augmentation and lateral window sinus augmentation with a common goal of increasing vertical bone dimensions. Both the procedures have shown high long-term implant survival rates following sinus augmentation [33]. Due to the healing and regenerative properties of PRF, it has been incorporated into sinus procedures: as a sole grafting material, in combination with allograft and xenograft material, as a membrane to cover the graft material, and to repair intra-operative Schneiderian membrane perforations [34–36]. PRF when used either as a sole grafting material or in combination with other materials have shown positive and promising results with respect to faster healing and maturation of bone [35]. The case demonstrated below (**Figure 5**) shows the use of

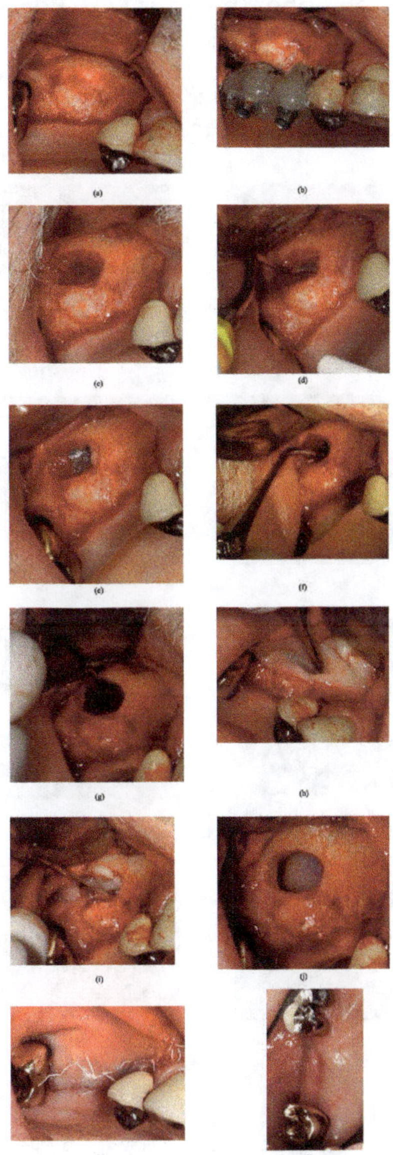

Figure 5. Lateral window sinus augmentation procedure to place implants at #3 and 4, due to insufficient vertical height. (a) Full thickness mucoperiosteal flap reflection, (b) surgical guide at place to guide lateral window position, (c) lateral window ostectomy created, (d) sinus elevator used to elevate Schneiderian membrane, (e) intact Schneiderian membrane, (f) accidental Schneiderian membrane perforation, (g) Schneiderian membrane perforation, (h) PRF membrane used to repair Schneiderian membrane, (i) second PRF membrane to provide stability and maintaining integrity of the perforated Schneiderian membrane, (j) Schneiderian membrane repaired, (k) primary closure achieved, (l) healing at 2-weeks.

PRF to reconstruct a Schneiderian membrane perforation, the most common intra-operative complication of the lateral window sinus augmentation technique [37].

2.4. Root coverage procedure with PRF

Another aspect of the periodontal therapy is the treatment of mucogingival defects which refers to gingival recession leading to root exposure. Gingival recession and root exposure can lead to sensitivity and esthetic concerns for the patient. A systematic review has shown predictable results with root coverage procedures for Miller Class I and Class II defects [21]. The most predictable results have been shown when SCTG is used as a material for root coverage procedure along with the coronal advancement of the flaps [21]. For harvesting connective tissue graft, a second surgical site (i.e. palate or tuberosity region) is needed in the oral cavity which leads to increased patient discomfort. Clinical studies have shown similar results to SCTG when PRF is used as a material for root coverage procedures [22, 23]. **Figure 6** shows a successful root

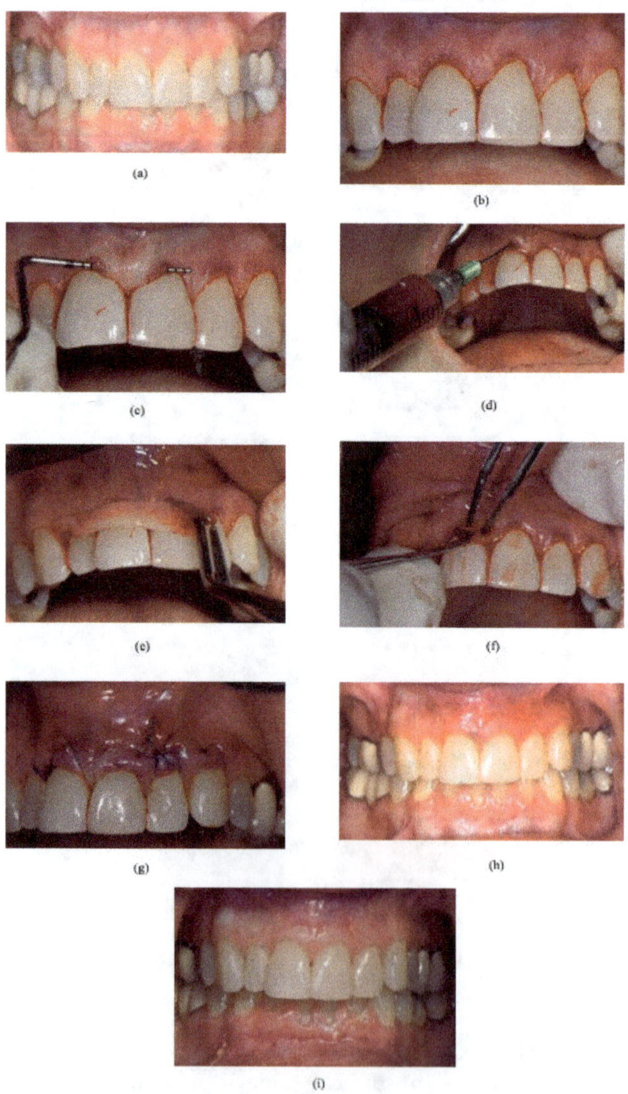

Figure 6. Root coverage procedure for #7–11. (a) Gingival recession shown from #7–11, (b, c) tunnel preparation shown for PRF placement, (d) Exudate collected after fibrin clot compression used to irrigate the site, (e) PRF membrane shown over the site, (f) PRF membrane placed in the tunnel, (g) soft tissue is coronally advanced with the help of sutures, (h) healing at 2 weeks, (i) stable root coverage at 3 months.

coverage procedure when PRF is tunneled and flap is coronally advanced. Healing and root coverage is stable at 3 months (**Figure 6i**).

3. Future scope and conclusion

The current research on PRF focuses on the clinical applications of the PRF in periodontology and implant dentistry and has shown promising results with better healing outcomes and less patient discomfort. At the same time, there is need to evaluate the properties of PRF which includes quantification of growth factors and the number of growth factors released from PRF over time. It is important to study the variables including age, sex, and the influence of any systemic disease on PRF quality. Further research is also needed on different formulation of the platelet concentrates to make it optimize its use for different procedures.

Overall, PRF can be utilized for many periodontal and implant procedures capitalizing on taking advantage of considering (1) the use of an autologous source, (2) enhanced healing and regeneration potential, and (3) a less expensive alternative to other commercially available biological modifiers.

Acknowledgements

We would like to acknowledge and thank Dr. Justin J. Villanueva, DMD, DHL and Dr. Srividya Prabhu, DMD for sharing the clinical cases and their valuable suggestions.

Author details

Apoorv Goel, Lester Jack Windsor* and Steven Blanchard

*Address all correspondence to: ljwindso@iu.edu

Indiana University School of Dentistry, Indianapolis, USA

References

[1] Gawaz M, Vogel S. Platelets in tissue repair: Control of apoptosis and interactions with regenerative cells. Blood. 2013;**122**(15):2550-2554

[2] Marx RE. Platelet-rich plasma: Evidence to support its use. Journal of Oral and Maxillofacial Surgery. 2004;**62**(4):489-496

[3] Dohan DM et al. Platelet-rich fibrin (PRF): A second-generation platelet concentrate. Part I: Technological concepts and evolution. Oral Surgery, Oral Medicine, Oral Pathology, Oral Radiology, and Endodontology. 2006;**101**(3):e37-e44

[4] Dohan Ehrenfest DM et al. Three-dimensional architecture and cell composition of a Choukroun's platelet-rich fibrin clot and membrane. Journal of Periodontology. 2010; **81**(4):546-555

[5] Ghanaati S et al. Advanced platelet-rich fibrin: A new concept for cell-based tissue engineering by means of inflammatory cells. The Journal of Oral Implantology. 2014;**40**(6):679-689

[6] Kobayashi E et al. Comparative release of growth factors from PRP, PRF, and advanced-PRF. Clinical Oral Investigations. 2016;**20**(9):2353-2360

[7] Choukroun J et al. Platelet-rich fibrin (PRF): A second-generation platelet concentrate. Part IV: Clinical effects on tissue healing. Oral Surgery, Oral Medicine, Oral Pathology, Oral Radiology, and Endodontology. 2006;**101**(3):e56-e60

[8] Basdra EK, Komposch G. Osteoblast-like properties of human periodontal ligament cells: An in vitro analysis. European Journal of Orthodontics. 1997;**19**(6):615-621

[9] Chang YC, Zhao JH. Effects of platelet-rich fibrin on human periodontal ligament fibroblasts and application for periodontal infrabony defects. Australian Dental Journal. 2011; **56**(4):365-371

[10] Vahabi S et al. Effects of plasma rich in growth factors and platelet-rich fibrin on proliferation and viability of human gingival fibroblasts. Journal of Dentistry (Tehran). 2015;**12**(7): 504-512

[11] Fujioka-Kobayashi M et al. Optimized platelet-rich fibrin with the low-speed concept: Growth factor release, biocompatibility, and cellular response. Journal of Periodontology. 2017;**88**(1):112-121

[12] Reynolds MA et al. Periodontal regeneration – intrabony defects: A consensus report from the AAP regeneration workshop. Journal of Periodontology. 2015;**86**(2 Suppl):S105-S107

[13] Reddy MS et al. Periodontal regeneration – furcation defects: A consensus report from the AAP regeneration workshop. Journal of Periodontology. 2015;**86**(2 Suppl):S131-S133

[14] Avila-Ortiz G, De Buitrago JG, Reddy MS. Periodontal regeneration – furcation defects: A systematic review from the AAP regeneration workshop. Journal of Periodontology. 2015; **86**(2 Suppl):S108-S130

[15] Wu YC et al. Comparisons of periodontal regenerative therapies: A meta-analysis on the long-term efficacy. Journal of Clinical Periodontology. 2017;**44**(5):511-519

[16] Nevins M et al. Platelet-derived growth factor promotes periodontal regeneration in localized osseous defects: 36-month extension results from a randomized, controlled, double-masked clinical trial. Journal of Periodontology. 2013;**84**(4):456-464

[17] Suarez-Lopez Del Amo F et al. Biologic agents for periodontal regeneration and implant site development. BioMed Research International. 2015;**2015**:957518

[18] Hauser F et al. Clinical and histological evaluation of postextraction platelet-rich fibrin socket filling: A prospective randomized controlled study. Implant Dentistry. 2013;**22**(3): 295-303

[19] Simonpieri A et al. Current knowledge and perspectives for the use of platelet-rich plasma (PRP) and platelet-rich fibrin (PRF) in oral and maxillofacial surgery part 2: Bone graft, implant and reconstructive surgery. Current Pharmaceutical Biotechnology. 2012;**13**(7): 1231-1256

[20] Chambrone L et al. Root-coverage procedures for the treatment of localized recession-type defects: A Cochrane systematic review. Journal of Periodontology. 2010;**81**(4):452-478

[21] Chambrone L, Tatakis DN. Periodontal soft tissue root coverage procedures: A systematic review from the AAP regeneration workshop. Journal of Periodontology. 2015;**86**(2-s): S8-S51

[22] Jankovic S et al. Use of platelet-rich fibrin membrane following treatment of gingival recession: A randomized clinical trial. The International Journal of Periodontics & Restorative Dentistry. 2012;**32**(2):e41-e50

[23] Oncu E. The use of platelet-rich fibrin versus subepithelial connective tissue graft in treatment of multiple gingival recessions: A randomized clinical trial. The International Journal of Periodontics & Restorative Dentistry. 2017;**37**(2):265-271

[24] Van der Weijden F, Dell'Acqua F, Slot DE. Alveolar bone dimensional changes of post-extraction sockets in humans: A systematic review. Journal of Clinical Periodontology. 2009;**36**(12):1048-1058

[25] Morjaria KR, Wilson R, Palmer RM. Bone healing after tooth extraction with or without an intervention: A systematic review of randomized controlled trials. Clinical Implant Dentistry and Related Research. 2014;**16**(1):1-20

[26] Temmerman A et al. The use of leucocyte and platelet-rich fibrin in socket management and ridge preservation: A split-mouth, randomized, controlled clinical trial. Journal of Clinical Periodontology. 2016;**43**(11):990-999

[27] Del Corso M et al. Current knowledge and perspectives for the use of platelet-rich plasma (PRP) and platelet-rich fibrin (PRF) in oral and maxillofacial surgery part 1: Periodontal and dentoalveolar surgery. Current Pharmaceutical Biotechnology. 2012; **13**(7):1207-1230

[28] Wessing B, Lettner S, Zechner W. Guided bone regeneration with collagen membranes and particulate graft materials: A systematic review and meta-analysis. The International Journal of Oral & Maxillofacial Implants. 2018;**33**(1):87-100

[29] Benic GI, Hammerle CH. Horizontal bone augmentation by means of guided bone regeneration. Periodontology 2000. 2014;**66**(1):13-40

[30] Jung RE et al. Long-term outcome of implants placed with guided bone regeneration (GBR) using resorbable and non-resorbable membranes after 12–14 years. Clinical Oral Implants Research. 2013;**24**(10):1065-1073

[31] Fu JH, Wang HL. Horizontal bone augmentation: The decision tree. The International Journal of Periodontics & Restorative Dentistry. 2011;**31**(4):429-436

[32] Lim G et al. Wound healing complications following guided bone regeneration for ridge augmentation: A systematic review and meta-analysis. The International Journal of Oral & Maxillofacial Implants. 2018;**33**(1):41-50

[33] Corbella S, Taschieri S, Del Fabbro M. Long-term outcomes for the treatment of atrophic posterior maxilla: A systematic review of literature. Clinical Implant Dentistry and Related Research. 2015;**17**(1):120-132

[34] Choukroun J et al. Platelet-rich fibrin (PRF): A second-generation platelet concentrate. Part V: Histologic evaluations of PRF effects on bone allograft maturation in sinus lift. Oral Surgery, Oral Medicine, Oral Pathology, Oral Radiology, and Endodontics. 2006;**101**(3): 299-303

[35] Ali S, Bakry SA, Abd-Elhakam H. Platelet-rich fibrin in maxillary sinus augmentation: A systematic review. The Journal of Oral Implantology. 2015;**41**(6):746-753

[36] Tajima N et al. Evaluation of sinus floor augmentation with simultaneous implant placement using platelet-rich fibrin as sole grafting material. The International Journal of Oral & Maxillofacial Implants. 2013;**28**(1):77-83

[37] Geminiani A et al. A meta-analysis of complications during sinus augmentation procedure. Quintessence International. 2017;**48**(3):231-240

2

Aggressive Periodontitis

Aysan Lektemur Alpan

Abstract

Aggressive periodontitis (AgP) is a disease characterized by rapid loss of periodontal tissues affecting systemically healthy individuals under age of 30 years. AgP classified into two categories named localized and generalized aggressive periodontitis. It differs from chronic periodontitis (CP) depending on age of onset of the disease, rate of progression of the disease, structure and composition of the associated subgingival microflora, changes in host response and familial predisposition. Tissue destruction in patients with AgP is not directly related to bacterial deposits also personal immune response plays a major role in severity of destruction. Surgical and non-surgical techniques can be applied in the treatment of AgP. It is important to treat and obtain frequent controls of individuals with AgP. The main purpose of the treatment is to create a clinical condition that can hold the largest number of teeth in the mouth. After the treatment performed and provided the health of periodontal tissues, patient should be included in the maintenance program.

Keywords: aggressive periodontitis, generalized aggressive periodontitis, genetics, familial predisposition, localized aggressive periodontitis

1. Introduction

Aggressive periodontitis (AgP) is a disease characterized by rapid loss of periodontal tissues affecting systemically healthy individuals during adolescence and adulthood, and forms a group of periodontal diseases [1]. It differs from chronic periodontitis (CP) depending on age of onset of the disease, rate of progression of the disease, structure and composition of the associated subgingival microflora, changes in host response and familial predisposition.

AgP classified into two categories named localized and generalized aggressive periodontitis [2] and took place prepubertal, juvenile, rapidly progressive periodontitis in the group that was defined as early onset periodontitis in 1999 International Workshop for a Classification of Periodontal Disease and Conditions [1]. This report defined some characteristic features of the AgP [2, 3].

- Patients are clinically healthy, except for the presence of periodontitis.
- Rapid attachment loss and bone destruction.
- Familial aggregation.

Secondary features that are often, but not always, present include the following:

- The amounts of microbial deposits are inconsistent with the severity of periodontal tissue destruction.
- Elevated proportions of *Actinobacillus actinomycetemcomitans* (*A. actinomycetemcomitans*) which is now termed *Aggregatibacter actinomycetemcomitans.*
- Elevated proportions of *Porphyromonas gingivalis* (*P. gingivalis*) in some populations.
- Phagocyte abnormalities.
- A hyper-responsive macrophage phenotype, including elevated levels of prostaglandin E2 and interleukin-1β.

2. Localized aggressive periodontitis (LAgP)

2.1. Clinical features

LAgP starts at a much earlier age than CP, but it is not right to go to a certain age limit. The age of onset of the disease can help us diagnose the disease [4]. There is no significant subgingival and supragingival calculus in patients with LAgP. Lesions are mostly associated with the biofilm layer. In the form of LAgP there is little or no inflammation of the gums [5, 6]. During this period gingival hyperplasia depending on dental plaque and/or calculus rarely appears [6]. It is characterized by rapid bone loss in the first molar and incisors [7]. In this disease, there are at least two permanent teeth involvement, one of them must be the first molar, and involving no more than two teeth other than first molars and incisors [8]. Powerful serum antibody response to infecting agents and circumpubertal onset are among disease features [3]. According to the workshop in 1999, if the involvement is less than 30%, the disease is localized, if it is not, considered as generalize [1]. During the disease bone loss in the first molar region is symmetric [9]. Patients with LAgP between the ages of 21–35 are those who have not been diagnosed and treated before, depending on the severity of the disease and previous treatments, tooth loss, bone defects and gingival recessions are observed [6, 7].

The following reasons have been proposed regarding the limited localization of lesions in AgP [8].

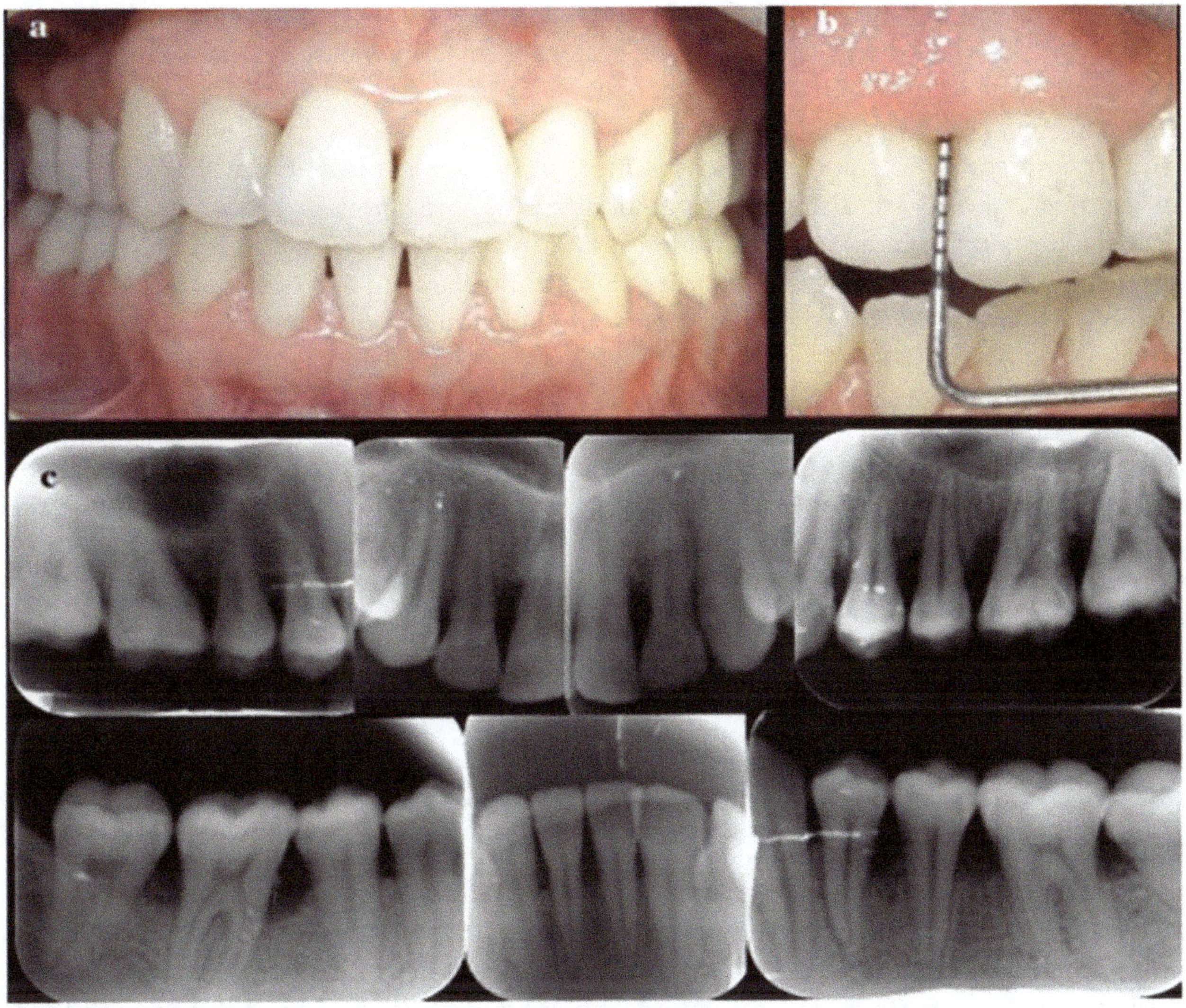

Figure 1. LAgP patient; (a)-clinical view of the LAgP patient, (b) 7 mm probing depth at distal of the incisor tooth, (c) radiographic view of the LAgP patient.

1. *A. actinomycetemcomitans* affects the host response in many ways after colonization in first molars and incisors:
    - *A actinomycetemcomitans* secretes a factor that inhibits Polymorphonuclear leukocytes (PMNL) chemotaxis.
    - *A actinomycetemcomitans* secretes some factors such as endotoxin, collagenase and leukotoxin to facilitate the colonization of bacteria in the periodontal pocket and cause destruction of periodontal tissues.
2. Antagonistic bacteria against to *A. actinomycetemcomitans*. Colonize the periodontal tissues and prevent the colonization of *A. actinomycetemcomitans* in other areas of the mouth. This situation leads the localization of infection and tissue destruction.
3. For unknown reasons, *A. actinomycetemcomitans* may lose its ability to produce leukotoxin. In this case, the disease progression slows down and colonization of new areas is prevented.

4. The possibility that the cement formation is defective and may also cause the lesions to be localized. The hypoplasia or aplastic cement formation was seen in the examinations performed on teeth withdrawn from patients with LAgP.

LAgP progresses rapidly and bone loss is three to four times greater than CP. Other clinical features of LAgP are distolabial migrations of the upper incisor teeth and consequent diestema formation, increased mobility in the first molars, tenderness on the uncovered root surfaces, deep pain spreading in every direction during chewing that does not last so long. In this phase, periodontal abscess and regional lymphadenopathy may occur [8].

2.2. Radiographic features

The classic feature of LAgP is the vertical bone loss seen in alveolar bone in the first molar and incisor teeth in healthy teenagers. Radiographic finding may include an arc shaped alveolar bone loss extending from the distal surface of the premolar to the mesial surface of the second molar. In this disease bone loss usually wider than CP [8] (**Figure 1**).

3. Generalized aggressive periodontitis (GAgP)

3.1. Clinical features

GAgP; is characterized by diffuse attachment and bone loss affecting at least three permanent teeth other than first molar and incisor teeth, usually seen in young adults, where poor serum antibody responses to infectious agents occur [10]. The GAgP may begin as localized and become more generalized as more teeth are affected over time. The disease remained active and passive periods. The rate of attachment and bone loss is not the same at these times. Dark red and ulcerated areas are characterized by severe acute inflammatory disease table is detected during the active phase. The condition is accompanied by bleeding which usually occurs with light stimulation and discharge of the pus. Severe attachment and bone loss occur during this period of the disease [10, 11]. GAgP sometimes accompanied by systemic findings such as weight loss, mental depression and fatigue [12]. Also, GAgP has been implicated in the pathogenesis of systemic diseases such as uncontrolled diabetes mellitus, AIDS, leukemia, neutropenia, histiocytosis X, syndromes such as Papillon-Lefevre or Cheidak-Higashi, rare inherited diseases such as hypophosphatasia and intraoral symptom of acquired disorders such as granulocytopenia [13]. In the passive period, the clinical image is especially similar to that of healthy individuals in terms of color, shape and consistency. However, deep periodontal pockets are encountered in the probing. It has been stated that Gram(−) microorganisms play a role mostly in microbial dental plaque (MDP). Pathogenic microorganisms, especially *P. gingivalis* and *Tannerella forsythensis* (*T. forsythensis*) are related to disease progression [10, 11]. Patients also had increased antibody response against *A. Actinomycetemcomitans*, *Prevotella intermedia* (*P. intermedia*) and *Campylobacter rectus (C. rectus)* [14].

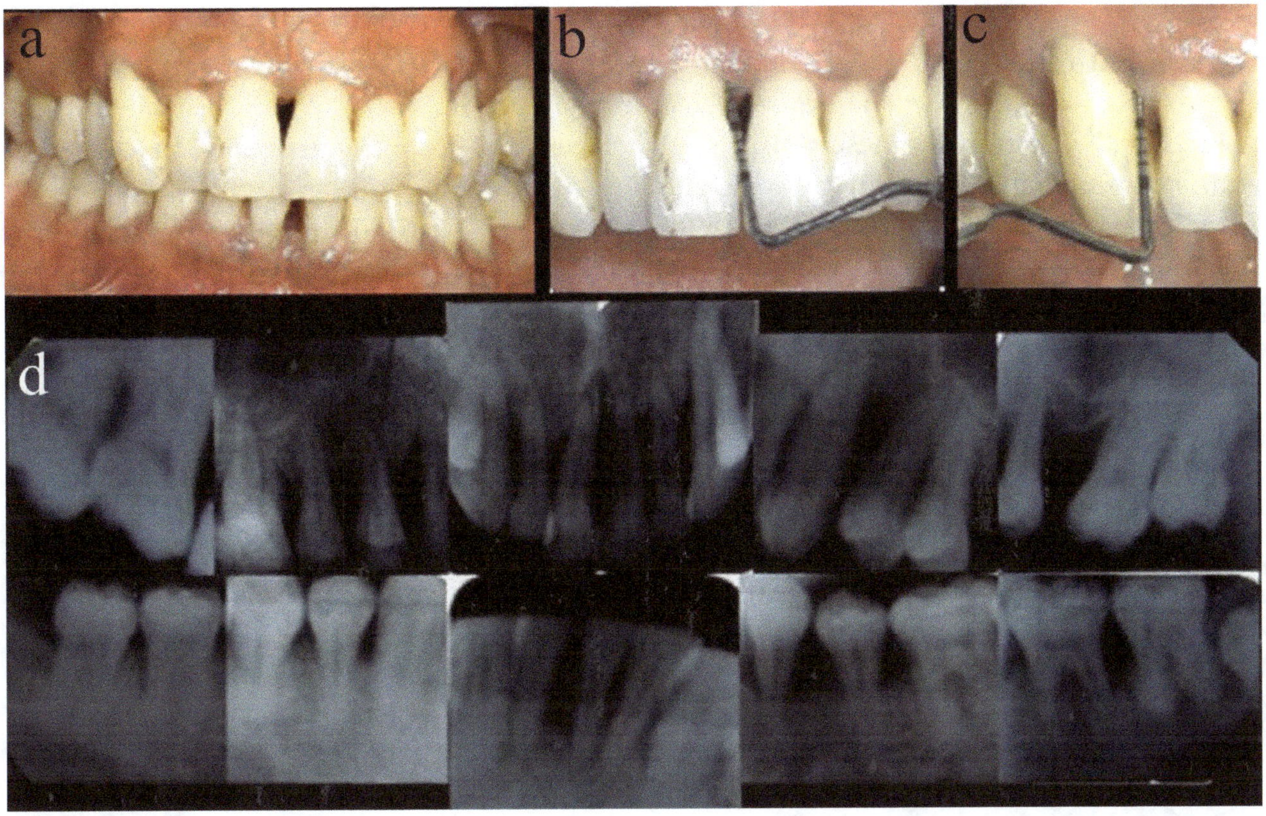

Figure 2. GAgP patient; (a) clinical view of the GAgP patient, (b, c) increased probing depth around the teeth, (d) radiographic view of the GAgP patient.

3.2. Radiographic features

The radiographic image of GAgP, characterized by severe horizontal and vertical alveolar bone loss especially in the first molar and incisors. This severe destruction can affect only a few teeth as well as the majority of the teeth in the mouth. The disease can progress so quickly that the aggressive nature, radiographs taken at different times, bone loss is easily recognizable [8]. Page et al. [12] reported that in patients with GAgP, the loss of alveolar bone in regions where periodontal destruction is more severe is increased from 25–60% over 9 weeks (**Figure 2**).

4. Epidemiology of AgP

The prevalence of AgP changes significantly different between geographical regions and between different racial/ethnic origins. For this reason, the prevalence of the disease in a given population can be determined by the distribution of the population according to the type and proportion of the race and ethnic group. In the studies, the methods which have been used to diagnosis of disease such as; whether radiographies is taken or not, differences in diagnostic equipment, different indexing systems etc. varies. According an epidemiologic study performed by Susin et al. [15] prevalence of AgP in Africa is between 1–5%, in North and mid-Europe Caucasians 0.1%, in South European ~0.5%, in North America ~0.1–0.2% of Caucasians, 0.5–1.0% of Hispanics and 2.6% of Black people, in South America 0.3–2.0%, in Asia 0.2–1.0%. According these results, AgP can be a health problem in some populations and/or races. In a national survey which include US school children aged 13–19 years, the prevalence of AgP was found 0.40% in 13–15 years, 0.80% in 16–19 years, 0.06% in whites, 2.60% in blacks and 0.50% in Hispanics [16]. Haubek et al. [17] found a high prevalence of AgP as 7.6% in Moroccan children aged 14–19 years. Also Albandar et al. [18] found AgP with a high prevalence 6.5%, in Uganda. Given the prevalence of AgP in Asia; it found 1.8% in Iraq, 0.86% in Israel, 0.47% in Japan and 0.42% in Saudi Arabia [19]. In South America, the prevalence of disease was vary among the countries: 0.32–2.6% in Brazil, 0.32% in Chile [19]. In Europe it has relatively low prevalence been observed; 0.1% in Denmark, 0.1% in Finland, 0.5% in Italy, 0.1–0.3% in Netherlands, 0% in Norway, 0.11–0.13% in Switzerland, 0.02–0.8% in United Kingdom [19]. The disease is most commonly seen in African-Caribbean (80%) and least Norwegian (0.2%) [20]. In terms of the prevalence of racial attachment, it was found that AgP was higher in black people (2.6%) than white people (0.17%) [21]. Most studies show comparable disease prevalence in both male and female patients. Gender factor and its role in development of AgP have not become clear. In some studies AgP was found to be more common in women than men with 3: 1 ratio [22–25]. However, researches are also available that indicates AgP more common in men than women [18, 21].

5. Pathogenesis of AgP

Periodontal destruction in AgP occurs pathogenic microorganisms and host immune system interaction [14, 26] and this interaction is influenced by many local and systemic factors [27]. Four basic factors play role in the pathogenesis of AgP [26].

- Microbial factors.
- Host factors.
- Environmental factors.
- Genetic factors.

5.1. Microbial factors

The presence of microorganisms is essential for the initiation of the inflammatory process in periodontal diseases and the factors related to the host are involved in the progress of the disease. The appearance of severe tissue destruction with a small amount of plaque in AgP suggests that microorganisms with high virulence in the etiology of the disease may play a role. *A. actinomycetemcomitans* is considered to be the most effective etiologic agent in AgP for about 30 years [28]. *A. actinomycetemcomitans,* short (0.4–1 μm), facultative anaerobic, immobile, Gram(−) rod. The virulence factor is serotypically variable and some serotypes are known to be invasive epithelial cells and gingival tissue. Tonetti and Mombelli (1999) listed the findings of *A. actinomycetemcomitans* in relation to LAgP [11].

1. In areas where periodontal tissue destruction occurs in aggressive periodontitis patients, 90% of *A. actinomycetemcomitans* are found.
2. In the areas where the destruction proceeds and continues, in high amounts, *A. actinomycetemcomitans* were detected.
3. High serum antibody levels against *A. actinomycetemcomitans* were observed in the majority of locally aggressive periodontitis patients.
4. Clinical trials have shown that improvement in clinical parameters with treatment is associated with a decrease in the level of *A. actinomycetemcomitans* in subgingival floras.
5. It is known that *A. actinomycetemcomitans* has virulence factors that can play a role in the development of the disease such as leukotoxin.

A. actinomycetemcomitans has been suggested to play a role in the onset of AgP by interacting with facultative anaerobic and capnophilic species such as the locally useful Capnocytophaga species and *Eikenella corrodens* (*E. corrodens*) [29]. Today, the microbiological profile of AgP has changed from the presence of specific microorganisms to the presence of more complex microbiota [30]. Some of the bacteria found in periodontal pockets related to gingivitis, while some are related to periodontitis. Dental plaque biofilm is a dynamic structure and changes over time. Different bacterial groups are complexed at different times in biofilm. Among these, orange complex bacteria: *P. intermedia, Prevotella nigrescense* (*P. nigrescense*), *Parvimonas micra* (*P. micra*), *Fusobacterium nucleatum* (*F. nucleatum*), *C. rectus, Eubacterium nodatum* (*E. nodatum*) and *Campylobacter showae* (*C. showae*) build a bridge between the pathogens seen in the early period of periodontal disease named red complex bacteria. Red complex bacteria named *P. gingivalis, T. forsythia* and *Treponema denticola* (*T. denticola)* were associated with periodontal tissue destruction [31]. In some studies, *P. gingivalis* and *T. Forsythia* have been shown to be an etiological agent for AgP [10, 11]. Patients also had increased antibody response against *A. Actinomycetemcomitans, P. intermedia* and *C. rectus* [14]. Electron microscopic studies performed on LAgP demonstrates that bacteria found in the connective tissue to the extending bone surface. When examined by more advanced techniques, the presence of *A. Actinomycetemcomitans, Capnocytophaga sputigena (C. sputigena),* mycoplasma strains and spirochetes has been defined [8]. In the extracted teeth affected by LAgP, electron microscopic observations showed that in the biofilm layer on the root surface formed Gram(−) cocci bacteria and other microorganisms [5]. In some studies, it has been reported that spirochetes are rarely or not present in LAgP lesions [32, 33], in contrast some authors reported that there is a high number of spirochetes in lesions [34, 35]. In a study performed in population of Chilean patients with GAgP and CP, *P. gingivalis, P. micra* and *C. rectus* isolated from subgingival plaque and found to be related to disease progression [36]. In a recent study performed with patients who affected by GAgP, the authors concluded that existence of a complex cooperative interaction promoted by *Herpes Simplex Virus Type-1* (HSV-1) infection, involving *Staphylococcus aureus* (*S. aureus*) and the periodontopathogens *P. gingivalis, T. forsythia,* and *Fusobacterium periodonticum (F. periodonticum),* that could promote an accelerate progression of lesions of GAgP [37]. Dogan et al. [38] compared subgingival flora in LAgP, GAgP, CP and healthy controls in 69 Turkish people. *T. forsythensis* and *C. rectus* found the lowest frequency in LAgP. *A. actinomycetemcomitans, P. gingivalis,* and *C. rectus* were higher in GAgP than in healthy controls. Yeasts also were found in samples. Lee et al. [39] found the bacteria in diseased sites in Korean AgP patients, descending percentages; *Fusobacterium sp., P. gingivalis, Treponema sp., T. forsythensis, P. intermedia and A. actinomycetemcomitans.* They also concluded *P. intermedia* was associated with GAgP. In a study red complex bacteria found in that of Generalized CP and GAgP. No significant differences found in term of 40 bacteria species in Generalized CP and GAgP [40]. *Human cytomegalovirus, Epstein–Barr virus type-1* and *HSV-1* are also involved in the progression of the disease [41, 42]. These differences may be related to variations in the societies living in the various regions of the world, as well as the difficulties in grouping diseases.

5.2. Host factors

AgP is a disease that shows significant differences from other periodontal diseases in terms of severity of destruction, rate of progression, response to treatment, etiologic factors and genetic susceptibility criteria. Defects of host defense system and complex factors like microbial flora play a role together in hostility and disease formation affecting severity of destruction, speed of disease progress and response to treatment. In the response to dental plaque accumulation, which leads to gingivitis, substantial evidence has been collected to propose large differences between individuals. In line with this concept, it has been shown from the initial research attempts on early-onset periodontitis forms that affected individuals, suffer from metabolic imbalance or hereditary host response defects.

The first step of periodontal defense is inflammation in innate immune response that provided a respond to bacterial plaque by neutrophils, macrophages, fibroblasts, epithelial and dendritic cells [43]. If this immune response is not capable to control the inflammation process, complex inflammatory cascades are activated. Second stage which is called adaptive immune response that resumed by antigen-presenting cells and predominantly B-cell lesions composed in periodontitis [43]. Tissue destruction in patients with AgP is not directly related to bacteria accumulation in root surface. Personal immune response plays a major role in severity of destruction [44].

PMNL is an important component of the immune system and found in gingival lesions and in root surfaces of AgP cases [45]. Some of neutrophil malfunctions such as increased adhesion, reduced chemotaxis, increased superoxide and nitric oxide production and reduced phagocytosis were thought to be responsible for disease progression [46–48]. Hyper-responsive macrophage phenotype including elevated prostaglandin E2 and interleukin-1β levels took place among the features of AgP in the 1999 Workshop [49]. According to Kantarci et al. [50] LAgP has been associated with various abnormalities of host cell function such as; neutrophil abnormalities, reduced chemotaxis, increased superoxide production, reduced receptor expression, reduced phagocytosis and killing of *A. Actinomycetemcomitans,* impaired leukotriene B_4 and signal transduction abnormalities. They suggest the PMNL is not hypofunctional or deficient, but it is hyperfunctional and excessed activity is responsible of the tissue damage. A constantly uncontrolled periodontal infection activates neutrophils and make them more effectively stimulated to counteract microbial episodes. Thus, differences in neutrophil functions in AgP are thought to be a combination of genetic and acquired properties of person [51]. Human leukocyte antigens (HLA) are antigens that regulate the immune response. HLA-9 and HLA-15 antigens have been shown to be associated with AgP [8, 52]. Another study has shown that HLA class I, HLA class II antigens are associated with periodontal disease [53] but no significant associations were found between HLA class II antigens and AgP. There is a positive association with HLA-A9 and negative relationship with HLA-A2 and HLA-B5 have shown in patients with AgP [54]. HLA class II antigens are capable bind peptides derived from bacterial antigens and present them to T cells while HLA class I antigens generally present peptides derived from viruses and self-antigens to cytotoxic T cells. In a theory, viral peptide binding and presentation to T cells via HLA-A9 or HLA-B15 is not sufficient for activating immune response properly resulting AgP with severe periodontal destruction [53]. IgA plays an important role in the host defense system and, locally dominant in saliva. IgA is important because of its antiinflammatory function and reduces inflammation by inhibiting IgG and IgM production. Studies have shown that the IgA ratio decreases significantly in AgP subjects [55]. Hwang et al. provides evidence against the 1999 Workshop's decision of weak serum antibody response in AgP. In their study, serum IgG levels to *A. Actinomycetemcomitans* in GAgP patients is not differ from LAgP, Localized CP and Generalized CP but it is significantly increased to several species, including *P. gingivalis, T. denticola,* and *C. rectus* [56]. CRP is an acute phase response molecule and increases in an inflammatory condition such as heat, infection, hypoxia and tissue damage. Elevated fibrinogen levels can activate the inflammatory cascades. Chandy et al. [57] investigated these two molecules in AgP patients. Elevated CRP and fibrinogen levels found in CP patients not in AgP and healthy controls. These results may explain the severity of the lesions by delaying the immunological response against to AgP. In some studies platelet size and function found to decrease in GAgP patients due to the consumption of large platelets at sites of periodontal inflammation. Platelets may play active role in host response in GAgP patients [58, 59].

5.3. Environmental factors

Environmental factors such as oral hygiene/bacterial plaque, smoking, stress and systemic factors may exacerbate the inflammation and play an important role in the periodontitis progression. Studies have shown that there is a positive correlation between AgP and stress [60]. In a controlled study patients in the GAgP group were significantly more depressed and lonely than patients in the CP and control groups [60]. Existing dental plaque is also very important to develop the periodontal disease. A positive correlation found between the amount of plaque and GAgP, but not in LAgP [61]. Smoking is also a risk factor for AgP [54]. In a study smoking found to related disease activity and progression in GAgP but it is not associated with LAgP [62]. Also smoking affects the cytokine profiles of patients with AgP and disturbs the host–parasite relationship [63]. AgP patients who are smoking showed poor clinical respond the periodontal treatment [64].

According to the 1999 workshop, the main feature in diagnosing of AgP is that the individual should be medically healthy [1]. However symptoms of the gum in some systemic diseases/

conditions may resemble AgP. This group of diseases includes; neutropenia, hypophosphatasia, leukemias, Cheidak-Higashi syndrome, leukocyte adhesion deficiency, Papillon-Lefevre syndrome, trisomy 21, histiocytosis and agranulocytosis [1].

5.4. Genetic factors

AgP is a multifactorial disease and many etiological factors are required for clinical presentation. Bacterial content and host defense clearly play an important role in the disease. Genetic variations may affect the host response to the disease. Once diagnosed, the sibling of the child or adolescent must also be investigated for the AgP. The genetic factors that may be involved in the pathogenesis of AgP, have been investigated by considering the immune system regulated by genetic factors and that certain genetic polymorphisms may disrupt the defense system against the agent that infects the immune system.

Interleukin-1 (IL-1) is a potent pro-inflammatory mediator that is mainly released by monocytes, macrophages and dendritic cells and genetic polymorphisms of IL1 have been studied in association with AgP. Three studies have reported no association between the carriage rates of the IL1A − 889 (+4845) C → T gene and AgP [65–67], but one study have found an association with this gene and AgP in Chinese Population [68]. IL1B + 3954 (+3953) C → T gene polymorphisms and carriage rate of the rare (R) allele in Caucasians found associated with AgP in a study [65]. In studies involving IL-4 which have anti-inflammatory properties, no association was found between AgP and genotype encoding this cytokine [69]. In a meta-analysis that conducted the evaluating IL-6 polymorphisms, there was concluded an associated with AgP and IL-6 polymorphisms [70]. IL-10 is an anti-inflammatory cytokine which down-regulates the pro-inflammatory immune response of monocytes and macrophages. The results of the studies investigating polymorphism on the gene that encoded IL-10 were not significant [71, 72]. IL-17 plays an important role in natural and acquired immune response; there is a study in mice demonstrating that IL-17 receptor trigger bone loss in infectious conditions [73]. In a recent metaanalysis authors concluded that there is no significant association between the polymorphisms rs2275913 and rs763780 in interleukins 17A and 17F genes and CP and AgP in the allelic evaluation [74]. IL-23 is a pro-inflammatory cytokine and found positively correlated with CP but existing studies how that there is no significant association of IL-23 polymorphisms with AgP [75]. IL-8 is a chemokine and plays role of chemoattractant for the neutrophils. Insufficient studies exist that correlate IL-8 polymorphisms with AgP. Existing studies in literature demonstrated that there is no significant association between IL-8 polymorphisms and AgP [75].

Tumor necrosis factor (TNF) is a pro-inflammatory cytokine which has the potential to stimulate the production of secondary mediators, including chemokines or cyclo-oxygenase products, amplifying the degree of inflammation. No associations between the TNFA polymorphisms and AgP in a meta-analysis [72]. An Fc receptor is a protein found on the surface of certain cells and part of immunoglobulin (FcγR) link cellular and humoral parts of the immune system that contribute to the protective functions of the immune system [76]. A Japanese study reported an association for a composite genotype of the Fc cRIIIa N allele and the Fc cRIIIb +141 R allele in AgP [77] in contrast in a stud performed with Caucasian population there is no association found in term of this gene [78]. There is limited information about polymorphism of FcγR and AgP. The vitamin D receptor was included various biological processes such as bone metabolism and the immune response to microbial infections. Nibali et al. [79] and Park et al. [80] found an association with AgP but Bret et al. [65] could not find any accociation.CD14 and Tolllike receptors (TLRs) are extra and intracellular receptors such as recognize pathogen-associated molecules on Gram(+) and Gram(−) bacteria and mediate the production of cytokines required for effective immune response. In studies that performed to find a relationship CD14 polymorphism and AgP received no association [81, 82]. About TLRs, there is limited information and studies are available.

Most studies performed about polymorphisms were limited by sample size and had variations in case inclusion criteria. Genetic studies can also be limited by geographic and ethnical differences. To understand the pathogenesis of this complex disease multicenter studies and large sample sizes are required.

6. General treatment strategy

AgP is a complex periodontal disease that causes rapid destruction of the periodonticum and even causes tooth loss. Complex pathogens are involved in the etiology of AgP. Therefore, it is important for clinicians to treat the disease and maintain periodontal health [83]. The treatment protocols are based on studies so far. Physicians can achieve very effective results if they are working with microbial tests during and after treatment. People with the same clinical characteristics may have different bacterial flora, or people with different clinical characteristics may have the same bacterial flora. In clinical trials, the success of treatment is assessed by considering the probing depth (PD), clinical attachment level (CAL) and bleeding on probing (BOP) using conventional periodontal instruments. All parameters for the patients should be assessed and the treatment decision should be given. Surgical and non-surgical techniques are applied in the treatment of AgP [84]. It is important to treat and obtain frequent controls of individuals with AgP which is seen in younger patients coexistent rapid attachment and alveolar bone loss. There are studies demonstrated that the post-treatment attachment level can be maintained despite the risk of recurrence of the disease [85, 86]. A study of 40-year follow-ups from patients with GAgP shows that even the most aggressive and most advanced periodontitis cases are treatable [87]. The motivation and adaptation of the patient is very important in order to control the disease. In this phase, the patient should be informed by the doctor about the role of the patient, the severity of the illness and the risk factors. The main purpose of the treatment is to create a clinical condition that can hold the largest number of teeth in the mouth for as long as possible. Periodontal treatment is considered in four main phases. First phase; initial therapy or non-surgical periodontal treatment. The second periodontal treatment phase is surgical periodontal treatment, third phase prosthetic treatment and fourth phase maintenance periodontal treatment.

6.1. Non-surgical treatment of AgP

Removal of agents causing periodontal disease, providing good oral hygiene to the patient, and reducing pre-existing gingival inflammation and periodontal pocket depths in advance of future phases are among the goals of non-surgical periodontal treatment. Mechanical treatment involves removal of plaque and its products from dental surfaces (supra/subgingival), as well as dental and other plaque-retaining local agents by hand or ultrasonic instruments. Root planning are also included. The responses of patients with LAgP to initial periodontal care vary in studies. In general, the least amount of work on this issue and it is not long to observe the final results. Based on the literature GAgP responds good clinical results to scaling and root planning (SRP) in the short term (up to 6 months). However, after 6 months despite frequent visits to the physician and strengthening oral hygiene, relapses and disease progression have been reported [88].

Studies have shown that the total supragingival and subgingival plaque mass is reduced by mechanical treatment. However, because some pathogens can invade into the tissue, or because periodontal instruments are not effective in deep and complex pockets, mechanical treatment is sometimes ineffective [89]. The success of periodontal treatment depends on the removal of dental plaque and therefore pathogenic microorganisms in the dental plaque. The anti-infective treatments applied in this context directly affect the success of the treatment. Anti-infective treatment includes both mechanical and chemotherapeutic approaches and aims to destroy or reduce the microbial dental plaque biofilm which is primary etiological agent of periodontal infections. The use of therapeutic agents especially systemic antibiotics have been widespread to be able to obtain predictable treatment responses due to conventional periodontal treatment and to support treatment for the specific microbial structure of the disease.

At this time there is a clear consensus that mechanical instrumentation should always precede antimicrobial therapy. To achieve effective levels of the drug on the day of the completion of SRP [90]. The subgingival bacterial load that will be inhibited by the antimicrobial agent must be reduced by mechanical treatment. Insufficient antimicrobial agent concentrations may cause the emergence of resistant bacterial strains [88]. The tetracycline group is considered first in systemic treatment. Tetracycline and SRP found to be more effective in term of elimination *A. actinomycetemcomitans, Capnocytophaga* and spirochetes comparing only SRP [91]. Tetracycline is known to have beneficial effects in wound healing regarding its anticollagenase activity [92] .

Doxycycline is a semisynthetic tetracycline and is effective in the treatment of periodontitis. It is easier to take doxycycline at lower doses and use it with daily foods. In a study 60 patients were divided into a placebo group and a group that received systemic doxycycline (loading dose of 200 mg and doses of 100 mg daily for 14 days) SRP was performed to all groups over an 8-week period, systemic antibiotic or placebo was only used during the first 2 weeks of the SRP. At the end of the study no significant differences were found in term of PD, BOP [93]. It was demonstrated in many studies, biofilm showed high levels of resistance against tetracycline, minocycline, amoxicillin, doxycycline and amoxicillin/clavulanate. In addition, high-degree of antibiotic tolerance has been demonstrated in mature biofilms [94] when tetracycline was unable to suppress *A. actinomycetemcomitans,* it has been raised a combined use of antibiotics for the treatment of AgP. Metronidazole is a nitroimidazole derivative antibiotic which has a strong bactericidal effect on obligate anaerob Gram(−) bacteria. It is highly effective on periodontopathogenic bacteria such as *P. gingivalis* and *P. intermedia* which in the "red complex" [95]. The combination of 250 mg of metronidazole and 375 mg of amoxicillin, three times a day for 7 days, as an adjunct to SRP, was found to be very effective in suppressing subgingival *A. actinomycetemcomitans* load [96]. Guerrero et al. [97] evaluated SRP plus systemic metronidazole and amoxicillin in use on clinical parameters, in total of 41 individuals with GAgP. Twenty randomly selected patients were given 500 mg metronidazole and 500 mg amoxicillin three times a day for 1 week in addition to mechanical treatment, and the remaining 21 patients were given placebo in addition to mechanical treatment. Two and six months re-evaluations were made. Additional metronidazole and amoxicillin may provide a statistically significant improvement in clinical parameters in the short term. Xajigeorgiou et al. [84] investigated metronidazole + amoxicillin, doxycycline, metronidazole efficacy in 43 GAgP patient clinically and microbiologically. Patients were randomly divided into 4 groups. First group was received SRP plus 500 mg metronidazole +500 mg amoxicillin three times a day for 1 week, second group was received 200 mg for the first day loading, 100 mg doxycycline for the following 14 days, third group was received 500 mg metronidazole three times a day for 1 week, and the fourth group was evaluated as the control group. After 6 weeks and 6 months patients were reevaluated in term of CAL, BOP, PD. Additional metronidazole + amoxicillin or metronidazole plus SRP have been effective comparing the other groups. Adjunctive use of metronidazole plus amoxicillin, metronidazole alone or clindamycin in patients with GAgP results in well clinical improvements comparing with the use of doxycycline for a similar amount of time or with SRP alone [88].

The use of azithromycin in recent years has become an issue in AgP treatment. Long half-life of and use of only once every 3 days of azithromycin, provides advantages for the patient and the physician. In a study clinical efficacy of the adjunctive use of azithromycin with SRP was investigated in AgP. Twelve months after treatment, approximately 1 mm reduction in PD and higher percentage of teeth with attachment gain was observed in test group [98]. There is no certain protocol for the use of adjunctive systemic antimicrobials with SRP, but in general suggests that antibiotic intake should start on the day of debridement completion; debridement should be completed within a short time (preferably <1 week) [94].

Local antibiotic applications may also used to complete the periodontal therapy. Several local antibiotic applications have been developed in addition to initial periodontal therapy. These include metronidazole, chlorhexidine, minocycline, doxycycline and tetracycline. The use of this systems in LAgP may be more beneficial effect in term of the nature of the disease. To achieve maximum efficacy, drugs must provide some criteria such as; the drug must reach the targeted site of action, remain at an effective concentration and last for an adequate period of time [99]. In a study, 26 patients with LAgP divided into a control group, a group receiving 1% chlorhexidine gel and a group receiving a 40% tetracycline gel. After 12 weeks, either of these antimicrobial agents provide significant additional improvement of the clinical parameters [100]. Kaner et al. compared local chlorhexidine chip and ministration and systemic amoxicillin plus metronidazole combination in addition to SRP on clinical parameters in GAgP patients. Systemic use of amoxicillin plus metronidazole combination found to be statistically significant clinical improvements comparing the local chlorhexidine chip [101]. In a similar study Purucker et al. [102] concluded that additional applied local (tetracycline fibers) and systemic (500 mg amoxicillin/clavulanic acid) antibiotics showed equally benefits in terms of clinical parameters. In conclusion, local antimicrobial adjuvant effects reported in the literature do not appear to improve on the adjunctive effect of systemic antibiotics in patients with AgP. When using such systems, cost-benefit and efficiency should be considered well.

6.2. Surgical treatment of AgP

Surgical treatment may require for the remaining pockets after initial periodontal treatment of AgP. The surgical approach has the advantages such as; reaching difficult anatomical formations of the teeth, cleaning the pocket epithelium from invaded *A. actinomycetemcomitans* and application of regenerative procedures.

Twenty-five periodontal lesions in seven patients with LAgP divided into three treatment groups: SRP; SRP plus soft tissue curettage; SRP plus modified Widman flap surgery. The microbiologic and clinical measurements were performed up to 16 weeks. At the end of the study SRP alone unable to suppress *A. actinomycetemcomitans* in periodontal lesions, in contrast SRP plus soft tissue curettage and modified Widman flap surgery succeeded [103]. Systemic antibiotic use can preferred with various surgical techniques in the treatment of AgP. Kornman and Robertson [104] found modified Widman flap surgery plus tetracycline was effective in areas where the black pigmented bacteroides and *A. actinomycetemcomitans* load was high. Lindhe and Liljenberg [105] treated 16 patients with modified Widman flAgP surgery plus tetracycline (14 days). As a result of 5-year follow-up, successful clinical results were obtained and radiological bone fill in angular bony defects. In a case series performed by Buchmann et al. [106], SRP and modified Widman flap surgery plus systemic amoxicillin/metronidazole combination provide periodontal tissue stabilization at a rate 95% over 5 years.

There are many methods to regain bone in vertical bone defects such as bone grafting, guided tissue regeneration by using membranes, the use of biologic modifiers and combinations of the above. Autografts are the gold standard and have been extensively used because of its osseoinductive, osseoconductive, and osteogenic properties but it has limitations like morbidity and mortality hence different graft materials are available in practice. Allografts (e.g. freeze-dried bone allograft), xenografts (bovine or corral derived) and alloplastic materials (e.g. bioactive glass, hydroxyapatite and beta-tricalcium phosphate) are alternatively used instead of autograft [107]. Yukna and Sepe [108] demonstrated an average defect fill (80%) in 12 LAgP patients using freeze-dried bone allografts. In a study different graft materials were evaluated in 10 patients with LAgP. 4:1 ratio combination of beta-tricalcium phosphate/tetracycline, hydroxyapatite/tetracycline or freeze-dried bone allograft/tetracycline were applied into these groups. Each graft material showed a decrease in defect and pocket depth although no significant differences between the different grafting materials were found in terms of hard-tissue or soft-tissue changes. But hydroxyapatite/tetracycline showed a greater percentage of defect fill was comparing with beta-tricalcium phosphate/tetracycline [109].

Membranes have been grouped into two major categories: nonresorbable (high-density polytetrafluoroethylene (PTFE) membranes reinforced or not with a titanium framework (e.g. Cytoplast ® TXT-200; Osteogenics Biomedical, Lubbock, Tex., USA) and resorbable membranes (polylactic acid (PLA) and its copolymers, tissue-derived collagen membranes) [110]. Nonresorbable membranes serve as a space maintenance which is needed for tissue regeneration and inert also biocompatible. Unfortunately, second surgery for removal or membrane exposure take place among its disadvantages. Although resorbable membranes show lack of sufficient strength, unpredictable degradation rate and cause a greater inflammatory response [110]. Usage of nonresorbable or resorbable membranes for treating intrabony defects in AgP has been shown to be effective in many studies [86, 111].

6.3. Other treatment modalities

Photodynamic antimicrobial therapy that photosensitizers (toluidine blue, methylene blue, malachite green) are used inside periodontal pockets for increasing the cytotoxic potential of laser light to potential periodontal pathogens. In a metaanalysis authors concluded that photodynamic antimicrobial therapy cannot be suggested as routine with nonsurgical treatment of patients with AgP according to lack of evidence based on the literature [112].

Enamel matrix proteins (amelogenin) which provides new cementum and the formation of new attachment in periodontal defects and growth factors/differentiation factors (platelet-derived growth factor, insulin-like growth factor, fibroblast growth factor, bone morphogenetic protein, transforming growth factor-beta) which play an import role in tissue development and healing are tools for gaining attachment. Their effectiveness on periodontium were demonstrated in many studies with CP but studies with AgP, mostly exist as case reports [113, 114]. Yılmaz et al. [115] treated patients with GAgP with a total of 12 intrabony defects with the combination of platelet rich plasma +bovine derived xenograft combination. PD, marginal recession, relative attachment, probing bone and radiographic bone levels were measured at the beginning and at 12 months reentry. The researchers noted that the combination of platelet rich plasma and bovine derived xenograft for the treatment of GAgP, provided successful clinical results in large intrabony defects and that prognosis was affected positively even for teeth that were thought to have hopeless prognosis.

Dental implants are a widely used treatment edentulism and provides functional and esthetic resolutions. Since tooth loss is frequently seen in AgP patients, dental implant applications can be applied. However, marginal bone loss and implant survival rates in AgP patients significantly higher than those of CP and healthy subjects [113, 114]. Care should be taken when considering dental implant in AgP patients. Frequent follow-ups should not be neglected in these patients.

6.4. Maintenance therapy

After the treatment performed and provided the health of periodontal tissues, patient should be included in the maintenance program. Due to the recurrence nature of AgP, maintenance is given to for prevention of additional tooth loss and disease recurrence. Regular controls are useful for controlling the progression of the disease. These controls should be lifelong, but there is no definitive protocol for frequency. Some researchers suggested monthly checks during the first 6 months after the treatment finished. Some researchers stated that 3–4 controls per year would suffice. In every control session; PD and CAL should be assessed. Also, when necessary, SRP should be performed. Radiographs should be taken separately from each tooth or area affected by the disease once a year. Local antibiotic administration may be preferred to risky areas [116]. The prognosis of teeth that affected AgP depends on many factors such as the amount of missing bone, the presence or absence of furcation region, the morphology of bone defects, the degree of mobility, crown/root ratio, occlusal contacts, oral hygiene and general health. Treatment should be evaluated according to the initial condition. It is also important to perform microbial testing at every control session whenever possible. Thus, the physician may be an idea about the activation of the disease.

7. Conclusion

AgP is a complex disease and has multifactorial etiology. While bacterial plaque is essential for initiation of disease, it is generally accepted that genetic factors and host immune response play a large role in the disease susceptibility. Also environmental and behavioral factors determine the final clinical outcome. The outcome of rapid and severe alveolar bone loss; gingival recession, pathological migration of teeth, mobility and eventual loss of teeth occur. Because of the clinical results, AgP patients suffer social problems due to esthetic, phonetic and nutritional problems and their quality of life diminishes. The treatment of these patients is quite challenging, due to the absence of a standard treatment protocol for this disease which its etiology is not fully understood, but also because of the rapid progression, severe periodontal tissue loss and recurrence of the disease. Non-surgical and surgical periodontal treatments combined with systemic antibiotics are recommended for the complete eradication of deep periodontal pockets. In long term, active periodontal treatment must followed by maintenance periodontal treatment for preventing attachment and tooth loss.

Author details

Aysan Lektemur Alpan

Address all correspondence to: ysnlpn@gmail.com

Faculty of Dentistry, Department of Periodontology, Pamukkale University, Denizli, Turkey

References

[1] Armitage GC. Development of a classification system for periodontal diseases and conditions. Annals of Periodontology. 1999 Dec;**4**(1):1-6. DOI: 10.1902/annals.1999.4.1.1

[2] Lang NBP, Cullinan M, Jeffcoat M, Mombelli A, Murakami S, Page R, Papapanou P, Tonetti M, Van Dyke T. Consensus report – aggressive periodontitis. Annals of Periodontology. 1999;**4**:53. DOI: 10.1902/annals.1999.4.1.53

[3] Albandar JM. Aggressive periodontitis: Case definition and diagnostic criteria. Periodontology 2000. Jun 2014;**65**(1):13-26. DOI: 10.1111/prd.12014

[4] Armitage GC, Cullinan MP. Comparison of the clinical features of chronic and aggressive periodontitis. Periodontology 2000. Jun 2010;**53**:12-27. DOI: 10.1111/j.1600-0757.2010.00353.x

[5] Armitage GC. Comparison of the microbiological features of chronic and aggressive periodontitis. Periodontol 2000. Jun 2010;**53**:70-88. DOI: 10.1111/j.1600-0757.2010.00357.x

[6] Nevins ML, Melloning JT. Periodontal Therapy Volume 1: Clinical Approaches and Evidence of Success. Germany: Quintessence Publishing; 1998. pp.101-116. ISBN 978-0-86715-309-5

[7] Dörfer CE. Antimicrobials for the treatment of aggressive periodontitis. Oral Diseases. 2003;**9**(Suppl 1):51-53. PMID: 12974531

[8] Newman MG, Takei H, Carranza FA, Klokkevold PR. Carranza's Clinical Periodontology. 10th ed. St. Louis, Missouri: Saunders Elsevier; 2006. pp. 506-512

[9] Mombelli A, Meier C. On the symmetry of periodontal disease. Journal of Clinical Periodontology. Aug 2001;**28**(8):741-745. PMID: 11442733

[10] Trevilatto PC, Tramontina VA, Machado MA, Goncalves RB, Sallum AW, Line SR. Clinical, genetic and microbiological findings in a Brazilian family with aggressive periodontitis. Journal of Clinical Periodontology. Mar 2002;**29**(3):233-239. DOI: 10.1034/j.1600-051x.2002.290309.x

[11] Tonetti MS, Mombelli A. Early-onset periodontitis. Annals of Periodontology. Dec 1999;**4**(1):39-53. DOI: 10.1902/annals.1999.4.1.39

[12] Page RC, Altman LC, Ebersole JL, Vandesteen GE, Dahlberg WH, Williams BL, et al. Rapidly progressive periodontitis. A distinct clinical condition. Journal of Periodontology. Apr 1983;**54**(4):197-209. DOI: 10.1902/jop.1983.54.4.197

[13] Tonetti MS, Mombelli A. Aggressive periodontitis. In: Lindhe J, Lang NP, Karring T, editors. Clinical Periodontology and Implant Dentistry. 5th ed. Oxford, Malden, Iowa, Copenhagen, Victoria, Berlin, Paris: Blackwell Munksgaard Publishing Co.; 2008. pp. 428-458

[14] Schenkein HA, Van Dyke TE. Early-onset periodontitis: Systemic aspects of etiology and pathogenesis. Periodontology 2000. Oct 1994;**6**:7-25. DOI: 10.1111/j.1600-0757.1994.tb00023.x

[15] Susin C, Haas AN, Albandar JM. Epidemiology and demographics of aggressive periodontitis. Periodontology 2000. Jun 2014;**65**(1):27-45. DOI: 10.1111/prd.12019

[16] Albandar JM, Brown LJ, Loe H. Clinical features of early-onset periodontitis. Journal of the American Dental Association (1939). Oct 1997;**128**(10):1393-1399. DOI: 10.14219/jada.archive.1997.0058

[17] Haubek D, Ennibi OK, Abdellaoui L, Benzarti N, Poulsen S. Attachment loss in Moroccan early onset periodontitis patients and infection with the JP2-type of Actinobacillus actinomycetemcomitans. Journal of Clinical Periodontology. Jul 2002;**29**(7):657-660. DOI: 10.1034/j.1600-051X.2002.290711.x

[18] Albandar JM, Muranga MB, Rams TE. Prevalence of aggressive periodontitis in school attendees in Uganda. Journal of Clinical Periodontology. Sep 2002;**29**(9):823-831. DOI: 10.1034/j.1600-051X.2002.290906.x

[19] Albandar JM, Tinoco EM. Global epidemiology of periodontal diseases in children and young persons. Periodontology 2000. 2002;**29**:153-176. DOI: 10.1034/j.1600-0757.2002.290108.x

[20] Ronderos M MB. Epidemiology of periodontal diseases and risk factors. In: Genco RJ, Cohen DW, editors. Periodontics Medicine, Surgery, and Implants. 4th ed. St.Louis: Elsevier Mosby; 2004. pp. 32-69

[21] Loe H, Brown LJ. Early onset periodontitis in the United States of America. Journal of Periodontology. Oct 1991;**62**(10):608-616. DOI: 10.1902/jop.1991.62.10.608

[22] Baer PN. The case for periodontosis as a clinical entity. Journal of Periodontology. Aug 1971;**42**(8):516-520. DOI: 10.1902/jop.1971.42.8.516

[23] Davies RM, Smith RG, Porter SR. Destructive forms of periodontal disease in adolescents and young adults. British Dental Journal. Jun 22, 1985;**158**(12):429-436. PMID: 3860226

[24] Genco RJ, Christersson LA, Zambon JJ. Juvenile periodontitis. International Dental Journal. Sep 1986;**36**(3):168-176. PMID: 3533789

[25] Hormand J, Frandsen A. Juvenile periodontitis. Localization of bone loss in relation to age, sex, and teeth. Journal of Clinical Periodontology. Dec 1979;**6**(6):407-416. DOI: 10.1111/j.1600-051X.1979.tb01939.x

[26] Kulkarni C, Kinane DF. Host response in aggressive periodontitis. Periodontology 2000. Jun 2014;**65**(1):79-91. DOI: 10.1111/prd.12017

[27] Albandar JM, Rams TE. Risk factors for periodontitis in children and young persons. Periodontology 2000. 2002;**29**:207-222. DOI: 10.1034/j.1600-0757.2002.290110.x

[28] Slots J. The predominant cultivable organisms in juvenile periodontitis. Scandinavian Journal of Dental Research. Jan 1976;**84**(1):1-10. DOI: 10.1111/j.1600-0722.1976.tb00454.x

[29] Delaney JE, Kornman KS. Microbiology of subgingival plaque from children with localized prepubertal periodontitis. Oral Microbiology and Immunology. Jun 1987;**2**(2):71-76. DOI: 10.1111/j.1399-302X.1987.tb00293.x

[30] Kononen E, Muller HP. Microbiology of aggressive periodontitis. Periodontology 2000. Jun 2014;**65**(1):46-78. DOI: 10.1111/prd.12016

[31] Socransky SS, Haffajee AD, Cugini MA, Smith C, Kent Jr RL. Microbial complexes in subgingival plaque. Journal of Clinical Periodontology. Feb 1998;**25**(2):134-144. DOI: 10.1111/j.1600-051X.1998.tb02419.x

[32] Liljenberg B, Lindhe J. Juvenile periodontitis. Some microbiological, histopathological and clinical characteristics. Journal of Clinical Periodontology. 1980 Feb;**7**(1):48-61. DOI: 10.1111/j.1600-051X.1980.tb01948.x

[33] Listgarten MA. Structure of the microbial flora associated with periodontal health and disease in man. A light and electron microscopic study. Journal of Periodontology. 1976 Jan;**47**(1):1-18. DOI: 10.1902/jop.1976.47.1.1

[34] Savitt ED, Socransky SS. Distribution of certain subgingival microbial species in selected periodontal conditions. Journal of Periodontal Research. Mar 1984;**19**(2):111-123. DOI: 10.1111/j.1600-0765.1984.tb00800.x

[35] Muller HP, Flores-de-Jacoby L. The composition of the subgingival microflora of young adults suffering from juvenile periodontitis. Journal of Clinical Periodontology. Feb 1985;**12**(2):113-123. DOI: 10.1111/j.1600-051X.1985.tb01370.x

[36] Gajardo M, Silva N, Gomez L, Leon R, Parra B, Contreras A, et al. Prevalence of periodontopathic bacteria in aggressive periodontitis patients in a Chilean population. Journal of Periodontology. Feb 2005;**76**(2):289-294. DOI: 10.1902/jop.2005.76.2.289

[37] Passariello C, Gigola P, Testarelli L, Puttini M, Schippa S, Petti S. Evaluation of microbiota associated with Herpesviruses in active sites of generalized aggressive periodontitis. Annali Di Stomatologia (Roma). Apr–Jun 2017;**8**(2):59-70. DOI: 10.11138/ads/2017.8.2.071

[38] Dogan B, Antinheimo J, Cetiner D, Bodur A, Emingil G, Buduneli E, et al. Subgingival microflora in Turkish patients with periodontitis. Journal of Periodontology. Jun 2003;**74**(6):803-814. DOI: 10.1902/jop.2003.74.6.803

[39] Lee JW, Choi BK, Yoo YJ, Choi SH, Cho KS, Chai JK, et al. Distribution of periodontal pathogens in Korean aggressive periodontitis. Journal of Periodontology. Sep 2003;**74**(9):1329-1335. DOI: 10.1902/jop.2003.74.9.1329

[40] Ximenez-Fyvie LA, Almaguer-Flores A, Jacobo-Soto V, Lara-Cordoba M, Moreno-Borjas JY, Alcantara-Maruri E. Subgingival microbiota of periodontally untreated Mexican subjects with generalized aggressive periodontitis. Journal of Clinical Periodontology. Dec 2006;**33**(12):869-877. DOI: 10.1111/j.1600-051X.2006.01006.x

[41] Kamma JJ, Slots J. Herpesviral-bacterial interactions in aggressive periodontitis. Journal of Clinical Periodontology. May 2003;**30**(5):420-426. DOI: 10.1034/j.1600-051X.2003.20002.x

[42] Parameter on Aggressive Periodontitis. American Academy of periodontology. Journal of Periodontology. May 2000;**71**(5 Suppl):867-869. DOI: 10.1902/jop.2000.71.5-S.867

[43] Kornman KS, Page RC, Tonetti MS. The host response to the microbial challenge in periodontitis: Assembling the players. Periodontology 2000. Jun 1997;**14**:33-53. DOI: 10.1111/j.1600-0757.1997.tb00191.x

[44] Meng H, Xu L, Li Q, Han J, Zhao Y. Determinants of host susceptibility in aggressive periodontitis. Periodontology 2000. 2007;**43**:133-159. DOI: 10.1111/j.1600-0757.2006.00204.x

[45] Fine DH, Oshrain R. Preliminary characterization of material eluted from roots affected by juvenile periodontitis. Journal of Periodontal Research. Mar 1984;**19**(2):146-151. DOI: 10.1111/j.1600-051X.1991.tb01118.x

[46] Shapira L, Borinski R, Sela MN, Soskolne A. Superoxide formation and chemiluminescence of peripheral polymorphonuclear leukocytes in rapidly progressive periodontitis patients. Journal of Clinical Periodontology. Jan 1991;**18**(1):44-48

[47] Leino L, Hurttia HM, Sorvajarvi K, Sewon LA. Increased respiratory burst activity is associated with normal expression of IgG-fc-receptors and complement receptors in peripheral neutrophils from patients with juvenile periodontitis. Journal of Periodontal Research. May 1994;**29**(3):179-184. DOI: 10.1111/j.1600-0765.1994.tb01211.x

[48] Shibata K, Warbington ML, Gordon BJ, Kurihara H, Van Dyke TE. Nitric oxide synthase activity in neutrophils from patients with localized aggressive periodontitis. Journal of Periodontology. Aug 2001;**72**(8):1052-1058. DOI: 10.1902/jop.2001.72.8.1052

[49] Armitage GC. Development of a classification system for periodontal diseases and conditions. Northwest Dentistry. Nov–Dec 2000;**79**(6):31-35. PMID: 11413609

[50] Kantarci A, Oyaizu K, Van Dyke TE. Neutrophil-mediated tissue injury in periodontal disease pathogenesis: Findings from localized aggressive periodontitis. Journal of Periodontology. Jan 2003;**74**(1):66-75. DOI: 10.1902/jop.2003.74.1.66

[51] Armitage GC, Cullinan MP, Seymour GJ. Comparative biology of chronic and agg-ressive periodontitis: Introduction. Periodontology 2000. Jun 2010;**53**:7-11. DOI: 10.1111/j. 1600-0757.2010.00359.x

[52] Stein J, Reichert S, Gautsch A, Machulla HK. Are there HLA combinations typical supporting for or making resistant against aggressive and/or chronic periodontitis? Journal of Periodontal Research. Oct 2003;**38**(5):508-517. DOI: 10.1034/j.1600-0765.2003.00683.x

[53] Stein JM, Machulla HK, Smeets R, Lampert F, Reichert S. Human leukocyte antigen polymorphism in chronic and aggressive periodontitis among Caucasians: A meta-analysis. Journal of Clinical Periodontology. Mar 2008;**35**(3):183-192. DOI: 10.1111/j.1600-051X. 2007.01189.x

[54] Stabholz A, Soskolne WA, Shapira L. Genetic and environmental risk factors for chronic periodontitis and aggressive periodontitis. Periodontology 2000. Jun 2010;**53**:138-153. DOI: 10.1111/j.1600-0757.2010.00340.x

[55] Hagewald S, Bernimoulin JP, Kottgen E, Kage A. Salivary IgA subclasses and bacteria-reactive IgA in patients with aggressive periodontitis. Journal of Periodontal Research. Oct 2002;**37**(5):333-339. DOI: 10.1034/j.1600-0765.2002.00337.x

[56] Hwang AM, Stoupel J, Celenti R, Demmer RT, Papapanou PN. Serum antibody responses to periodontal microbiota in chronic and aggressive periodontitis: A postulate revisited. Journal of Periodontology. Apr 2014;**85**(4):592-600. DOI: 10.1902/jop.2013.130172

[57] Chandy S, Joseph K, Sankaranarayanan A, Issac A, Babu G, Wilson B, et al. Evaluation of C-reactive protein and fibrinogen in patients with chronic and aggressive periodontitis: A clinico-biochemical study. Journal of Clinical and Diagnostic Research. Mar 2017;**11**(3):ZC41-ZZC5. DOI: 10.7860/JCDR/2017/23100.9552

[58] Zhan Y, Lu R, Meng H, Wang X, Sun X, Hou J. The role of platelets in inflammatory immune responses in generalized aggressive periodontitis. Journal of Clinical Periodontology. Feb 2017;**44**(2):150-157. DOI: 10.1111/jcpe.12657

[59] Duan F, Guo Y, Zhang L, Chen P, Wang X, Liu Z, Hu Y, Chen S, Chen D. Association of KCNQ1 polymorphisms with gliclazide efficacy in Chinese type 2 diabetic patients. Pharmacogenetics and Genomics. Apr 2016;**26**(4):178-183. PMID: 26866747 DOI: 10.1097/ FPC.0000000000000204

[60] Monteiro da Silva AM, Oakley DA, Newman HN, Nohl FS, Lloyd HM. Psychosocial factors and adult onset rapidly progressive periodontitis. Journal of Clinical Periodontology. 1996 Aug;**23**(8):789-794. DOI: 10.1111/j.1600-051X.1996.tb00611.x

[61] Tanner AC, Kent Jr R, Van Dyke T, Sonis ST, Murray LA. Clinical and other risk indicators for early periodontitis in adults. Journal of Periodontology. Apr 2005;**76**(4):573-581. DOI: 10.1902/jop.2005.76.4.573

[62] Schenkein HA, Gunsolley JC, Koertge TE, Schenkein JG, Tew JG. Smoking and its effects on early-onset periodontitis. Journal of the American Dental Association (1939). Aug 1995;**126**(8):1107-1113. PMID: 7560567

[63] Kamma JJ, Giannopoulou C, Vasdekis VG, Mombelli A. Cytokine profile in gingival crevicular fluid of aggressive periodontitis: Influence of smoking and stress. Journal of Clinical Periodontology. Oct 2004;**31**(10):894-902. DOI: 10.1111/j.1600-051X.2004.00585.x

[64] Darby IB, Hodge PJ, Riggio MP, Kinane DF. Clinical and microbiological effect of scaling and root planing in smoker and non-smoker chronic and aggressive periodontitis patients. Journal of Clinical Periodontology. Feb 2005;**32**(2):200-206. DOI: 10.1111/j.1600-051X.2005.00644.x

[65] Brett PM, Zygogianni P, Griffiths GS, Tomaz M, Parkar M, D'Aiuto F, et al. Functional gene polymorphisms in aggressive and chronic periodontitis. Journal of Dental Research. Dec 2005;**84**(12):1149-1153. DOI: 10.1177/154405910508401211

[66] Fiebig A, Jepsen S, Loos BG, Scholz C, Schafer C, Ruhling A, et al. Polymorphisms in the interleukin-1 (IL1) gene cluster are not associated with aggressive periodontitis in a large Caucasian population. Genomics. Nov 2008;**92**(5):309-315. DOI: 10.1016/j.ygeno.2008.07.004

[67] Walker SJ, Van Dyke TE, Rich S, Kornman KS, di Giovine FS, Hart TC. Genetic polymorphisms of the IL-1alpha and IL-1beta genes in African-American LJP patients and an African-American control population. Journal of Periodontology. May 2000;**71**(5):723-728. DOI: 10.1902/jop.2000.71.5.723

[68] Li QY, Zhao HS, Meng HX, Zhang L, Xu L, Chen ZB, et al. Association analysis between interleukin-1 family polymorphisms and generalized aggressive periodontitis in a Chinese population. Journal of Periodontology. 2004 Dec;**75**(12):1627-1635. DOI: 10.1902/jop.2004.75.12.1627

[69] Gonzales JR, Kobayashi T, Michel J, Mann M, Yoshie H, Meyle J. Interleukin-4 gene polymorphisms in Japanese and Caucasian patients with aggressive periodontitis. Journal of Clinical Periodontology. May 2004;**31**(5):384-389. DOI: 10.1111/j.1600-051X.2004.00492.x

[70] Shao MY, Huang P, Cheng R, Hu T. Interleukin-6 polymorphisms modify the risk of periodontitis: A systematic review and meta-analysis. Journal of Zhejiang University. Science. B. 2009 Dec;**10**(12):920-927. DOI: 10.1631/jzus.B0920279

[71] Jaradat SM, Ababneh KT, Jaradat SA, Abbadi MS, Taha AH, Karasneh JA, et al. Association of interleukin-10 gene promoter polymorphisms with chronic and aggressive periodontitis. Oral Diseases. Apr 2012;**18**(3):271-279. DOI: 10.1111/j.1601-0825.2011.01872.x

[72] Laine ML, Crielaard W, Loos BG. Genetic susceptibility to periodontitis. Periodontol 2000. Feb 2012;**58**(1):37-68. DOI: 10.1111/j.1600-0757.2011.00415.x

[73] Yu JJ, Ruddy MJ, Wong GC, Sfintescu C, Baker PJ, Smith JB, et al. An essential role for IL-17 in preventing pathogen-initiated bone destruction: Recruitment of neutrophils to inflamed bone requires IL-17 receptor-dependent signals. Blood. May 1, 2007;**109**(9):3794-3802. DOI: 10.1182/blood-2005-09-010116

[74] da Silva FRP, Pessoa LDS, Vasconcelos A, de Aquino Lima W, Alves EHP, Vasconcelos DFP. Polymorphisms in interleukins 17A and 17F genes and periodontitis: Results from a meta-analysis. Molecular Biology Reports. Dec 2017;**44**(6):443-453. DOI: 10.1007/s11033-017-4128-x

[75] Maney P, Owens JL. Interleukin polymorphisms in aggressive periodontitis: A literature review. Journal of Indian Society of Periodontology. Mar–Apr 2015;**19**(2):131-141. DOI: 10.4103/0972-124X.145787

[76] Yuan ZN, Schreurs O, Gjermo P, Helgeland K, Schenck K. Topical distribution of fc gammaRI, FcgammaRII and FcgammaRIII in inflamed human gingiva. Journal of Clinical Periodontology. Jul 1999;**26**(7):441-447. DOI: 10.1034/j.1600-051X.1999.260705.x

[77] Kobayashi T, Sugita N, van der Pol WL, Nunokawa Y, Westerdaal NA, Yamamoto K, et al. The Fcgamma receptor genotype as a risk factor for generalized early-onset periodontitis in Japanese patients. Journal of Periodontology. Sep 2000;**71**(9):1425-1432. DOI: 10.1902/jop.2000.71.9.1425

[78] Nibali L, Parkar M, Brett P, Knight J, Tonetti MS, Griffiths GS. NADPH oxidase (CYBA) and FcgammaR polymorphisms as risk factors for aggressive periodontitis: A case-control association study. Journal of Clinical Periodontology. Aug 2006;**33**(8):529-539. DOI: 10.1111/j.1600-051X.2006.00952.x

[79] Nibali L, Parkar M, D'Aiuto F, Suvan JE, Brett PM, Griffiths GS, et al. Vitamin D receptor polymorphism (−1056 Taq-I) interacts with smoking for the presence and progression of periodontitis. Journal of Clinical Periodontology. Jul 2008;**35**(7):561-567. DOI: 10.1111/j.1600-051X.2008.01233.x

[80] Park KS, Nam JH, Choi J. The short vitamin D receptor is associated with increased risk for generalized aggressive periodontitis. Journal of Clinical Periodontology. Aug 2006;**33**(8):524-528. DOI: 10.1111/j.1600-051X.2006.00944.x

[81] Holla LI, Buckova D, Fassmann A, Halabala T, Vasku A, Vacha J. Promoter polymorphisms in the CD14 receptor gene and their potential association with the severity of chronic periodontitis. Journal of Medical Genetics. Nov 2002;**39**(11):844-848. DOI: 10.1136/jmg.39.11.844

[82] James JA, Poulton KV, Haworth SE, Payne D, McKay IJ, Clarke FM, et al. Polymorphisms of TLR4 but not CD14 are associated with a decreased risk of aggressive periodontitis. Journal of Clinical Periodontology. Feb 2007;**34**(2):111-117. DOI: 10.1111/j.1600-051X.2006.01030.x

[83] Yek EC, Cintan S, Topcuoglu N, Kulekci G, Issever H, Kantarci A. Efficacy of amoxicillin and metronidazole combination for the management of generalized aggressive periodontitis. Journal of Periodontology. Jul 2010;**81**(7):964-974. DOI: 10.1902/jop.2010.090522

[84] Xajigeorgiou C, Sakellari D, Slini T, Baka A, Konstantinidis A. Clinical and microbiological effects of different antimicrobials on generalized aggressive periodontitis. Journal of Clinical Periodontology. Apr 2006;**33**(4):254-264. DOI: 10.1111/j.1600-051X.2006.00905.x

[85] Kamma JJ, Baehni PC. Five-year maintenance follow-up of early-onset periodontitis patients. Journal of Clinical Periodontology. Jun 2003;**30**(6):562-572. DOI: 10.1034/j.1600-051X.2003.00289.x

[86] Zucchelli G, Brini C, De Sanctis M. GTR treatment of intrabony defects in patients with early-onset and chronic adult periodontitis. The International Journal of Periodontics & Restorative Dentistry. Aug 2002;**22**(4):323-333. PMID: 12212679

[87] Nevins M, Kim DM. Classical versus contemporary treatment planning for aggressive periodontal disease. Journal of Periodontology. May 2010;**81**(5):767-775. DOI: 10.1902/jop.2010.090537

[88] Teughels W, Dhondt R, Dekeyser C, Quirynen M. Treatment of aggressive periodontitis. Periodontology 2000. Jun 2014;**65**(1):107-133. DOI: 10.1111/prd.12020

[89] Shaddox LM, Walker C. Microbial testing in periodontics: Value, limitations and future directions. Periodontology 2000. 2009;**50**:25-38. DOI: 10.1111/j.1600-0757.2008.00285.x

[90] Sanz M, Teughels W. Innovations in non-surgical periodontal therapy: Consensus Report of the Sixth European Workshop on Periodontology. Journal of Clinical Periodontology. Sep 2008;**35**(8 Suppl):3-7. DOI: 10.1111/j.1600-051X.2008.01256.x

[91] Slots J, Rosling BG. Suppression of the periodontopathic microflora in localized juvenile periodontitis by systemic tetracycline. Journal of Clinical Periodontology. Sep 1983;**10**(5):465-486. DOI: 10.1111/j.1600-051X.1983.tb02179.x

[92] Drisko CH. Nonsurgical periodontal therapy. Periodontology 2000. 2001;**25**:77-88. DOI: 10.1034/j.1600-0757.2001.22250106.x

[93] Asikainen S, Jousimies-Somer H, Kanervo A, Saxen L. The immediate efficacy of adjunctive doxycycline in treatment of localized juvenile periodontitis. Archives of Oral Biology. 1990;**35**(Suppl):231S-234S. PMID: 2088233

[94] Herrera D, Alonso B, Leon R, Roldan S, Sanz M. Antimicrobial therapy in periodontitis: The use of systemic antimicrobials against the subgingival biofilm. Journal of Clinical Periodontology. Sep 2008;**35**(8 Suppl):45-66. DOI: 10.1111/j.1600-051X.2008.01260.x

[95] Haffajee AD, Socransky SS, Gunsolley JC. Systemic anti-infective periodontal therapy. A systematic review. Annals of Periodontology. Dec 2003;**8**(1):115-181. DOI: 10.1902/annals.2003.8.1.115

[96] van Winkelhoff AJ, Tijhof CJ, de Graaff J. Microbiological and clinical results of metronidazole plus amoxicillin therapy in Actinobacillus actinomycetemcomitans-associated periodontitis. Journal of Periodontology. Jan 1992;**63**(1):52-57. DOI: 10.1902/jop.1992.63.1.52

[97] Guerrero A, Griffiths GS, Nibali L, Suvan J, Moles DR, Laurell L, et al. Adjunctive benefits of systemic amoxicillin and metronidazole in non-surgical treatment of generalized aggressive periodontitis: A randomized placebo-controlled clinical trial. Journal of Clinical Periodontology. Oct 2005;**32**(10):1096-1107. DOI: 10.1111/j.1600-051X.2005.00814.x

[98] Haas AN, de Castro GD, Moreno T, Susin C, Albandar JM, Oppermann RV, et al. Azithromycin as an adjunctive treatment of aggressive periodontitis: 12-months randomized clinical trial. Journal of Clinical Periodontology. Aug 2008;**35**(8):696-704. DOI: 10.1111/j.1600-051X.2008.01254.x

[99] Da Rocha HA, Silva CF, Santiago FL, Martins LG, Dias PC, De Magalhaes D. Local drug delivery systems in the treatment of periodontitis: A literature review. Journal of the International Academy of Periodontology. Jul 2015;**17**(3):82-90. PMID: 26373225

[100] Unsal E, Walsh TF, Akkaya M. The effect of a single application of subgingival antimicrobial or mechanical therapy on the clinical parameters of juvenile periodontitis. Journal of Periodontology. Jan 1995;**66**(1):47-51. DOI: 10.1902/jop.1995.66.1.47

[101] Kaner D, Bernimoulin JP, Hopfenmuller W, Kleber BM, Friedmann A. Controlled-delivery chlorhexidine chip versus amoxicillin/metronidazole as adjunctive antimicrobial therapy for generalized aggressive periodontitis: A randomized controlled clinical trial. Journal of Clinical Periodontology. Oct 2007;**34**(10):880-891. DOI: 10.1111/j.1600-051X.2007.01122.x

[102] Purucker P, Mertes H, Goodson JM, Bernimoulin JP. Local versus systemic adjunctive antibiotic therapy in 28 patients with generalized aggressive periodontitis. Journal of Periodontology. Sep 2001;**72**(9):1241-1245. DOI: 10.1902/jop.2000.72.9.1241

[103] Christersson LA, Slots J, Rosling BG, Genco RJ. Microbiological and clinical effects of surgical treatment of localized juvenile periodontitis. Journal of Clinical Periodontology. Jul 1985;**12**(6):465-476. DOI: 10.1111/j.1600-051X.1985.tb01382.x

[104] Kornman KS, Robertson PB. Clinical and microbiological evaluation of therapy for juvenile periodontitis. Journal of Periodontology. Aug 1985;**56**(8):443-446. DOI: 10.1902/jop.1985.56.8.443

[105] Lindhe J, Liljenberg B. Treatment of localized juvenile periodontitis. Results after 5 years. Journal of Clinical Periodontology. Jul 1984;**11**(6):399-410. DOI: 10.1111/j.1600-051X.1984.tb01338.x

[106] Buchmann R, Nunn ME, Van Dyke TE, Lange DE. Aggressive periodontitis: 5-year follow-up of treatment. Journal of Periodontology. Jun 2002;**73**(6):675-683. DOI: 10.1902/jop.2002.73.6.675

[107] Khojasteh A, Kheiri L, Motamedian SR, Khoshkam V. Guided bone regeneration for the reconstruction of alveolar bone defects. Annals of Maxillofacial Surgery. Jul–Dec 2017;**7**(2):263-277. DOI: 10.4103/ams.ams_76_17

[108] Yukna RA, Sepe WW. Clinical evaluation of localized periodontosis defects treated with freeze-dried bone allografts combined with local and systemic tetracyclines. The International Journal of Periodontics & Restorative Dentistry. 1982;**2**(5):8-21. PMID: 6757167

[109] Evans GH, Yukna RA, Sepe WW, Mabry TW, Mayer ET. Effect of various graft materials with tetracycline in localized juvenile periodontitis. Journal of Periodontology. Sep 1989;**60**(9):491-497. DOI: 10.1902/jop.1989.60.9.491

[110] Bottino MC, Thomas V. Membranes for periodontal regeneration--a materials perspective. Frontiers of Oral Biology. 2015;**17**:90-100. DOI: 10.1159/000381699

[111] Sirirat M, Kasetsuwan J, Jeffcoat MK. Comparison between 2 surgical techniques for the treatment of early-onset periodontitis. Journal of Periodontology. Jun 1996;**67**(6):603-607. DOI: 10.1902/jop.1996.67.6.603

[112] Souza E, Medeiros AC, Gurgel BC, Sarmento C. Antimicrobial photodynamic therapy in the treatment of aggressive periodontitis: A systematic review and meta-analysis. Lasers in Medical Science. Jan 2016;**31**(1):187-196. DOI: 10.1007/s10103-015-1836-0

[113] Bonta H, Llambes F, Moretti AJ, Mathur H, Bouwsma OJ. The use of enamel matrix protein in the treatment of localized aggressive periodontitis: A case report. Quintessence International. Apr 2003;**34**(4):247-252. PMID: 12731609

[114] Kaner D, Bernimoulin JP, Kleber BM, Friedmann A. Minimally invasive flap surgery and enamel matrix derivative in the treatment of localized aggressive periodontitis: Case report. The International Journal of Periodontics & Restorative Dentistry. Feb 2009;**29**(1):89-97. PMID: 19244886

[115] Yilmaz S, Cakar G, Kuru BE, Yildirim B. Platelet-rich plasma in combination with bovine derived xenograft in the treatment of generalized aggressive periodontitis: A case report with re-entry. Platelets. Nov 2007;**18**(7):535-539. DOI: 10.1080/09537100701481393

[116] Deas DE, Mealey BL. Response of chronic and aggressive periodontitis to treatment. Periodontology 2000. Jun 2010;**53**:154-166. DOI: 10.1111/j.1600-0757.2009.00334.x

3

The Periodontal-Endodontic Relationship: What do we Know?

Kai Ling Siew, Victor Goh, Chui Ling Goo,
Esmonde Francis Corbet and Wai Keung Leung

Abstract

Diagnosis and management of periodontal-endodontic lesions are often complicated by the close interrelationship between periodontal tissues and dental pulps. Communications between both biological entities may occur through the apical foramen, accessory canals or exposed dentinal tubules, allowing bi-directional spread of infection and/or inflam mation. Endodontic and periodontal lesions may occur distinctly or in tandem. Infected pulps may provoke an inflammatory response in adjoining periodontal tissues, and induce tissue destruction, and likewise, periodontal infection may elicit progressive pulpal pathoses. Solely periodontal or solely endodontic lesions are often clinically recognizable as distinct pathologies. However reported pain from pulpal or periodontal tissues may be similar, especially in combined lesions in which both endodontic and periodontal infection co-exist. When combined lesions develop, signs and symptoms such as toothache, tooth mobility, increased probing pocket depths and localized swelling may develop concurrently. As such, appropriate diagnostic tests and detailed clinical examination are required to differentiate periodontal, endodontic and combined pathologies and to arrive at correct diagnoses. Successful treatment outcomes for any periodontal and/or endodontic lesion depend on correct diagnosis and timely implementation of appropriate therapies. In this chapter, available evidence on periodontal-endodontic lesions will be reviewed with classification, clinical presentations, prognoses and treat ment modalities discussed collectively.

Keywords: diagnosis, oral disease, endodontics, periodontal diseases, periodontics

1. Introduction

The close inter-relationship between the periodontium and root canal systems has resulted in concomitant lesions from both entities, leading to periodontal-endodontic (perio-endo) infections that, to date, remain a challenge for the dental professional to both diagnose and manage. An in-depth understanding of the anatomy and disease pathogenesis is of utmost importance in assisting clinicians to establish a prognosis, derive a rational treatment plan and troubleshoot complicated cases grounded on sound biological and clinical bases. In this chapter, evidence-based and contemporary approaches to managing periodontal and/or end odontic lesions will be discussed collectively.

2. Relationship between the periodontium and root canal systems

2.1. Influence of pulpal pathologies on the periodontium

Periodontal disease is an inflammatory disease of the tooth supporting structures initiated by bacteria that form a biofilm on the tooth/root surfaces [1]. Root canal infections (i.e. api cal periodontitis) are multi-microbial, biofilm-associated diseases [2, 3]. Apical ramifications, lateral canals, and isthmuses connecting main root canals may harbor biofilm-like microbial structures [2]. The communications between the pulp and the periodontium occur primarily through: exposed dentinal tubules, small portal of exits - e.g. accessory canals and lateral canals - and via the apical foramen [4, 5]. As such, it is unsurprising that pathogens infect ing the periodontium and root canal systems are highly similar, indicative of an inseparable relationship between the root canal system and the periodontium [6].

In chronic apical abscesses caused by endodontic infections, a localized collection of pus with a draining sinus may track through the periodontium, forming a deep, narrow and isolated periodontal pocket, adjacent to, or alongside, the gingival sulcus. For molars or multi-rooted teeth, radiographic examination may reveal a radiolucent area at the furcation of an infected tooth, indicating presence of accessory canals which drain into the furcation area [4].

Jansson et al. [7] reported that teeth in periodontitis-prone patients lost more attachment when a continuous root canal infection was present compared to teeth with no periapical lesions. Such findings were also observed by Ehnevid et al. [8] who concluded that a root-canal infec tion, if left untreated, may impair periodontal healing following non-surgical periodontal therapy. When the pulp is the source of infection, considerations should be given towards treating the endodontic infections prior to periodontal treatment [5, 9]. Such an approach is aimed at eliminating the source of pulpal infection prior to periodontal therapy, as root instrumentation may remove the protective cementum layer [10] and communicate residual infection through exposed dentinal tubules or accessory canals [11, 12].

2.2. Influence of periodontal inflammation on the pulp

An inflamed periodontium resulting from a periodontal infection may affect the vitality of the pulp. Seltzer and Bender [13], reported that periodontal lesions could potentially infect the pulp through numerous lateral and accessory canals in the furcation area. The authors found that 79% of periodontally involved teeth, without caries and restorations, exhibited histological evidence of pulpal pathology. In periodontal disease affected teeth, localized pulpal necrosis adjacent to accessory canals was found [13].

Langeland et al. [14] reported that the effect of periodontal disease on the pulp was degenerative in nature, resulting in pulpal inflammation, calcifications and resorption. Such insults from periodontal disease to the pulp were cumulative over time [14]. Similarly, Wan et al. [15] reported that the severity of periodontitis had substantial effect on pulpal health. They speculated that denuded root surfaces could induce more pathological changes within the pulp [15]. Root surfaces may be denuded of the protective cementum layer as a result of periodontal treatment [16], developmental defects [17] or even due to direct bacterial invasion [18]. Denuded surfaces are thought to allow passage of microorganisms between the pulp and periodontal tissues through patent dentinal tubules, lateral or accessory canals [18]. Furthermore, if the microvasculature of the apical foramen remains intact, the pulp may maintain its vitality [14].

2.3. Communications between the periodontium and dental pulp

The dental pulp and periodontium are closely related both anatomically and functionally, through three different channels of communication – as discussed below.

2.3.1. Apical foramen

The root canal system is a complicated system with the apical foramen as the principal route of communication between the pulp and the periodontium. A single apical foramen is the exception rather than the rule. Multiple foramina, fins, deltas, loops, and furcations are usually present at the apical end of the root canal [19]. Bacteria, bacterial toxins, inflammatory by-products and mediators pass readily through the apical foramen into the root canal eliciting inflammation of the pulp and subsequently pulpal necrosis [20].

If periodontal disease reaches the apical foramen, such inflammatory reactions may spread both ways leading to perio-endo pathologies. Similarly, infection from an infected pulp may exit the apical foramen, track through the periodontium, eliciting tissue destruction and formation of what registers clinically as a periodontal pocket.

2.3.2. Lateral and accessory canals

Accessory or lateral canals from the dental pulp may be formed during formation of the root sheath. A break develops in the continuity of the sheath, producing a small gap, which results in a small "accessory" canal between the dental sac and the pulp. Accessory and lateral canals can be seen anywhere along the root, creating a potential perio-endo pathway of communication [21]. Studies have reported that nerve fiber and blood vessels are commonly present in these lateral canals. They are found to traverse the periodontal ligament, course through the portal on cementum wall, root dentin and connect to the main root canal system [22]. Approximately 17% of teeth may present with multiple canal systems in the apical third of the root, about 9% in the middle third and fewer than 2% in the coronal third [23]. It has been reported that debridement at molar furcation areas may increase the risk of bacterial contamination of the pulp by 39% through exposed dentin or furcation canals [24].

2.3.3. Dentinal tubules

As periodontitis gradually destroys the periodontal ligament between the cementum and bone, cementum becomes exposed to the oral environment via periodontal pockets and through gingiva recession. Destruction of Sharpey's fibers leaves a sieve-like surface on the cementum, full of canals which may be contaminated by bacteria and their toxins that may transverse the protective cemental layer into the patent dentinal tubules [10]. Furthermore, iatrogenic removal of cementum during periodontal treatment, various developmental fissures, grooves and incomplete calcifications on cementum may all permit penetration by bacteria into the underlying dentinal tubules [10].

Dentin is highly permeable with dentinal tubules as the major channels for diffusion of material across dentin. Bergenholtz and Lindhe [25] reported that the application of soluble material from bacterial plaque readily caused pulpal inflammation, suggesting there was a pathway of communication between the dentinal tubules, periodontium and the pulp. Such findings were again confirmed by Bergenholtz [26], who found that bacterial products applied to exposed dentin initiated inflammatory reactions in the dental pulp whilst occlusion of such exposed dentin had a protective effect with respect to the pulp.

2.4. The etiological agents

The source of perio-endo infection is no doubt from within the mouth yet there is no comprehensive report on the microbiota involved compare with periodontal or endodontic infection occurring independently. More than 460 bacterial, almost 10 fungal and 1 archaeal taxa [27] plus predominantly herpesviruses detectable at periradicular lesions [28] were reported associated with endodontic infection. Such observations were rather similar to microbiology of periodontitis [29]. Microbiology of failed endodontic treatment [30] and persisting periradicular endodontic infection (i.e. L-phase bacteria) [28], however exhibit unique microbiology. Taking that into consideration, the exact microbiological nature of perio-endo lesion remained to be elucidated.

3. Contributing factors to perio-endo lesions

3.1. Inadequate endodontic treatment

The primary aim of endodontic treatment is to disinfect the root canal system through chemomechanical debridement and cleaning so that the canal space can be freed of infected organic materials and obturated with an inert material [31]. Endodontic failures are caused by inadequate disinfection of the root canal system or reinfection of the root canal system due to failure to obtain a hermetic seal [32]. Endodontic infection may spread to the periodontium leading to perio-endo pathologies.

Endodontic failure may be caused by various biological and procedural factors e.g. (i) persistence intra- and extra-canal infection; (ii) inadequate or poorly condensed filling of the canal; (iii) overextensions of root filling materials; (iv) leakage due to inadequate coronal seal; (v) missed and thus undebrided canals; (vi) iatrogenic procedural errors such as poor access cavity design; and (vii) improper instrumentation (inadequate chemo-mechanical cleaning, ledges, perforations, or separated instruments). As it stands, proper access cavity design, thorough chemo-mechanical debridement and complete sealing of the root canal system to obliterate infection and prevent reinfection are key in prevention of endodontic failure.

3.2. Poor restorations

Poor restorations can be a major culprit for periodontal conditions and endodontic failure. Poor contours due to overhanging restorations, which impinge upon and thus violate the biological width, can contribute to localized periodontal defects [33, 34].

Poorly adapted restorations predispose to coronal leakage, allowing for recontamination of the root canal system and subsequent endodontic failure [35, 36]. Ray and Trope [36] reported that defective restorations with adequate root fillings had a higher failure rate in comparison to teeth with inadequate root fillings but with adequate restoration [36]. Similarly, a systematic review by Gillen et al. [35] reported that adequate root canal treatment (RCT) and good coronal seal increased the odds for healing of periapical lesions. In cases with adequate root filling-inadequate coronal restoration and inadequate root filling-adequate coronal restoration, poorer resolution of periapical infections are to be expected [35].

In short, sufficient disinfection and filling of the root canal system and a well-adapted coronal restoration which respects the biological width are paramount in ensuring long-term endodontic success and maintenance of a healthy periodontium around the treated tooth.

3.3. Perforations

Root perforation is a mechanical or pathological, communication between the root canal system and the external tooth surface [37]. Misalignment of instruments during endodontic access, negotiation and preparation of the root canals, and preparation of post space can cause iatrogenic perforations. Pathological root perforation, on the other hand, is caused by root resorption and/or caries.

In perforations, bacterial infections emanating from either the root canal or periodontal tissues, or both, could prevent healing and bring about inflammation. Down-growth of the gingival epithelium to the perforation site can follow, resulting in accelerated periodontal breakdown [38]. Ideally, any perforation should be repaired immediately. Treatment outcomes of endodontic perforations at the apical part of roots have been reported to be more successful than those located more coronally [39, 40]. Mineral trioxide aggregate (MTA) is often used for perforation repair [41] as it can stimulate hard tissue deposition [42], is biocompatible [43], provides excellent seal [44] and sets in the presence of moisture [45].

3.4. Developmental malformations

Developmental malformations both affect the periodontium and complicate conventional RCT. One of the most common dental malformations seen is the palatal-radicular groove, which has a reported prevalence of 4.6% appearing in maxillary incisors [46]. Its presence is a locus of plaque accumulation and provides potential pathway for microorganisms to penetrate into deeper parts of the periodontium, causing local inflammation and subsequent periodontal breakdown. Attachment loss may extend apically until it adversely affects the viability of the pulp, which is typical of the pathogenesis of a primary periodontal lesion with secondary endodontic involvement. RCT may be needed first if the patient complains of toothache. This may then be followed by periodontal surgical debridement or regenerative periodontal therapy when indicated [47].

Cemental tear is a rare periodontal condition characterized by partial or total separation of the cementum. The detachment normally happens at the cementum-dentin junction predisposing the tooth to plaque-induced periodontitis. Clinically, a cemental tear may present as a localized deep periodontal pocket, with or without other symptoms such as a sinus tract or pain. Probing at the affected site may detect root surface roughness or an obstruction, different to the expected typical tactile sense of calculus [48]. Treatment of cemental tear includes conventional periodontal therapy, combined periodontal and endodontic treatment when pulpal status of the affected tooth is compromised and/or surgery to remove the tear.

Cervical enamel projections and enamel pearls are development anomalies presenting as ectopic globules of enamel on the root surface. Enamel projections are small continuous or discontinuous extensions of enamel that occur in the molar furcations while enamel pearls are larger masses of enamel that have a predilection for molars [49]. It has been reported that 82.5% of molars with furcation attachment loss exhibited cervical enamel projections [50]. Enamel pearls are a rarity and occur mostly on permanent molars with an incidence rate of 1.1–9.7% [51]. Cervical enamel projections and enamel pearls predispose to periodontitis because Sharpey's fiber insertion is not developmentally possible, allowing only a hemidesmosomal attachment, which may be less resistant to periodontal breakdown. Both entities may also prevent effective oral hygiene procedures when exposed to the oral environment and may serve as a nidus for periodonto-pathogenic bacteria to grow and populate their surface [49]. In longstanding conditions, down-growth of epithelial attachment may cause a perio-endo lesion, especially if exposed accessory canals in the furcation area allow bacteria invasion into the pulp [24]. A combination of treatments may be warranted, such as RCT if pulpal symptoms are present, followed by periodontal surgery to recontour locally the affected root to allow for root debridement and to facilitate proper oral hygiene measures and periodontal maintenance measures.

3.5. Resorptions

Dental resorption is the loss of dental hard tissues as a result of resorptive activities by clastic cells (aptly known as odontoclasts) [52]. Root resorption may occur as a physiologic or pathologic phenomenon. Root resorption is classified into two types, external and internal.

3.5.1. *External inflammatory resorption*

External inflammatory resorption (EIR) is often a result of root avulsion injuries [53]. Traumatic dental injuries (e.g., intrusion, lateral luxation, and avulsion) and subsequent replantation often result in contusion injuries to the periodontal ligament (PDL). Damage to the pre-cementum, with a resultant breach in its integrity, is the precipitating factor in all types of external resorption [53]. In the wound healing process that follows, necrotic PDL tissues, damaged cementum and even root dentin may be actively removed by macrophages and osteoclasts, although the underlining mechanism is still unclear [52].

The diagnosis of EIR in clinical situations is often based on radiographic findings [54]. However, in two-dimentional radiographic imaging EIR may be obscured by overlapping images, or may not detectably show early signs of EIR, resulting in late diagnosis of EIR. Chronic inflammation seen in periodontal disease has been regarded as a cause for root resorption [55, 56], and such resorptive processes are associated with the severity of periodontitis [55]. The exact mechanism of periodontal disease-associated resorption is not known, but such a process may be a sequela of tooth mobility due to attachment loss [55]. When mobile teeth are subjected to occlusal forces, traumatic assault of the radicular surface may ensue, causing formation of cemental tears or lesions which may become colonized by odontoclastic cells or even periodontal pathogens that may resorb the root [55].

Treatment of EIR is based on effective removal of the cause, which is to institute a RCT with removal of the infected necrotic pulpal tissue [57]. Although the treatment of such lesions in periodontal disease is inconclusive, conventional mechanical debridement [56] may suppress inflammation and arrest the resorptive process. The earlier EIR is diagnosed and treated, the better the prognosis is for the affected tooth [58].

3.5.2. *External cervical resorption*

External cervical resorption (ECR) is a form of root resorption that originates on the external root surface but may invade root dentin in any direction and to varying degrees. ECR generally develops immediately apical to the epithelial attachment to the tooth. However, in teeth that have developed gingival recession and lost periodontal support and/or have developed a long junctional epithelium, the resorptive defect may arise at a more apical location [59]. The difference between EIR and ECR is that the pulp remains vital in ECR lesions unless the lesion is extensive and erodes into the pulpal space, while EIR always presents with necrotic pulp with or without any periapical lesion.

The exact etiology and pathogenesis of ECR have not been fully elucidated but may be regarded as the same for EIR. Infected or denuded cementum surfaces allow binding of multinucleated clastic cells which perpetuate the resorptive process [52]. Orthodontic treatment, dental trauma, oral surgery, periodontal therapy, bruxism, delayed eruption, and dental developmental defects were all identified as potential predisposing factors to ECR [60, 61]. In patients with periodontal disease, ECR may occur if the root-protective junctional epithelium (JE) did not develop. In such instances periodonto-pathogen initiated inflammation and dietary acid may extend into the root surfaces to cause ECR [56]. Although not fully understood, such a situation may explain why resorption occurs only in the cervical region, where JE is absent and dietary acid easily gains access and may accumulate over a long period.

The clinical features of ECR may vary depending on etiology. However, the process is very often quiescent and asymptomatic initially. Its diagnosis is commonly made from a chance radiographic finding. A pink or red discoloration may later develop at the cervical region due to fibrovascular granulation tissue occupying the resorptive defect [59]. Inflammatory periodontal destruction may occur in the region of the resorption, resulting in a periodontal pocket that bleeds profusely on probing.

In recent years, CBCT has allowed three-dimensional assessment of the nature, position, and extent of resorptive defects, eliminating diagnostic confusion and providing essential information about the restorability and subsequent management of affected teeth [62–64]. A CBCT scan (at the smallest voxel size – 0.2 mm) provides a more site-focused and clearer radiographic image [65], thus reducing the need for exploratory treatment (usually surgical exploration), allowing timely intervention and reduced patient morbidity.

The fundamental treatment objectives in ECR are to access and excavate the resorptive defect (usually by raising a mucoperiosteal flap), halt the resorptive process (through application of 90% trichloroacetic acid), restore the hard tissue defect [66], and regular monitoring of the affected tooth for ECR recurrence, and the same for all other teeth which may be predisposed to the same resorptive event. This is especially true for ECRs related to periodontal diseases as multiple ECRs may occur in the same patient [56]. In cases where perforation of the root canal wall has occurred, RCT should be carried out as soon as possible to avoid pain. In periodontal disease-associated ECR, treatment was primarily aimed at suppressing periodontal pathogens through mechanical debridement, oral hygiene instruction and systemic antibiotics. This was supplemented with diet counseling and monitoring to lower the patients daily acid intake. High acidic intake may have contributed to the initiation of the resorptive process by retarding the proliferative capacity of the protective junctional epithelium [56].

3.6. Vertical root fractures

A vertical root fracture (VRF) is a longitudinally oriented complete or incomplete fracture initiated in the root at any level and is usually directed buccolingually [67]. The diagnosis of a VRF is somehow difficult in the early phase with patients complaining of dull pain, tooth sensitivity and discomfort while chewing. Early detection of VRF is unlikely radiographically due to various obstructions and overlapping structures, making proper diagnosis difficult. In of long-standing VRFs, a sinus tract may develop at a location more coronal than a sinus tract associated with chronic apical abscess [68]. This hints that the source of infection is not likely from an apical lesion [69, 70]. A deep, narrow, isolated periodontal pocket may be present, which is usually pathognomonic of a VRF. Radiographically, a typical J-shaped or halo radiolucency, with bone loss seen apically and extends alongside the involved root is highly indicative of VRF [71].

Over time, the pocket along the fracture line, which was initially tight and narrow, may become wider and easier to detect. When the fracture line propagates coronally, extending to the cervical root area, bacteria may penetrate and biofilm can attach along the fracture line, triggering local host immune response which destroys the local periodontium. The fracture line allows the leakage of oral bacteria into the clean and previously sealed root canal system causing contamination. As reported by Tamse et al. [68], a typical VRF pocket could be observed in 67% of the cases. In periodontitis patients, vertical root fractures and cracks may serve to communicate the dental pulp with the periodontium. If the periodontium is infected or inflamed, pulp necrosis may ensue due to bacterial and bacterial product dissemination through such crevices [72].

Treatment for VRF differs greatly. VRF does not usually respond to non-surgical RCT or retreatment or to periodontal treatments instituted. In most cases, extraction of the tooth, especially for single-rooted teeth, is required. As for multi-rooted teeth, a root-resective approach may sometimes be considered.

3.7. Advanced periodontal disease

Untreated periodontal disease may progress and cause extensive damage to the tooth supporting structures. As the disease extends along the root surface, infection and/or inflammation can spread through the various communications between the pulp and the periodontium [28] until periodontal disease progression reaches the apical foramen leading to a primary periodontal lesion with secondary endodontic involvement [4]. Classification and management of such lesions will be discussed in the segments below.

4. Classification of periodontal and endodontic lesions

Many classifications for perio-endo lesions have been suggested [4, 72–74]. However, the proposed classification by Simon et al. [4] is still espoused by many, despite more rational later classifications, for many cases of perio-endo infections, and shall form the framework for the following discussion below.

4.1. Primary endodontic lesions

A necrotic pulp with its infected root canal system elicits inflammation of the adjacent periodontium through leaking of bacteria and bacterial by-products through the apical foramen and/or lateral canals causing tooth-supporting bone destruction [4, 72]. In multi-rooted teeth, infection from the apical foramen or the numerous accessory canals located in the molar bifurcation area, may track into the bifurcation area giving a radiographic and often clinical appearance of periodontal furcation involvement [21]. To consider solely endodontic lesions as having a component attributable to periodontitis is a diagnostic and conceptual error.

As such, when differentiating endodontic or periodontal lesions, one should be suspicious of a pulpally/endodontically induced lesion when the crestal bone levels on the mesial and distal aspects of the offending tooth appear relatively normal radiographically, despite a radiographically evident furcation radiolucency, and when clinical attachment loss is localized. Moreover, when the pulp is non-responsive to sensibility testing, it is likely that a necrotic pulp may be the infectious source. Adequate RCT with adequate coronal restoration should usually resolve a primary endodontic lesion without any periodontal therapy, for such lesions are solely endodontic in origin. If solely affected by pulpal pathology, such teeth are only endodontically involved, and the so-called "primary endodontic lesion" is solely an endodontic lesion, and thus really should not be a component of any perio-endo classification. **Figure 1** illustrates a pure endodontic lesion managed by endodontic retreatment alone.

4.2. Primary endodontic lesions with secondary periodontal involvement

Over time, an untreated primary endodontic lesion may result in secondary consequential periodontal breakdown, which, if this reaches the gingival sulcus or a periodontal pocket, may become infected by periodonto-pathogens which subsequently trigger further periodontitis-associated periodontal tissue destruction, pocket formation, crestal bone loss and plaque (and calculus) contamination of root surfaces.

A tooth so affected requires both endodontic and periodontal treatments. In general, healing of tissues damaged by infection from the pulp can be anticipated after adequate RCT. The prognosis of the tooth will then largely depend on the outcome of periodontal therapy [4].

4.3. Primary periodontal lesions

Pure periodontal lesions are bacterial-induced inflammatory destructions of the tooth supporting apparatus due to periodonto-pathogens [75]. Diagnosis is based on periodontal examination such as probing pocket depths at 6 sites of each tooth, plaque accumulation and gingival bleeding scores [75, 76], on teeth having normal pulpal sensibility test outcomes. Teeth affected by solely periodontitis, which should respond to adequate periodontal therapy alone, are not endodontically involved.

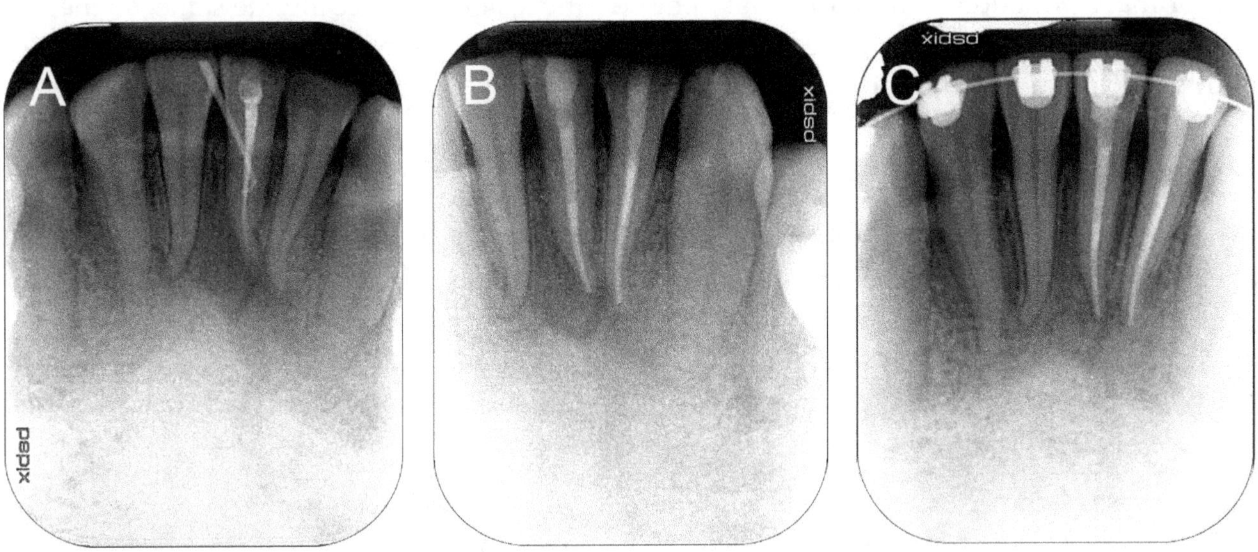

Figure 1. Endodontic lesion managed by endodontic retreatment. (A) Periapical radiograph of previously root treated tooth 31 exhibiting a large periapical lesion and infection draining through buccal gingival sulcus; (B) retreatment of 31 and RCT of a non-vital 32 completed; (C) radiograph of 31 and 32 showing bone fill 6 months post treatment.

In periodontitis, probing usually reveals plaque and calculus of varying quantity and quality along the root surface. In periodontitis many teeth are usually. The pulp typically responds positively to endodontic sensibility tests unless periodontitis has progressed towards the root apex. Prognosis of purely periodontally affected teeth depends largely upon the amount of bony destruction, the overall management of the patient, including non-surgical and surgical periodontal therapy, practice of adequate oral hygiene measures and adherence to supportive periodontal care [76, 77]. Once more, if a tooth is affected by only periodontitis which would respond to adequate periodontal treatment alone, then it is free from any endodontic involvement, and as such the so-called "primary periodontal lesion" should not form any part of a classification of perio-endo lesions.

4.4. Primary periodontal lesions with secondary endodontic involvement

If periodontitis progresses apically along the root surface, bacterial infiltrates from the periodontium may penetrate the pulp through exposed accessory and lateral canals, canaliculi of the furcation area, and eventually the apical foramen [72]. Pulpal necrosis can also result from periodontal procedures where the blood supply, through an accessory canal or the apex is severed during instrumentation. Lateral canals and dentinal tubules may be exposed to the oral environment during periodontal treatment allowing microorganism to pass freely to, or be pushed into, the pulpal tissue space [4].

Primary periodontal lesions with secondary endodontic involvement differ from primary endodontic lesion with secondary periodontal involvement only by the temporal sequence of the disease processes. Regardless of the primary cause of disease, RCT should precede periodontal therapy to prevent excessive removal of the protective root cementum and to alleviate any pulpal pain [5, 9, 22]. The tooth prognosis depends on adequate endodontic therapy, adequate coronal restoration and continuing periodontal care subsequent to endodontic therapy. The sequencing of treatment for both primary endodontic with secondary periodontal lesions and primary periodontal with secondary endodontic lesions is basically the same, so there is not a therapeutic distinction to be drawn from the differentiation between these two types of both periodontal and endodontic lesions affecting a tooth.

4.5. "True" combined lesions

True combined lesions occur where a primary endodontic lesion exists on a tooth that is also affected by periodontitis. These lesions are created when an infected periodontal pocket progresses apically to join with the endodontic lesion progressing coronally. Once the endodontic and periodontal lesions coalesce, they may be clinically and radiographically indistinguishable. The degree of attachment loss is usually quite substantial and the prognosis of such lesion is often very guarded [4].

In most cases, apical healing is often evident following successful endodontic treatment. The periodontal lesion, however, should respond well to adequate periodontal treatment and the prognosis may well depend on the severity of the periodontitis-induced periodontal attachment loss and the extent and pattern of alveolar bony destruction. The radiographic appearance of combined endodontic–periodontal disease may be similar to that of a VRF [4, 78].

4.6. Changes in the classification of perio-endo lesions

The primary endodontic lesion and the primary periodontal lesion are solely endodontic or periodontal in origin and should not be confused as perio-endo lesions where both entities are assumed to be associated with one another. To clarify such relationships, Abbott and Salgado [11] proposed a classification that limits the diagnosis of perio-endo lesions to teeth that have both endodontic and periodontal diseases occurring simultaneously. They proposed that such teeth should be classified into:

i. *Concurrent endodontic and periodontal diseases without communication*: Implying that a tooth has an infection from the root canal system and concomitant alveolar bone loss due to periodontal disease but the periapical and periodontal lesions do not communicate with each other.

ii. *Concurrent endodontic and periodontal diseases with communication*: Such a diagnosis applies to a tooth that has an infection from the root canal system and concomitant alveolar bone loss due to periodontal disease and the periapical and periodontal lesions communicate with each other. Radiographically, the periapical radiolucency and the marginal periodontal bone loss appear as one continuous radiolucent lesion.

Al-Fouzan [72] in their discussion on perio-endo lesions agreed largely with the classification by Simon et al. [4] but proposed a modification to the primary endodontic lesion. They classified an endodontic lesion with a deep narrow probing defect as "retrograde periodontal disease", with two subdivisions:

i. *Primary endodontic lesion with drainage through the periodontal ligament*: Which applies to an infected tooth with an apical lesion that drains coronally through a sinus tract that tracks along the periodontal ligament, mimicking a periodontal defect. There is usually a single deep and narrow periodontal pocket which heals upon endodontic treatment alone.

ii. *Primary endodontic lesion with secondary periodontal involvement*: Such lesions exhibit extensive periodontal destruction as a result of drainage of infection from a necrotic root canal system. As the chronic communication persists, plaque and calculus accumulate within the periodontal pocket and contribute to the advancement of periodontal disease, necessitating periodontal treatment.

Al-Fouzan [72] also added an additional classification termed "iatrogenic periodontal lesions" which included: root perforation, coronal leakage, dental injuries or trauma, damage from chemicals used in dentistry and vertical root fractures. Although such lesions are not exactly periodontal lesions, such a classification allowed separate definition of perio-endo pathologies associated with trauma or iatrogenic injuries to the root surface itself. This was important as extensive damage to the root greatly diminishes a tooth's long-term prognosis. This distinction may aid clinicians in identifying perio-endo lesions with direct and extensive damage to the root surface as opposed to lesions initiated by root canal infections and/or periodontal infections. Perio-endo lesions arising from root canal and/or periodontal infections are basically inflammatory lesions initiated by a wide array of microbiota such as bacteria, viruses or fungi.

These are usually presented clinically without detectable damage to the root itself. Such lesions are treated differently from those with significant root damage and will be discussed below.

Evidently, various opinions and controversies have emerged over the classification of perio-endo lesions. Future research or discussion may bring about a more comprehensive classification for such lesions that can clearly define the etiology of such pathologies and serve as a guide to adequately treat them.

5. Treatment modalities

Combined perio-endo lesions are a challenge to manage. RCT, or at least its initiation with mechanical and chemical cleaning of the pulp canal spaces, and effective intra-canal medication, is usually advocated as the first step in treatment of teeth with combined perio-endo lesions presenting with increased PPD and for teeth are unresponsive to pulp sensibility testing. Non-surgical periodontal therapy can proceed. Once RCT has been completed, adequate time for healing of the endodontic lesion should be given before further advanced periodontal therapy is considered [9]. Treatment modalities aimed at removal of bacterial irritants result in tooth prognosis which has been shown to improve over time [47]. This section summarized the treatment sequence for perio-endo lesions (**Figure 2**).

5.1. Non-surgical management

In the management of perio-endo lesions, it is important to recall that infected or necrotic pulps may lead to a narrow sinus tract undistinguishable clinically from a periodontal pocket. Because the primary cause of such lesions is pulpal in origin, the indicated treatment is solely RCT followed by adequate coronal seal, with long-term follow-up and monitoring to assess healing.

Similarly, if a vital tooth affected by solely periodontal disease develops mild pulpal symptoms, periodontal treatment should be the only intervention, followed by long-term follow-up. This will allow the mild and usually reversible inflammatory reaction of the pulp (which may transiently increase after periodontal therapy) to resolve as the vital pulp resists the spread of inflammation from the periodontal lesion [12].

With regards to concurrent perio-endo infections, although these separate entities may not be communicating, RCT should be carried out, or at least initiated, first to eliminate pulpal infection and relieve pain. This may then be followed by root surface debridement. Such a treatment sequence will allow removal of infectious source from the pulp and control of any possible communication between the infected root canal system and the adjacent periodontium. With this, even if the protective cementum layer is removed during root surface debridement, there should be no pulpal infection that can spread towards the periodontium through open dentinal tubules or accessory canals [11, 12]. Such a treatment philosophy is applied to true perio-endo lesions as well, to allow the affected tooth to undergo infection control in its entirety, sequentially and as effectively as possible [12].

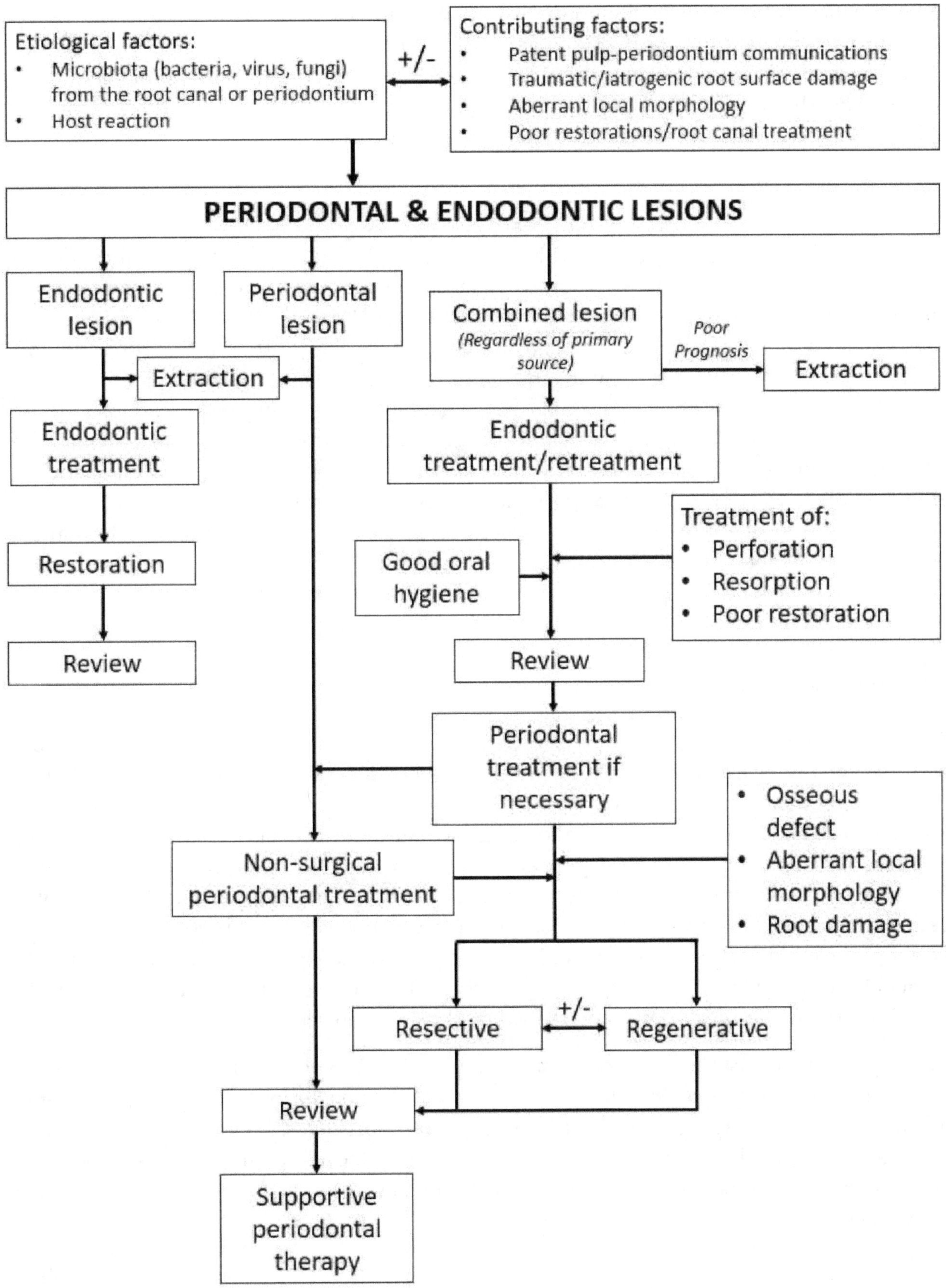

Figure 2. Flow chart summarizing treatment sequence for perio-endo lesions.

Indeed, in any patient with periodontal disease, management should include plaque control, non-surgical scaling and root debridement; periodontal surgery (with or with regenerative periodontal therapies) when indicated; and subsequent supportive periodontal care (SPC) [76, 79]. SPC should allow any teeth with pathologies, periodontal, endodontic or combined, to be well maintained within the oral cavity in the long term.

5.2. Surgical management

Conventional non-surgical periodontal and endodontic therapy may be predictably used to treat mild to moderate bony defects caused by perio-endo lesions. However, these non-surgical therapies alone might be inadequate for the treatment of lesions characterized by deep pockets, or wide circumferential apical defects caused by non-healing endodontic lesions, previous endodontic surgery [80], or those with substantial root surface damage such as root fracture of resorption. An endodontic lesion may be considered non-healing if the periapical lesion increases in size or remains unchanged after RCT. A decision to provide alternative treatment modalities will depend largely on the signs and symptoms experienced by the patient and judgment of the treating clinician, as periapical lesions can take up to four years [32] or longer [81] to heal. Surgical options for perio-endo lesions can be divided into surgical debridement, periodontal- or root- resective, or regenerative, approaches. The extent of periodontal tissue destruction or the failure of adequately delivered treatment to resolve the lesions, or any component thereof, may leave tooth extraction as the only practical treatment option.

5.2.1. Root-resective therapy

Root resection is the removal of a root (or roots, or root with coronal tooth structure) along with accompanying odontoplasty, before or preferably after endodontic treatment. Such tooth respective modalities are advocated to treat specific non-furcation and furcation defects that unlikely to be managed by non-surgical or surgical debridement alone [82]. The indications for root resection include root fracture, perforation, root caries, dehiscence, fenestration, external root resorption involving one root, incomplete endodontic treatment of a particular root, severe periodontitis affecting only one or two roots with at least one good sized root with proper/sufficient periodontal support to remain [83], or and severe grade II or grade III furcation involvement of multi-rooted teeth in the treatment of which clinicians attempt to create 'single rooted' situations to remove affect root(s) and to facilitate oral hygiene and SPC measures [84, 85].

Factors such as occlusal forces, tooth restorability, residual periodontal support and strategic value of the remaining root(s) should be taken into consideration during the planning stage before treatment. Proper reshaping of the occlusal table and appropriate restoration of the clinical crown are essential [83]. Additionally, the root surface at the site of the amputation must be recontoured after removal of the root stump to allow reestablishment of soft and hard tissue morphology favorable for oral hygiene measures by the patient and SPC measures by treating clinicians [86].

Hemisection is the surgical separation of a multirooted tooth. This is usually only a treatment option for mandibular molars with severe furcation involvement and periodontal attachment loss having affected one root more severely than the other (**Figure 3**). The tooth was sectioned

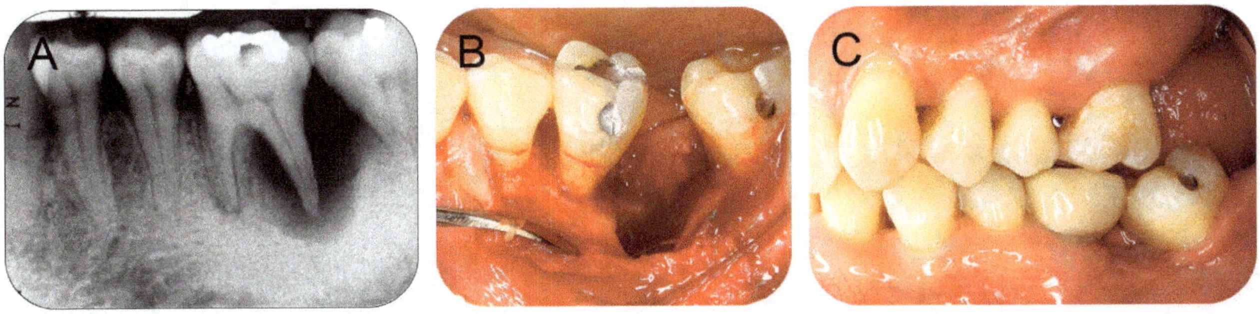

Figure 3. Management of a mandibular left first molar with severe furcation involvement and periodontal attachment loss. (A) Radiographic bone loss observable at distal root of a non-vital 36; (B) RCT was completed and 36 was hemisected distally; (C) 36 was subsequently crowned to coronally seal the treated root canal, re-establish occlusion and prevent further mesial drift of the second molar.

through the furcation, and the respective root and associated portion of the crown may be removed while another moiety is retained [87]. In most instances, an elective RCT should be performed before or as soon as possible after the hemisection to avoid any future pulpal complications. Hemisection allows retention of natural tooth structure, especially the root, which helps preserve surrounding alveolar bone, and may facilitate the placement of fixed prostheses [87].

The restorative aspects of the tooth to be so treated must be carefully assessed and integrated into the anticipated surgical procedure to ensure proper positioning of restorative margins relative to the osseous crest, and also to manage the anticipated changes in occlusal relationships and masticatory forces. In certain occasions, splinting of a resected tooth to neighboring teeth or the use of such teeth as abutments for fixed partial dentures may confer some reinforcement towards its long-term survival [83]. Although factors such as older age at time of resection, grade II mobility or above, and reduced pre-operative radiographic bone heights around roots seem to reduce the survival of resected teeth, the major cause of failure of resective procedures is often due to endodontic failure or vertical root fractures [88]. This is especially true if periodontal treatment had been properly carried out and the patient adheres to strict SPC [83, 88]. In most situations, the residual periodontal support of the treated tooth dictates the prognosis of the tooth. However, teeth with reduced periodontal support may still be maintained if proper SPC is provided [76, 89].

5.2.2. Regenerative therapy

Regenerative therapy has been shown to yield greater attachment gain and re-establish more favorable tissue morphology for oral hygiene measures compared to conventional periodontal therapy [90]. Pre-surgical assessment includes assessment of the pulp status and the severity of periodontal destruction. Once the therapeutic prognosis for the periodontal regenerative procedure is determined to be favorable, endodontic therapy is provided and the endodontic lesion is allowed to heal. Unsatisfactory healing after RCT might be further addressed with a surgical endodontic therapy approach (apicectomy) [78]. After a successful RCT, tooth mobility is reassessed to determine the necessity for splinting, as tooth mobility may reduce the success of regenerative therapy [91]. The intrasurgical assessment includes morphology of the

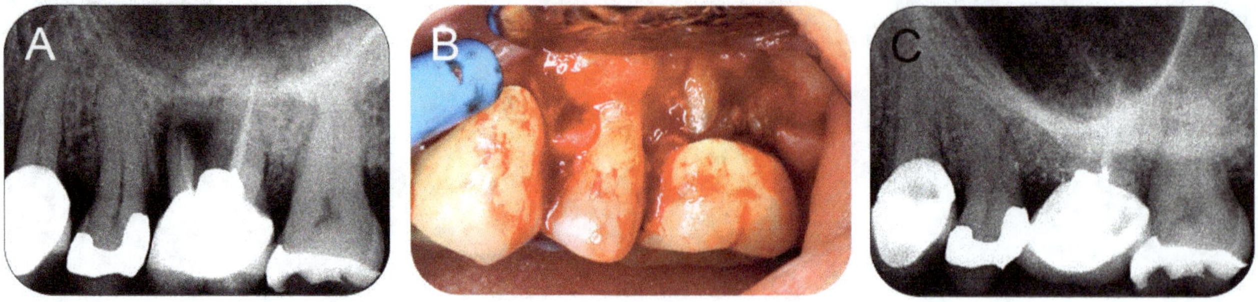

Figure 4. Periodontal surgical management of an upper left first molar with a root fracture. (A) Radiograph of root treated 26 with suspected mesio-buccal root fracture; (B) intra-operative view of 26 confirming initial diagnosis; (C) 26 MB root was resected and the defect regenerated with xenograft and a collagen barrier membrane. Radiograph taken at 6 months post treatment.

periodontal defect, material of choice to manage the defect, control of patient's oral hygiene, wound and tooth stabilization [78]. The defect, patient, and surgery-specific factors associated with favorable periodontal regeneration are [80]:

- **i.** Defect considerations: Deep (≥4 mm), narrow (<45 degrees), vertical, two to three wall defects with no/minimal furcation involvement, adequate soft tissue thickness (>1.1 mm) and keratinization (2 mm).
- **ii.** Patient considerations: Good oral hygiene, compliance towards periodontal care, abstinence from smoking/non-smoking and good systematic health/properly controlled systemic conditions.
- **iii.** Surgical considerations: Atraumatic incisions and flap elevation, primary closure, passive wound tension, uncontaminated wound during surgery (and post-surgical healing) and no occlusal trauma

In perio-endo lesions, regenerative periodontal therapies, such as use of biologically active products or guided tissue regeneration (GTR), may be used to promote periodontal regeneration and crestal intra-osseous defect bone-fill after endodontic treatment. In GTR, a barrier membrane is used to prevent contact of connective tissue with the osseous walls of an intra-osseous defect, to protect the underlying blood clot and to encourage growth of key tissues, while excluding unwanted cells such as epithelial cells [80]. When the intra-osseous defect is large, bone substitutes may be placed in the defect to support the overlying membrane and to maintain a space in which healing may occur [80]. Sometimes both root-resective and regenerative treatment may be carried out simultaneously to retain a tooth in function. **Figure 4** shows treatment of an upper first molar with a root fracture.

6. Summary

An in-depth understanding of the biology underlying perio-endo inter-relationships guides a clinician in diagnosing and subsequently deriving a sensible and timely treatment plan. Conventional endodontic and periodontal therapy have been shown to be successful in managing such lesions [47] with endodontic therapy, or at least its initiation, being the first line of treatment in most cases [9]. The use of regenerative approaches to manage perio-endo lesions has advantages especially in terms of enhanced attachment gain and better long-term outcome of treated teeth. Various other treatment modalities for managing the periodontal component of perio-endo lesions, such as the application of enamel matrix derivatives [92] or platelet-rich fibrins [93] may offer good results. However, more research is warranted in this field with hope that retention of perio-endo involved teeth may become more predictable in the near future.

Acknowledgements

The work described in this chapter was substantially supported by the Young Researcher's Incentive Grants (GGPM-2016-062 and GGPM-2017-109), The National University of Malaysia, and the Research Grants Council of the Hong Kong Special Administrative Region, China (HKU 772110 M).

Author details

Kai Ling Siew[1], Victor Goh[1,2], Chui Ling Goo[2], Esmonde Francis Corbet[1] and Wai Keung Leung[1]*

*Address all correspondence to: ewkleung@hku.hk

1 Faculty of Dentistry, The University of Hong Kong, Hong Kong SAR, China

2 Faculty of Dentistry, The National University of Malaysia, Malaysia

References

[1] Offenbacher S, Barros SP, Singer RE, Moss K, Williams RC, Beck JD. Periodontal disease at the biofilm–gingival interface. Journal of Periodontology. 2007;**78**(10):1911-1925

[2] Ricucci D, Siqueira Jr JF. Biofilms and apical periodontitis: Study of prevalence and association with clinical and histopathologic findings. Journal of Endodontics. 2010;**36**(8): 1277-1288

[3] Ricucci D, Siqueira Jr JF. Fate of the tissue in lateral canals and apical ramifications in response to pathologic conditions and treatment procedures. Journal of Endodontics. 2010;**36**(1):1-15

[4] Simon JH, Glick DH, Frank AL. The relationship of endodontic-periodontic lesions. Journal of Periodontology. 1972;**43**(4):202-208

[5] Chen SY, Wang HL, Glickman GN. The influence of endodontic treatment upon peri odontal wound healing. Journal of Clinical Periodontology. 1997;**24**(7):449-456

[6] Parahitiyawa NB, Chu FC, Leung WK, Yam WC, Jin LJ, Samaranayake LP. Clonality of bacterial consortia in root canals and subjacent gingival crevices. Journal of Investigative and Clinical Dentistry. 2015;**6**(1):32-39

[7] Jansson L, Ehnevid H, Lindskog S, Blomlof L. The influence of endodontic infection on progression of marginal bone loss in periodontitis. Journal of Clinical Periodontology. 1995;**22**(10):729-734

[8] Ehnevid H, Jansson L, Lindskog S, Blomlof L. Periodontal healing in teeth with periapical lesions. A clinical retrospective study. Journal of Clinical Periodontology. 1993;**20**(4): 254-258

[9] Schmidt JC, Walter C, Amato M, Weiger R. Treatment of periodontal-endodontic lesions – A systematic review. Journal of Clinical Periodontology. 2014;**41**(8):779-790

[10] Hiatt WH. Pulpal periodontal disease. Journal of Periodontology. 1977;**48**(9):598-609

[11] Abbott PV, Salgado JC. Strategies for the endodontic management of concurrent endodontic and periodontal diseases. Australian Dental Journal. 2009;**54**(Suppl 1):S70-S85

[12] Heasman PA. An endodontic conundrum: The association between pulpal infection and periodontal disease. British Dental Journal. 2014;**216**(6):275-279

[13] Seltzer S, Bender IB, Ziontz M. The interrelationship of pulp and periodontal disease. Oral Surgery, Oral Medicine, and Oral Pathology. 1963;**16**:1474-1490

[14] Langeland K, Rodrigues H, Dowden W. Periodontal disease, bacteria, and pulpal histo pathology. Oral Surgery, Oral Medicine, and Oral Pathology. 1974;**37**(2):257-270

[15] Wan L, Lu HB, Xuan DY, Yan YX, Zhang JC. Histological changes within dental pulps in teeth with moderate-to-severe chronic periodontitis. International Endodontic Journal. 2015;**48**(1):95-102

[16] Goh V, Corbet EF, Leung WK. Impact of dentine hypersensitivity on oral health-related quality of life in individuals receiving supportive periodontal care. Journal of Clinical Periodontology. 2016;**43**(7):595-602

[17] Jeffcoat MK, Jeffcoat RL, Jens SC, Captain K. A new periodontal probe with automated cemento-enamel junction detection. Journal of Clinical Periodontology. 1986;**13**(4):276-280

[18] Adriaens PA, Edwards CA, De Boever JA, Loesche WJ. Ultrastructural observations on bacterial invasion in cementum and radicular dentin of periodontally diseased human teeth. Journal of Periodontology. 1988;**59**(8):493-503

[19] Herbranson E. The anatomy of the root canal system as a challenge to effective disinfection. In: Cohenca N, editor. Disinfection of Root Canal Systems. John Wiley & Sons, Inc. Ames, IA, USA; 2014. pp. 15-28

[20] Graunaite I, Lodiene G, Maciulskiene V. Pathogenesis of apical periodontitis: A literature review. Journal of Oral and Maxillofacial Research. 2012;**2**(4):e1

[21] Gutmann JL. Prevalence, location, and patency of accessory canals in the furcation region of permanent molars. Journal of Periodontology. 1978;**49**(1):21-26

[22] Dongari A, Lambrianidis T. Periodontally derived pulpal lesions. Endodontics and Dental Traumatology. 1988;**4**(2):49-54

[23] De Deus QD. Frequency, location, and direction of the lateral, secondary, and accessory canals. Journal of Endodontics. 1975;**1**(11):361-366

[24] Shambarger S, Johnson D, Versulius-Tantbirojin D, Bowles WR, McClanahan SB. The incidence of furcation region patency in molars before and after simulated periodontal therapy. Northwest Dentistry. 2015;**94**(2):27-32

[25] Bergenholtz G, Lindhe J. Effect of soluble plaque factors on inflammatory reactions in the dental pulp. Scandinavian Journal of Dental Research. 1975;**83**(3):153-158

[26] Bergenholtz G, Reit C. Reactions of the dental pulp to microbial provocation of calcium hydroxide treated dentin. Scandinavian Journal of Dental Research. 1980;**88**(3):187-192

[27] Siqueira Jr JF, Rôças IN. Diversity of endodontic microbiota revisted. Journal of Dental Research. 2009;**88**(11):969-981

[28] Rotstein I. Interaction between endodontics and periodontics. Periodontology 2000. 2017;**74**(1):11-39

[29] Paster BJ, Olsen I, Aas JA, Dewhirst FE. The breadth of bacterial diversity in the human periodontal pocket and other oral sites. Periodontology 2000. 2006;**42**(1):80-87

[30] Wade WG. The oral microbiome in health and disease. Pharmacological Research. 2013; **69**(1):137-143

[31] Tabassum S, Khan FR. Failure of endodontic treatment: The usual suspects. European Journal of Dentistry. 2016;**10**(1):144-147

[32] Quality guidelines for endodontic treatment. Consensus report of the european society of endodontology. International Endodontic Journal. 2006;**39**(12):921-930

[33] Albandar JM, Buischi YA, Axelsson P. Caries lesions and dental restorations as predisposing factors in the progression of periodontal diseases in adolescents. A 3-year longitudinal study. Journal of Periodontology. 1995;**66**(4):249-254

[34] Lang NP, Kiel RA, Anderhalden K. Clinical and microbiological effects of subgingival restorations with overhanging or clinically perfect margins. Journal of Clinical Periodontology. 1983;**10**(6):563-578

[35] Gillen BM, Looney SW, Gu LS, Loushine BA, Weller RN, Loushine RJ, et al. Impact of the quality of coronal restoration versus the quality of root canal fillings on success of root canal treatment: A systematic review and meta-analysis. Journal of Endodontics. 2011;**37**(7):895-902

[36] Ray HA, Trope M. Periapical status of endodontically treated teeth in relation to the technical quality of the root filling and the coronal restoration. International Endodontic Journal. 1995;**28**(1):12-18

[37] American Association of Endodontists. Glossary of Endodontic Terms. 9th ed. Chicago: AAE; 2015

[38] Tsesis I, Rosen E, Schwartz-Arad D, Fuss Z. Retrospective evaluation of surgical endodontic treatment: Traditional versus modern technique. Journal of Endodontics. 2006; **32**(5):412-416

[39] Kvinnsland I, Oswald RJ, Halse A, Gronningsaeter AG. A clinical and roentgenological study of 55 cases of root perforation. International Endodontic Journal. 1989;**22**(2):75-84

[40] Siew K, Lee AH, Cheung GS. Treatment outcome of repaired root perforation: A systematic review and meta-analysis. Journal of Endodontics. 2015;**41**(11):1795-1804

[41] Torabinejad M, Parirokh M, Dummer PMH. Mineral trioxide aggregate and other bioactive endodontic cements: An updated overview – Part ii: Other clinical applications and complications. International Endodontic Journal. 2018;**51**(3):284-317

[42] Economides N, Pantelidou O, Kokkas A, Tziafas D. Short-term periradicular tissue response to mineral trioxide aggregate (mta) as root-end filling material. International Endodontic Journal. 2003;**36**(1):44-48

[43] Torabinejad M, Parirokh M. Mineral trioxide aggregate: A comprehensive literature review – Part ii: Leakage and biocompatibility investigations. Journal of Endodontics. 2010;**36**(2):190-202

[44] Torabinejad M, Watson TF, Pitt Ford TR. Sealing ability of a mineral trioxide aggregate when used as a root end filling material. Journal of Endodontics. 1993;**19**(12):591-595

[45] Parirokh M, Torabinejad M. Mineral trioxide aggregate: A comprehensive literature review – Part iii: Clinical applications, drawbacks, and mechanism of action. Journal of Endodontics. 2010;**36**(3):400-413

[46] Kogon SL. The prevalence, location and conformation of palato-radicular grooves in maxillary incisors. Journal of Periodontology. 1986;**57**(4):231-234

[47] Cho YD, Lee JE, Chung Y, Lee WC, Seol YJ, Lee YM, et al. Collaborative management of combined periodontal-endodontic lesions with a palatogingival groove: A case series. Journal of Endodontics. 2017;**43**(2):332-337

[48] Xie C, Wang L, Yang P, Ge S. Cemental tears: A report of four cases and literature review. Oral Health and Preventive Dentistry. 2017;**15**(4):337-345

[49] Matthews DC, Tabesh M. Detection of localized tooth-related factors that predispose to periodontal infections. Periodontology 2000. 2004;**34**:136-150

[50] Hou GL, Tsai CC. Relationship between periodontal furcation involvement and molar cervical enamel projections. Journal of Periodontology. 1987;**58**(10):715-721

[51] Moskow BS, Canut PM. Studies on root enamel (2). Enamel pearls. A review of their morphology, localization, nomenclature, occurrence, classification, histogenesis and incidence. Journal of Clinical Periodontology. 1990;**17**(5):275-281

[52] Arana-Chavez VE, Bradaschia-Correa V. Clastic cells: Mineralized tissue resorption in health and disease. The International Journal of Biochemistry and Cell Biology. 2009; **41**(3):446-450

[53] Andreasen FM, Pedersen BV. Prognosis of luxated permanent teeth – The development of pulp necrosis. Endodontics and Dental Traumatology. 1985;**1**(6):207-220

[54] Andreasen FM, Sewerin I, Mandel U, Andreasen JO. Radiographic assessment of simulated root resorption cavities. Endodontics and Dental Traumatology. 1987;**3**(1):21-27

[55] Mahajan AC, Kolte AP, Kolte RA, Agrawal AA. Dimensional evaluation of root resorption areas in differing severity of chronic periodontitis: A scanning electron microscopic study. Contemporary Clinical Dentistry. 2017;**8**(3):433-438

[56] Beertsen W, Piscaer M, Van Winkelhoff AJ, Everts V. Generalized cervical root resorption associated with periodontal disease. Journal of Clinical Periodontology. 2001;**28**(11): 1067-1073

[57] Barnett F. The role of endodontics in the treatment of luxated permanent teeth. Dental Traumatology. 2002;**18**(2):47-56

[58] Moule AJ, Moule CA. The endodontic management of traumatized permanent anterior teeth: A review. Australian Dental Journal. 2007;**52**:S122-SS37

[59] Heithersay GS. Clinical, radiologic, and histopathologic features of invasive cervical resorption. Quintessence International. 1999;**30**(1):27-37

[60] Heithersay GS. Invasive cervical resorption: An analysis of potential predisposing factors. Quintessence International. 1999;**30**(2):83-95

[61] Heithersay GS. Invasive cervical resorption following trauma. Australian Endodontic Journal. 1999;**25**(2):79-85

[62] Vaz de Souza D, Schirru E, Mannocci F, Foschi F, Patel S. External cervical resorption: A comparison of the diagnostic efficacy using 2 different cone-beam computed tomographic units and periapical radiographs. Journal of Endodontics. 2017;**43**(1):121-125

[63] Patel S, Dawood A. The use of cone beam computed tomography in the management of external cervical resorption lesions. International Endodontic Journal. 2007;**40**(9):730-737

[64] Gunst V, Mavridou A, Huybrechts B, Van Gorp G, Bergmans L, Lambrechts P. External cervical resorption: An analysis using cone beam and microfocus computed tomography and scanning electron microscopy. International Endodontic Journal. 2013;**46**(9):877-887

[65] Talwar S, Utneja S, Nawal RR, Kaushik A, Srivastava D, Oberoy SS. Role of cone-beam computed tomography in diagnosis of vertical root fractures: A systematic review and meta-analysis. Journal of Endodontics. 2016;**42**(1):12-24

[66] Heithersay GS. Treatment of invasive cervical resorption: An analysis of results using topical application of trichloracetic acid, curettage, and restoration. Quintessence International. 1999;**30**(2):96-110

[67] Liao WC, Tsai YL, Wang CY, Chang MC, Huang WL, Lin HJ, et al. Clinical and radiographic characteristics of vertical root fractures in endodontically and nonendodontically treated teeth. Journal of Endodontics. 2017;**43**(5):687-693

[68] Tamse A, Fuss Z, Lustig J, Kaplavi J. An evaluation of endodontically treated vertically fractured teeth. Journal of Endodontics. 1999;**25**(7):506-508

[69] Meister Jr F, Lommel TJ, Gerstein H. Diagnosis and possible causes of vertical root fractures. Oral Surgery, Oral Medicine, and Oral Pathology. 1980;**49**(3):243-253

[70] Testori T, Badino M, Castagnola M. Vertical root fractures in endodontically treated teeth: A clinical survey of 36 cases. Journal of Endodontics. 1993;**19**(2):87-91

[71] Tamse A, Fuss Z, Lustig J, Ganor Y, Kaffe I. Radiographic features of vertically fractured, endodontically treated maxillary premolars. Oral Surgery, Oral Medicine, Oral Pathology, Oral Radiology, and Endodontics. 1999;**88**(3):348-352

[72] Al-Fouzan KS. A new classification of endodontic-periodontal lesions. International Journal of Dentistry. 2014;**2014**:919173

[73] Benenati FW, Roane JB, Waldrop TC. The perio-pulpal connection: An analysis of the periodontic-endodontic lesion. General Dentistry. 1981;**29**(6):515-520

[74] Guldener PH. The relationship between periodontal and pulpal disease. International Endodontic Journal. 1985;**18**(1):41-54

[75] Armitage GC. Periodontal diagnoses and classification of periodontal diseases. Periodontology 2000. 2004;**34**:9-21

[76] Goh V, Hackmack PP, Corbet EF, Leung WK. Moderate- to long-term periodontal outcomes of subjects failing to complete a course of periodontal therapy. Australian Dental Journal. 2017;**62**(2):152-160

[77] Leung WK, Ng DK, Jin L, Corbet EF. Tooth loss in treated periodontitis patients responsible for their supportive care arrangements. Journal of Clinical Periodontology. 2006;**33**(4): 265-275

[78] Oh SL, Fouad AF, Park SH. Treatment strategy for guided tissue regeneration in combined endodontic-periodontal lesions: Case report and review. Journal of Endodontics. 2009;**35**(10):1331-1336

[79] Goh V, Nihalani D, Yeung KWS, Corbet EF, Leung WK. Moderate- to long-term therapeutic outcomes of treated aggressive periodontitis patients without regular supportive care. Journal of Periodontal Research. 2018;**53**(3):324-333

[80] Bashutski JD, Wang HL. Periodontal and endodontic regeneration. Journal of Endodontics. 2009;**35**(3):321-328

[81] Molven O, Halse A, Fristad I, MacDonald-Jankowski D. Periapical changes following root-canal treatment observed 20-27 years postoperatively. International Endodontic Journal. 2002;**35**(9):784-790

[82] DeSanctis M, Murphy KG. The role of resective periodontal surgery in the treatment of furcation defects. Periodontology 2000. 2000;**22**:154-168

[83] Lee KL, Corbet EF, Leung WK. Survival of molar teeth after resective periodontal therapy – A retrospective study. Journal of Clinical Periodontology. 2012;**39**(9):850-860

[84] Svardstrom G, Wennstrom JL. Periodontal treatment decisions for molars: An analysis of influencing factors and long-term outcome. Journal of Periodontology. 2000;**71**(4):579-585

[85] Walter C, Weiger R, Zitzmann NU. Periodontal surgery in furcation-involved maxillary molars revisited – An introduction of guidelines for comprehensive treatment. Clinical Oral Investigations. 2011;**15**(1):9-20

[86] Carnevale G, Pontoriero R, di Febo G. Long-term effects of root-resective therapy in furcation-involved molars. A 10-year longitudinal study. Journal of Clinical Periodontology. 1998;**25**(3):209-214

[87] Sharma S, Sharma R, Ahad A, Gupta ND, Mishra SK. Hemisection as a conservative management of grossly carious permanent mandibular first molar. Journal of Natural Science, Biology, and Medicine. 2018;**9**(1):97-99

[88] Huynh-Ba G, Kuonen P, Hofer D, Schmid J, Lang NP, Salvi GE. The effect of periodontal therapy on the survival rate and incidence of complications of multirooted teeth with furcation involvement after an observation period of at least 5 years: A systematic review. Journal of Clinical Periodontology. 2009;**36**(2):164-176

[89] Graetz C, Dorfer CE, Kahl M, Kocher T, Fawzy El-Sayed K, Wiebe JF, et al. Retention of questionable and hopeless teeth in compliant patients treated for aggressive periodontitis. Journal of Clinical Periodontology. 2011;**38**(8):707-714

[90] Jepsen S, Eberhard J, Herrera D, Needleman I. A systematic review of guided tissue regeneration for periodontal furcation defects. What is the effect of guided tissue regeneration compared with surgical debridement in the treatment of furcation defects? Journal of Clinical Periodontology. 2002;**29**(Suppl 3):103-116 (discussion 60-2)

[91] Cortellini P, Tonetti MS, Lang NP, Suvan JE, Zucchelli G, Vangsted T, et al. The simplified papilla preservation flap in the regenerative treatment of deep intrabony defects: Clinical outcomes and postoperative morbidity. Journal of Periodontology. 2001;**72**(12):1702-1712

[92] Azaripour A, Willershausen I, Kammerer P, Willershausen B. Post-endodontic treatment periodontal surgery: A case report. Quintessence International. 2013;**44**(2):123-126

[93] Karunakaran JV, Fenn SM, Jayaprakash N, Ragavendran N. Successful surgical management of palatogingival groove using platelet-rich fibrin and guided tissue regeneration: A novel approach. Journal of Pharmacy and Bioallied Sciences. 2017;**9**(Suppl 1):S268-S273

4

Post-Operative Pain Following Non-Surgical and Surgical Periodontal Procedures

David G. Gillam and Dominiki Chatzopoulou

Abstract

Post-operative sensitivity may occur following restorative procedures including periodontal therapy affecting both the hard and soft tissues of the oral cavity and can have a major effect on the quality of life (QoL) of the individual. Ideally, the clinician needs to prevent or minimise these effects to reduce any unnecessary discomfort for the patient and this may be accomplished through preventive strategies, the provision of the required information about the procedures both pre- and post-treatment as well as reassuring the patient in the event of any subsequent discomfort. Furthermore, it is important for the clinician to be able to correctly diagnose the exact cause of the patient's discomfort and have the confidence to successfully manage the problem. The aim of this chapter is to provide an overview on the management and treatment of post-operative sensitivity following both non-surgical and surgical periodontal procedures and will be primarily concerned about the discomfort associated with dentine hypersensitivity/root sensitivity following these procedures.

Keywords: post-operative sensitivity, non-surgical and surgical procedures, gingival recession, root surface coverage, quality of life and pain assessment, management strategies

1. Introduction

Traditionally, pain arising from the exposed dentine in response to chemical, thermal, tactile or osmotic stimuli which cannot be explained as arising from any other dental defect or disease has been termed dentine hypersensitivity (DH) [1].

The pain associated with DH is generally considered to be transient in nature and will resolve once the initiating stimulus, such as cold air from a dental air syringe, has been removed.

Other terminology has been used to describe the condition, for example, cervical dentine sensitivity (CDS) or cervical dentine hypersensitivity (CDH) or dentine sensitivity (DS) and root dentine sensitivity (RDS)/root dentine hypersensitivity (RDH). Although there may be some justification in using these terms to describe the condition, Addy [2] advocated the retention of the term dentine hypersensitivity for traditional reasons and perhaps more importantly to enable the clinician to distinguish between those individuals complaining of DH who have relatively healthy mouths with individuals who complain of DH from the effects of periodontal disease and/or its treatment. The term root (dentine) sensitivity (RS/RDS) or root dentine hypersensitivity (RDH) has been used in recent years to describe sensitivity arising from the effects of periodontal disease and/or its treatment (e.g. non-surgical and surgical procedures) [3]. The basis for recommending this terminology was that any sensitivity following periodontal therapy may be a distinct condition from that of DH occurring following the hydrodynamic stimulation, for example, the penetration of bacteria into the dentinal tubules [3, 4] although there appears to be limited epidemiological data to justify this distinction. The prevalence of RS/RDS/RDH in individuals in periodontal problems appears to be higher than those individuals with DH [5–7]. Post-operative sensitivity following non-surgical and surgical periodontal procedures has been reported to affect both the hard and soft tissues of the oral cavity and can have a major effect on the quality of life (QoL) of the individual [8]. The perception of this discomfort varies from individual to individual and the intensity of the discomfort may range from mild/moderate to severe requiring pain relief (analgesics) [9]. Management of this discomfort may range from the professional applications of varnishes or a desensitising prophylaxis paste following the treatment session to the recommendation of over-the-counter (OTC) products such as desensitising toothpaste/gel formulations [10]. The aim of this chapter is to provide an overview on the management and treatment of post-operative sensitivity following both non-surgical and surgical periodontal procedures.

2. Prevalence, mechanisms, aetiology and clinical features of dentine hypersensitivity/root sensitivity

2.1. Prevalence

Most of the published literature relates to the prevalence of DH and as such there are limited data specifically on the prevalence of root dentine hypersensitivity (RDH) or root sensitivity (RS) following periodontal procedures [4, 6–7]. According to Cuhna-Cruz and Watana [11] a reasonable estimate of the prevalence of DH was 10% with an average of 33% across the published studies. By way of contrast, the prevalence of RS reported in the literature was considerably higher (60–98%) [6]. According to Gillam and Orchardson [6], DH/RS may affect individuals of all ages, although the peak prevalence appears to be between the ages of 30 and 60 years. Females appear to be numerically more affected than males although this difference does not appear to be significant. Evidence from the published epidemiological studies would suggest that the buccal (facial) tooth surfaces in individuals with DH/RS are generally affected. A study by Kamal et al. [12] also reported an association with gingival recession and DH in a Jordanian population with a prevalence of DH (23.6%) in patients with gingival recession. These findings would suggest that not all patients who exhibit exposed dentine will experience DH. Several systematic reviews have indicated that the prevalence of DH/RS prior to treatment ranged from 9–23% whereas the prevalence increased following non-surgical therapy (54–55%) [4]. A similar study by Lin and Gillam [7] reported that the prevalence ranged from 62.5 to 90% following treatment but decreased progressively to approximately 52.6–55% after 1 week. In a similar fashion, the prevalence of DH/RS following surgical therapy ranged from 76.8 to 80.4% after 1 day and subsequently decreased over time to 36.8% after 1 week, 33.4% after 2 weeks, 29.6% after 4 weeks and 21.7% after 8 weeks, respectively [7].

2.2. Mechanisms involved in dentine hypersensitivity and root sensitivity

The prevailing view in the published literature is that the mechanisms associated with DH are primarily based on the hydrodynamic theory, as proposed by Brännström and Åström [13]. According to Gillam [14] this theory promotes two basic approaches for treating hypersensitive dentine, namely: (a) by occluding the exposed open dentine tubules, which in turn reduce any stimulus-evoked fluid movements within the dentinal tubules and effectively prevent the transmission of the external stimulus (such as a cold stimulus) to the pulp and (b) by the diffusion of the potassium ion from desensitising products such as toothpaste formulations within the dentinal tubule to reduce intra-dental nerve excitability and prevent any nerve activation.

There is, however, some controversy regarding whether the mechanism associated with root sensitivity is also based on the hydrodynamic. Some investigators have suggested that as RS may have a plaque-related aetiology associated with the bacterial penetration of the dentinal tubules, an alternative mechanism must be involved. The relation between bacterial penetration, pulpal inflammatory changes and symptoms arising from DH/RS however is unclear. Furthermore, the existence of plaque covering the exposed root surface does not in itself suggest that other mechanisms of stimuli transmission other than Brännström's hydrodynamic theory are responsible for RS [6].

2.3. Aetiology

The aetiology of DH/RS is multi-factorial in nature and despite an extensive publication record is not fully understood, although it is recognised that the structure of dentine in the affected areas is changed resulting in areas of sensitive dentine with a greater number of open dentinal tubules compared to non-sensitive areas in unaffected teeth. For DH/RS to occur, both the overlying hard and soft tissues must be removed to expose the underlying dentine surface. There are several aetiological and predisposing factors that are implicated in this process and include gingival recession associated with overzealous or incorrect toothbrushing as well as factors associated with the effects of periodontal disease and its treatment (**Table 1**). As mentioned in the prevalence section there is epidemiological evidence of an association between gingival recession and DH. For example, a study by West et al. [15] reported that

- Loss of enamel
- Denudation of cementum
- Attrition
- Abrasion
- Abfraction
- Erosion (intrinsic and extrinsic)
- Tooth malposition
- Thinning, fenestrationand absent buccal alveolar bone plate
- Gingival recession
- Thin gingival biotype
- Restorative factors such as poorly fitting partial dentures, overhanging restorations and subgingival crown margins
- Periodontal disease and/or its treatment (non-surgical and surgical periodontal procedures)
- Plaque-related factors
- Wound healing following treatment
- Self-inflicted trauma—habits such as finger nail stripping
- Physical (over-enthusiastic and/or incorrect toothbrushing) and chemical trauma
- Smoking (risk factor for periodontal disease)

Table 1. Aetiological and predisposing factors associated with dentine hypersensitivity/root sensitivity and gingival recession (modified from Chabanski and Gillam) [16].

there was a link between a healthy erosive diet and lifestyle and toothwear with DH in young adults aged 18–35 years.

2.4. Clinical features

The clinical features of DH have been well documented in several published reviews [6, 16]; however, these reviews primarily deal with the features associated with DH in patients with well-maintained oral hygiene rather than clinical features associated with RS *per se*. It is reasonable to acknowledge that some of the aetiological and predisposing factors will be similar (**Figure 1**).

The intra-oral distribution of teeth in patients with DH generally involves all the buccal (facial) surfaces of canine, premolar and molar teeth although the condition can also be detected in the incisor teeth. The association of DH and gingival recession has been previously noted and approximately one in three teeth may be affected. The distribution of teeth with RS will generally affect the same tooth type but may also affect the palatal and lingual surfaces particularly following periodontal treatment. It is essential that the clinician undertakes a thorough clinical examination together with both medical and dental histories to obtain an overall picture of the history of the condition as well as the presenting clinical features and any precipitating and predisposing aetiological features [14]. For example, a patient who has recently received dental treatment such as the restoration of a tooth or had their teeth professionally cleaned

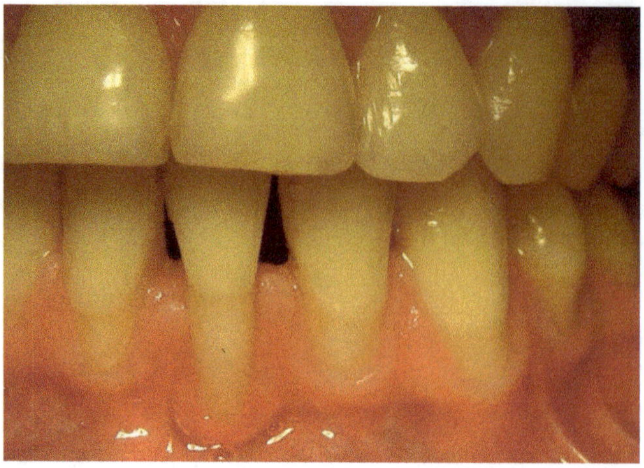

Figure 1. Clinical features of a patient with gingival recession and dentine hypersensitivity (acknowledgement G Belibasakis).

may be experiencing discomfort from these procedures and it would be relatively easy to resolve the problem by obtaining a history that included recent dental treatment. Patients with a more obscure orofacial problem, such as a persistent idiopathic facial pain (PIFP), may require more extensive examination and subsequent referral to an oral medicine/pain clinic.

2.4.1. Clinical diagnosis of DH (including a differential diagnosis)

According to Gillam [17], it is important for clinicians to identify patients with DH correctly by excluding any confounding factors from other orofacial pain conditions prior to the successful management of the condition. It is important to note that the original definition of DH was essentially a definition of exclusion and as such should encourage the clinician to exclude any other potential orofacial condition(s) to determine a definitive diagnosis of DH, for example, from dental disease such as caries, fractures of the tooth due to trauma and mechanical failure of restorations and the effects of restorative and cosmetic treatment such as restorations, whitening procedures and periodontal treatment.

Traditionally clinicians have used a dental explorer probe and air from a triple-air syringe to identify any sensitive areas on the exposed root surface to elicit a response from the patient [6]. This is a relatively simple and straightforward way to examine teeth which may be sensitive as the discomfort from the testing should be transient in nature and should resolve once the stimulus has been removed. The problem arises however, of how the patient can describe this pain since pain is highly subjective and will vary from individual to individual. A simple measure to quantify this response would be the use of a rating score such as a visual analogue scale [VAS (0–10)] and this would provide the clinician with an indication of how the patient rates his/her own pain. Other means of testing are also available such as an ice stick, ethyl chloride, pulp testers, etc., but these may be more relevant in testing for pulp vitality rather than for DH/RS *per se*. More recently quality of life (QoL) questionnaires have been utilised to determine the impact of DH/RS on the patient's quality of life [18]. Although these questionnaires have been mainly used for research purposes in clinical trials, nevertheless, they do provide an insight into how a clinical condition may affect an individual's daily activities as well as determine whether providing a desensitising product may relieve this impact on their QoL. Once a definitive diagnosis has been determined, the clinician can then formulate a management strategy to treat the condition.

2.5. Clinical management of dentine hypersensitivity and root sensitivity

According to Gillam and Orchardson [6] it is important for the clinician to recognise that a simple 'one-fit-all' solution to resolve a patient's pain associated with DH/RS may not necessarily meet the expectation of both the clinician and patient. Ideally a specific management strategy for the successful management of DH/RS should be based on the presenting clinical features. For example, a patient presenting with DH/RS associated with gingival recession can benefit from the clinician educating them regarding the relevant aetiological causes that may have precipitated their clinical problem as well as identifying the sites where the damage to the gingivae has occurred. In other words, simply providing a professionally applied product or procedure or recommending an OTC product without firstly resolving the aetiological factors responsible for the problem would be inappropriate management. Providing information and advice on the type of toothbrush (soft, medium and hard texture), demonstrating an atraumatic brushing technique (by reducing the brushing force) and modifying their dietary intake to avoid any erosive component in the diet should enable the patient to modify their lifestyle accordingly and reduce any future reoccurrence of the problem. The clinician should be aware of the various in-office and OTC products readily available to treat DH/RS and this information is available from a number of reviews [6, 19] (**Table 2**) but clinicians should be aware that currently there does not appear to be agreement on a universally accepted gold standard product or technique to resolve DH/RS and therefore he/she may need a number of different management strategies to resolve an individual patient's problem such as a combination of in-office and OTC products.

The rationale for the successful treatment of periodontal disease(s) can be accomplished through good oral hygiene measures by the patient and through professionally performed non-surgical mechanical debridement and surgical procedures [20]. Both non-surgical and surgical procedures are equally effective in the treatment of chronic periodontitis in terms of attachment level gain and reduction in gingival inflammation [21]. Reduction in pocket depth (PPD) and a gain in the clinical attachment level, however, are generally obtained through surgical procedures such as open flap debridement [21]. Unfortunately, these procedures may have unwanted side effects including gingival recession following the tissue shrinkage of the periodontal pocket, exposure of the underlying dentine following root cementum denudation with the risk of experiencing DH/RDS to both tactile and thermal stimuli as well as (in the anterior region) aesthetic problems (the so-called black triangles).

2.5.1. DH/RS from non-surgical dental procedures

Several studies have reported on the effects of periodontal therapy in the form of non-surgical and surgical procedures in dental practice, and it is evident that patients often report experiencing discomfort (in the form of DH/RS) immediately following these procedures or once the local anaesthesia has worn off [4, 7, 22]. According to these studies there are limited

Gingival recession	Periodontal treatment
Clinical evaluation	**Clinical evaluation**
• Clinical measurement of the gingival recession defect • Take study casts and clinical photographs to monitor the condition over time • Check and monitor periodontal health • Identification and correction of predisposing or precipitating factors • Use of pain scores to assess and monitor DH/RS (e.g. visual analogue scores [VAS])	• Periodontal disease or periodontal treatment as the primary cause of exposure of dentine and associated DH/RS • Check and monitor periodontal health (6-point pocket charting) • Use of pain scores to assess and monitor DH/RS (e.g. visual analogue scores [VAS])
Patient education (including preventive advice)	**Patient education (including preventive advice)**
• Show patient the affected site(s) • Explain probable cause for recession. • Explain factors triggering sensitive teeth episodes • Encourage patients to modify their oral hygiene regimen in order to reduce damage to gingivae (e.g. reducing brushing forceand correction of toothbrush technique) • Reduce excessive consumption of acid foods and drinks	• Reinforce the need for good oral hygiene • Show patient the site(s) affected by periodontal disease and explain probable cause of the exposed dentine • Guide the patient to improve 'at home' oral hygiene regimen • Instruction on measures of reducing periodontal risk factors such as diabetes, smoking, obesity
Corrective clinical outcomes	**Corrective clinical outcomes**
• Reduce excessive consumption of acid foods and drinks • The manufacture of silicone gingival veneers to mask the so-called black triangle appearance following the loss of the interdental papilla/apical displacement of the gingival margin • Orthodontic treatment • Restorative correction of recession defect and subgingival margins of fillings and crowns • Polymers: sealants/varnishes/resins/dentine-bonding agents • Laser obturation of dentinal tubules • Use of desensitising polishing pastes • Pulpal extirpation (root canal treatment) • For local recession defects soft tissue grafting (root coverage) surgical procedures can be considered (see section under periodontal treatment)	**Initial phase** • Non-surgical periodontal procedure(s) • DH treatment (including desensitising polishing pastes/fluoride varnishes) **Re-evaluation** • Follow-up assessment on periodontal status and DH/RS **Corrective phase** • Surgical periodontal procedure(s), for example, guided tissue regeneration, coronally advanced flap + enamel matrix derivatives with/without root conditioning, connective tissue graft (flap)and free gingival graft (acellular dermal matrix allograft) Combination therapy of the above techniques: • DH treatment (including desensitising polishing pastes/fluoride varnishes) **Follow-up management maintenance phase** • Supportive periodontal therapy • On-going monitoring of periodontal health • Dentine hypersensitivity treatment (including desensitising polishing pastes/ fluoride varnishes) • Oral hygiene advice

Recommendations for home use (including toothpaste/mouthrinses)	Recommendations for home use (including toothpaste/mouthrinses)
• Oral hygiene implementation as per recommendation • Strontium chloride/strontium acetate • Potassium nitrate/chloride/citrate/oxalate • Calcium compounds • Calcium carbonate and arginine and casein phosphopeptide+amorphous calcium phosphate • Bioactive glass • Nano/hydroxyapatite • Fluoride in higher concentration (2800/5000 ppm F[prescription]) • Amine/stannous fluoride	• Oral hygiene implementation as per recommendations • Regular brushing with an anti-bacterial toothpaste to aid plaque control • Short period, the use of a 0.2% chlorhexidine solution for plaque control • Use of a desensitising mouthrinse twice daily for DH/RS control (when appropriate) until resolution of the problem

Table 2. Examples of non-surgical and surgical approaches on the management of DH (modified from Gillam [10]).

epidemiological data available in terms of both prevalence and intensity of DH/RS following periodontal therapy (such as scaling, root surface debridement and surgical procedures) as well the lack of data in relation to the impact on the quality of life of those individuals who suffer from DH/RS following these procedures. Although using periodontal instrumentation may remove the biofilm, calculus and subsequently expose the dentinal tubules thereby initiating DH/RS, the same procedures may also create a smear layer on the exposed root surface which can be supplemented by the natural mineralisation processes from the saliva effectively preventing DH/RS. It is evident from the available literature that any discomfort initiated from non-surgical periodontal procedures is relatively short lived and will gradually diminish over time. The clinician is, therefore, in a position to reassure the patient, both prior to and after the treatment, regarding the duration of this discomfort. Several investigators have recommended the application of a prophylaxis desensitising polishing paste (see **Table 2**) immediately following treatment to reduce any discomfort from these procedures [6, 14, 23]. At the same time, the clinician may recommend a desensitising toothpaste as well as implementing a maintenance programme that would include some of the preventative strategies as outlined earlier as well as the monitoring of the condition (**Table 2**). It is also reasonable to suggest to the patient that if the discomfort does not resolve after 2 weeks or that the intensity of the discomfort does not diminish then they should contact the clinician for a re-evaluation of the treatment.

2.5.2. DH/RS following surgical procedures

As mentioned in Section 2.5 both non-surgical and periodontal surgical procedures while providing beneficial outcomes to the patient, including chewing ability, improved aesthetics, and patient satisfaction may also have unwanted side effects such as the exposure of the root surface, gingival recession through over-instrumentation of shallow pockets ≤4 mm or repositioning of the gingival margin following an apical repositioned flap procedure. Tonetti et al. [24] in a multi-centre randomised controlled clinical trial (n = 166 completed subjects) reported on post-surgical outcomes such as post-surgical oedema and hematoma, wound dehiscence, granulation tissue as well as DH/RS. Infection of both the recipient and donor sites or the rejection of the graft material may also occur depending on the surgical techniques used. According to Tonetti et al. [24] the most common post-operative outcome reported in the study was RS which affected 45% of the test and 35% of control groups, respectively, the prevalence of which peaked at 3 weeks and decreased below the baseline frequency by week 6. It should be noted, however, that 40–50% of the subjects in both groups did not report any post-operative sensitivity. In the other reported post-operative complications (post-surgical oedema and hematoma, wound dehiscence and granulation tissue), the prevalence of discomfort was highest at week 1 and rapidly decreased over a 6-week period.

One of the treatment options that have been reported in the literature to resolve the problem of both aesthetics and associated DH/RS was the use of root coverage procedures, which have been shown to reduce or completely abolish DH/RS over time [6–7, 24]. According to Douglas de Oliveira et al. [25] root coverage procedures (both partial and complete coverage) have been reported to decrease pain and improve a patient's quality of life, although currently there appears to be insufficient scientific evidence to associate root coverage procedures with the complete resolution of DH/RS [26].

Patients should, therefore, be warned about the aesthetic outcome anticipated from both non-surgical and surgical treatment, since aesthetic outcome(s) is a primary feature to consider when planning any surgical intervention. Furthermore, it is reasonable to inform the patient that some relapse of the gingival tissues may occur over time [27–28]. For example, the more resective procedures, such as an apically repositioned flap, are more likely to exhibit more exposure of the root surface following periodontal surgery compared to the other surgical techniques. A 14-year follow-up of 10 patients by Pini Prato et al. [28] reported that gingival recession reoccurred in 39% of the treated sites using a coronally advanced flap procedure (CAF).

2.5.3. Specific management strategies for post-operative sensitivity from non-surgical and surgical periodontal procedures

According to Gillam et al. [29], patients who experience DH/RS, as a result of periodontal disease or following treatment, should receive a multi-phase treatment and prevention plan that address both the periodontal health of the patient as well as the associated discomfort from DH/RS. Patient education is therefore an essential component of the strategy and it is vital that the patient understands their responsibility in maintaining their own oral hygiene at home (compliance) as well as recognising the importance of reducing any periodontal risk factors by maintaining good control of systemic disease conditions such as diabetes as well as the need for involvement in smoking cessation programmes (lifestyle and behavioural changes). The clinician also has a responsibility in providing a management strategy that includes the effective monitoring of the patient's periodontal health as well as monitoring any detrimental outcomes following periodontal treatment [24]. It is also important for the clinician to acknowledge that any aetiological or predisposing features that precipitated the clinical problem should be resolved rather than simply providing a desensitising toothpaste, gel or mouthrinse for home use or applying professional products in the clinic.

For patients that exhibit good oral hygiene with minimal or no gingivitis and no evidence of periodontitis but concerned about the appearance of their teeth (aesthetics) showing the root surface, the initial phase of treatment would be by showing the areas in the mouth at risk and discussing ways of how to minimise or prevent further damage to the hard and soft tissues. This may include modifying the toothbrush technique and determining which type of toothbrush would beneficial to the patient, for example, a powered toothbrush. It would also be useful to discuss the impact on the teeth of the frequent consumption of acidic food and/or drink, which may be in association with brushing after consumption. This activity may subsequently remove the protective smear layer on the tooth and expose the underlying dentinal tubules which will instigate DH/RS. One simple recommendation for the clinician would be to use a professionally desensitising polishing paste to any sensitive site both prior to and post-treatment. This will have the advantage of (a) providing instant or reduced relief of the patient's discomfort and (b) helping to reduce the stress associated with the dental procedure as well as the overall patient satisfaction (see **Table 2**).

When developing a strategy for managing patients who require periodontal surgery following the initial phase of non-surgical treatment it is important to recognise (as in the management of DH/RS following non-surgical procedures) to explain that this treatment may initiate a degree of post-therapeutic sensitivity. The evidence from the published literature would suggest that any post-surgical sensitivity is transient in nature and should resolve within 1–2 weeks depending on the extent and severity of the problem. Therefore, it is essential that the patient is made aware of the short nature of the problem, which can be successfully managed by a combination of professionally applied products and home-use toothpastes, mouthrinses and gels (see **Table 2**). One of the key recommendations from Gillam et al. [29] was the implementation of a management strategy that would include the monitoring of both the periodontal tissues and any associated DH/RS from the initial stages of treatment into the maintenance phase [24].

The following case report may highlight some of the elements in implementing a management strategy from the successful resolution of a patient with a periodontal condition with marked gingival recession and associated DH/RS. A 40-year old patient with generalised mild periodontitis and a Miller II gingival recession defect at the lower left central incisor (LL1) was referred for treatment complaining of the poor aesthetics and associated DH/RS. The initial phase of treatment included oral hygiene instruction, modification of the toothbrushing technique and the use of a desensitising toothpaste to relieve discomfort as well as a full-mouth supra- and subgingival debridement (incorporating the use of a prophylaxis polishing paste). Corrective surgery for the LL1 was planned as a two-stage surgery. The initial surgery (**Figures 2–6**) was to relieve the fraenum and deepen the sulcus with the incorporation of a porcine collagen xenograft (Mucograft®) to thicken and widen the band of keratinised tissue. A second-stage surgery using a coronally advanced flap procedure and a connective tissue graft to improve the coverage of the root surface will be completed at a later stage. Following surgery, a desensitising product was applied around the tooth and the patient was provided with a mouthwash. A zone of attached keratinised gingiva of 2 mm was clearly visible after 2 months and no further deterioration of the recession site was noted after 6 months (**Figures 2–6**). A recession defect of 3 mm, however, remained but this will be corrected during the second phase of corrective treatment. Regarding patient outcomes, the patient was happy with the current outcome and noticed a significant reduction in DH/RS which has improved her QoL and also reported that she observed less bleeding on brushing.

The selection and recommendation of desensitising products for the management of post-surgical sensitivity from non-surgical and surgical periodontal treatment should be evidenced based; however, there does not appear to be a universally accepted gold standard product to recommend to clinicians and therefore it may be expedient to use a range and/or combination of professionally applied and at-home products to treat DH/RS (**Table 2**). To some extent this will depend on the extent (localised/generalised) and severity of the problem (mild/moderate or severe) as well as the impact of the QoL of the individual patient. It is important for the clinician to note that it may not always be possible to fully resolve the problem of DH/RS and

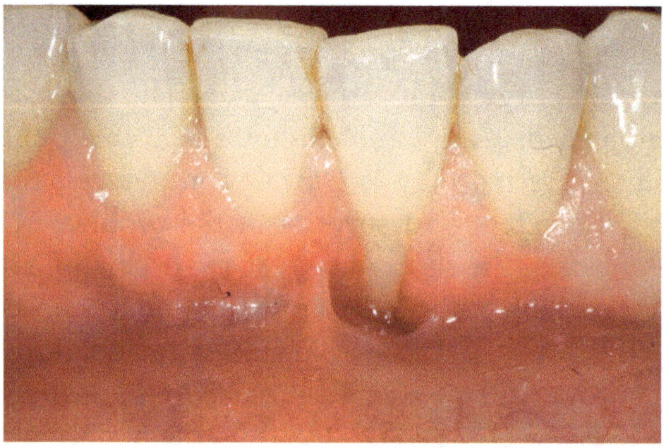

Figure 2. Pre-operative appearance of LL1 with a shallow vestibule present.

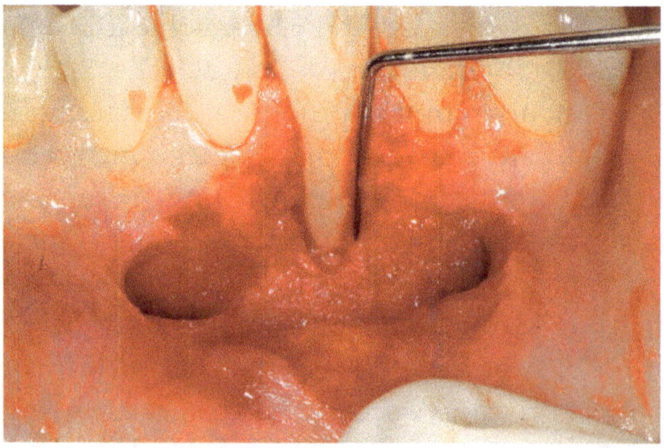

Figure 3. Peri-operative view illustrating the separation of the fraenum and deepening of the vestibule through the horizontal incision. The full extent of attachment loss is clearly evident.

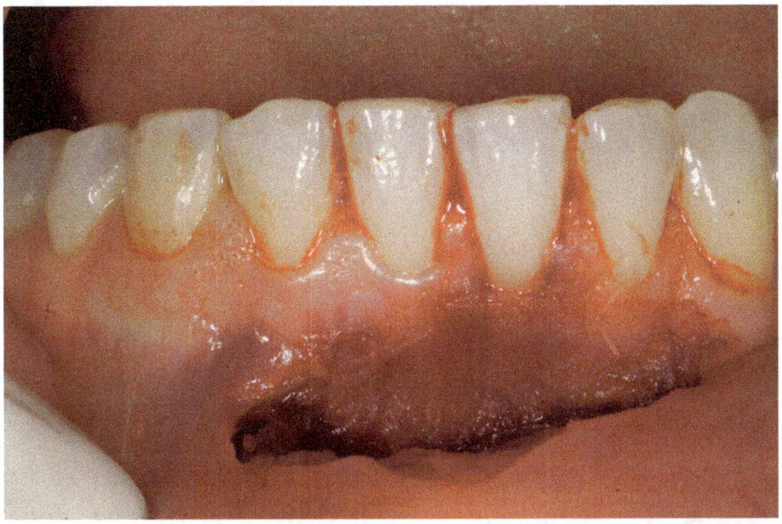

Figure 4. The gingival tissues adjacent to LL1 were de-epithelialised and the placement of the grafting material (Mucograft) with securing sutures was accomplished.

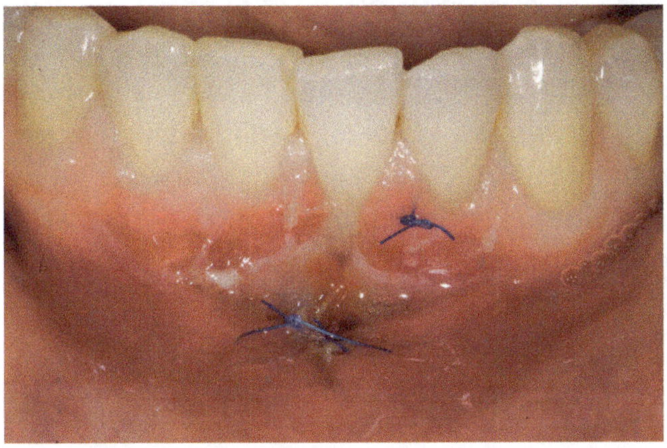

Figure 5. Post-operative view of uneventful soft tissue healing at 2 weeks. Closure of the incision was achieved by secondary intention and the graft was incorporated into the surrounding tissues.

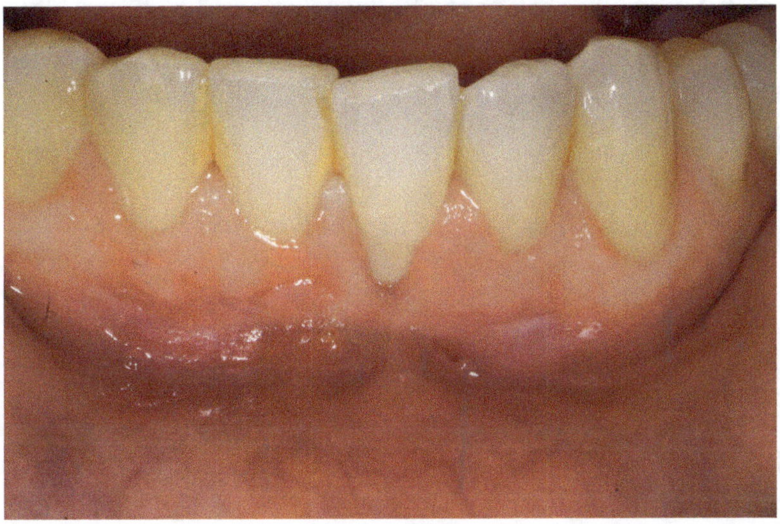

Figure 6. Post-operative view at the 6 months review. Complete healing of the soft tissues had occurred as well as the thickening of the gingiva with a widened band of keratinised tissue.

as such one should manage the expectations of both the clinician and patient. It may be more realistic to accept that if the treatment can minimise the impact of the problem on the QoL of the individual patient to allow them to complete a range of their normal daily activities, then this may be a successful treatment outcome.

3. Conclusions

Both non-surgical and surgical periodontal procedures together with the effects of periodon tal disease on the teeth and their supporting structures may have impact on the patient's aes thetics and quality of life due to the pain associated with DH/RS. Ideally the clinician needs to prevent or minimise these effects to reduce any unnecessary discomfort for the patient and this may be accomplished through preventive strategies such as patient education, lifestyle, behavioural changes, the provision of the required information about the procedures both pre- and post-treatment as well as reassuring the patient in the event of any subsequent dis comfort. The implementation of a management strategy that utilises a range of professionally applied products and techniques and procedures as well as home-use products depending on the extent and severity of the problemis an essential step to the successful treatment in resolving DH/RS following non-surgical and surgical periodontal procedures. This strategy should include the monitoring of both the periodontal tissues and any associated DH/RS from the initial stages of treatment (following a definitive diagnosis) to the maintenance phase of treatment.

Acknowledgements

The authors are grateful to Professor George Belibasakis and Dr. Hiten Halai for the provision of the clinical photographs in **Figures 1–6**.

Author details

David G. Gillam[1*] and Dominiki Chatzopoulou[2]

*Address all correspondence to: d.g.gillam@qmul.ac.uk

1 Centre for Oral Bioengineering, Institute of Dentistry, Barts and the London School of Medicine and Dentistry QMUL, London, UK

2 Oral Immunobiology and Regenerative Medicine, Institute of Dentistry, Barts and the London School of Medicine and Dentistry QMUL, London, UK

References

[1] Canadian Advisory Board on Dentin Hypersensitivity. Consensus based recommendations for the diagnosis and management of dentin hypersensitivity. Journal of the Canadian Dental Association. 2003;**2003**(69):221-226

[2] Addy M. Dentine hypersensitivity: Definition, prevalence distribution and aetiology. In: Addy M, Embery G, Edgar WM, Orchardson R, editors. Tooth Wear and Sensitivity. London, UK: Martin Dunitz; 2000. pp. 239-248

[3] Sanz M, Addy M. Group D summary. Journal of Clinical Periodontology. 2002;**29**(Suppl 3): 195-196

[4] Troll BV, Needleman I, Sanz M. A systematic review of the prevalence of root sensitivity following periodontal therapy. Journal of Clinical Periodontology. 2002;**29**(Suppl. 3): 173-177

[5] Chabanski MB, Gillam DG, Bulman JS, Newman HN. Prevalence of cervical dentine sensitivity in a population of patients referred to a specialist periodontology department. Journal of Clinical Periodontology. 1996;**23**:989-992

[6] Gillam DG, Orchardson R. Advances in the treatment of root dentine sensitivity: Mechanisms and treatment principles. Endodontic Topics. 2006;**13**:13-33

[7] Lin YH, Gillam DG. The prevalence of root sensitivity following periodontal therapy: A systematic review. International Journal of Dentistry. 2012;Article ID 407023;**2012**:12. DOI: 10.1155/2012/407023

[8] Ozcelik O, CenkHaytac M, Seydaoglu G. Immediate post-operative effects of different periodontal treatment modalities on oral health-related quality of life: A randomized clinical trial. Journal of Clinical Periodontology. 2007;**34**:788-796

[9] Pihlstrom BL, Hargreaves KM, Bouwsma OJ, Myers WR, Goodale MB, Doyle MJ. Pain after periodontal scaling and root planing. Journal of the American Dental Association (1939). 1999;**1999**(130):801-807

[10] Gillam DG. A new perspective on dentine hypersensitivity–guidelines for general dental practice. Dental Update. 2017;**44**:33-42

[11] Cunha-Cruz J, Wataha JC. The burden of dentine hypersensitivity. In: Robinson PG, editor. Dentine Hypersensitivity: Developing a Person-Centred Approach to Oral Health. Oxford, UK: Academic Press, Elsevier Inc.; 2014. pp. 34-44

[12] Kamal H, Abu Hantash RO, Taani DQ, Hammad MM. The prevalence of dentine hypersensitivity and gingival recession among Jordanian patients at JUST dental teaching center. Open Journal of Stomatology. 2014;**4**:497-506

[13] Brännström M, Åström A. The hydrodynamics of the dentin; its possible relationship to dentinal pain. International Dental Journal. 1972;**22**:219-227

[14] Gillam DG. A new perspective on dentine hypersensitivity – guidelines for general dental practice. Dental Update. 2017;**44**:33-42

[15] West NX, Sanz M, Lussi A, Bartlett D, Bouchard P, Bourgeois D. Prevalence of dentine hypersensitivity and study of associated factors: A European population based cross-sectional study. Journal of Dentistry. 2013;**41**:841-851

[16] Chabanski MB, Gillam DG. Aetiology, prevalence and clinical feature of cervical dentine sensitivity. Journal of Oral Rehabilitation. 1997;**24**:15-19

[17] Gillam DG. Current diagnosis of dentin hypersensitivity in the dental office: An overview. Clinical Oral Investigations. 2013;**17**(Suppl 1):S21-S29

[18] Gibson B, Boiko OV, Baker S, Robinson PG, Barlow A, Player T, Locker D. The everyday impact of dentine sensitivity: Personal and functional aspects. Social Science and Dentistry. 2010;**1**:11-20

[19] West NX, Seong J, Davies M. Management of dentine hypersensitivity: Efficacy of professionally and self-administered agents. Journal of Clinical Periodontology. 2015;**42**(Suppl 15):S256-S302

[20] Tammaro S, Wennstrom JL, Bergenholtz G. Root-dentin sensitivity following non-surgical periodontal treatment. Journal of Clinical Periodontology. 2000;**27**:690-697

[21] Heitz-Mayfield LJ, Trombelli L, Heitz F, Needleman I, Moles DA. Systematic review of the effect of surgical debridement vs non-surgical debridement for the treatment of chronic periodontitis. Journal of Clinical Periodontology. 2002;**29**(Suppl 3):92-102

[22] Draenert ME, Jakob M, Kunzelmann KH, Hickel R. The prevalence of tooth hypersensitivity following periodontal therapy with special reference to root scaling. A systematic review of the literature. American Journal of Dentistry. 2013;**26**(1):21-27

[23] Fiocchi MF, Moretti AJ, Powers JM, Rives T, Strassler HE. Commentary on the treatment of root sensitivity after periodontal therapy. American Journal of Dentistry. 2007;**20**(4):217-220. Inside Dentistry 2008, 3(3). Accessed from www.aegisdentalnetwork.com/.../treatment-of-root-sensitivity-after-periodontaltherapy

[24] Tonetti MS, Fourmousis I, Suvan J, Cortellini P, Brägger U, Lang NP. Healing, postoperative mobidity and patient perception of outcomes following regenerative therapy of deep intrabony defects. Journal of Clinical Periodontology. 2004;**31**:1092-1098

[25] Douglas de Oliveira DW, Marques DP, Aguiar-Cantuária IC, Flecha OD, Gonçalves PF. Effect of surgical defect coverage on cervical dentin hypersensitivity and quality of life. Journal of Periodontology. 2013 Jun;**84**(6):768-775. DOI: 10.1902/jop.2012.120479: Epub 2012 Aug 16

[26] Douglas de Oliveira DW, Oliveira-Ferreira F, Flecha OD, Gonçalves PF. Is surgical root coverage effective for the treatment of cervical dentin hypersensitivity? A systematic review. Journal of Periodontology. 2013;**84**(3):295-306. DOI: 10.1902/jop.2012.120143. Epub 2012 May 1

[27] Pini-Prato GP, Cairo F, Nieri M, Franceschi D, Rotundo R, Cortellini P. Coronally advanced flap versus connective tissue graft in the treatment of multiple gingival recessions: A split-mouth study with a 5-year follow up. Journal of Clinical Periodontology. 2010;**37**: 644-650

[28] Pini Prato G, Rotundo R, Franceschi D, Cairo F, Cortellini P, Nieri M. Fourteen-year outcomes of coronally advanced flap for root coverage: Follow-up from a randomized trial. Journal of Clinical Periodontology. 2011;**38**:715-720

[29] Gillam D, Chesters R, Attrill D, Brunton P, Slater M, Strand P, Whelton H, Bartlett D. Dentine hypersensitivity–guidelines for the management of a common oral health problem. Dental Update. 2013;**40**(7):514-516, 518-520, 523-524

5

Immunomodulatory Properties of Dental-Derived Mesenchymal Stem Cells

Oleh Andrukhov, Christian Behm,
Alice Blufstein and Xiaohui Rausch-Fan

Abstract

Mesenchymal stem cells are considered as an attractive tool for tissue regeneration. Almost all dental tissues contain a population of MSC-like cells, which were extensively studied within the last few years. Besides their ability to differentiate into different cell types, dental MSCs also possess strong immunomodulatory properties. Dental MSCs modulate both innate and adaptive immune response and influence the activity of almost all components of the immune system. The interaction between dental MSCs and the immune system is reciprocal because immunomodulatory activity of MSCs is strongly regulated by cytokines produced by immune cells. MSCs isolated from inflamed tissues might exhibit impaired immunomodulatory capacity, suggesting a potential role of these cells in inflammatory diseases and particularly periodontitis. Recent studies suggest that immunomodulatory properties of MSCs can also play an important role in their tissue regenerative capacity. The therapeutic effects of MSCs, including their immunomodulatory capacity, are largely explained by their tropic activity, including production of immunomodulatory proteins and growth factors. Summarizing, dental MSCs play an important role in tissue homeostasis under healthy and diseased conditions.

Keywords: mesenchymal stem cells, immune response, immunomodulation, T cells, dendritic cells, natural killer cells, B cells, macrophages, polymorphonuclear neutrophils

1. Introduction

Mesenchymal stem cells (MSC) are defined as cells that fulfill at least three criteria: adherence to culture plastic under standard cell culture condition; surface expression of mesenchymal markers CD73, CD90 and CD105 as well as lacking expression of hematopoietic markers CD11b, CD14, CD34, CD45 and HLA-DR; ability to differentiate into osteoblasts, adipocytes and chondrocytes *in vitro* [1]. Originally, MSCs were isolated from bone marrow, but later MSC-like cells were found in different postnatal tissues [2]. MSC-like cells were isolated from numerous dental tissues: dental pulp stem cells (DPSCs) [3]; stem cells of human exfoliated deciduous teeth (SHED) [4]; periodontal ligament stem cells (PDLSCs) [5]; stem cells from apical papilla (SCAP) [6]; dental follicle stem cells (DFSCs) [7]; gingival mesenchymal stem cells (GMSCs) [8] and bone marrow MSCs from orofacial bones [9]. One peculiarity of most dental tissue-derived MSCs is that these cells express several neural lineage markers, which can be explained by their neural crest origin [10, 11].

MSCs in dental tissues reside in perivascular niches, where they are maintained in quiescent nondifferentiated state by specific microenvironment [12]. Upon tissue injury, these cells are recruited to the damaged area and participate in wound healing by proliferation and differentiation into tissue-specific cells [13]. Another important function of MSCs is modulation of immune and inflammatory response. Perivascular localization of MSCs is an essential factor, which enables their interaction with a wide range of cells during the process of their recruiting *in vivo*, as well as transvascular migration and modulation of the functional acticity of these cells. Furthermore, inflammation is characterized by chemotaxis of MSCs to inflamed area where they can perform their immunomodulatory function.

Although the exact mechanisms underlying immunomodulatory properties of MSCs are not fully understood, it is known that they depend on expression of enzymes, production of soluble factors and cell-to-cell contact. The most important factor involved in MSC-mediated immunosuppression is indolamine-2,3-dioxygenase (IDO). This intracellular enzyme catalyzes the catabolism of tryptophan into kynurenine. The resulted tryptophan depletion leads to suppression of different immune cells [14]. The expression of IDO is very low in resting MSCs and is drastically upregulated by interferon (IFN)-γ [15, 16]. The most important soluble factors mediating immunomodulatory effects of MSCs are prostaglandin E2 (PGE-2), transforming growth factor (TGF)-β, and interleukin (IL)-10. PGE-2 is a metabolic product of arachidonic acid cascade, which production is controlled by cyclooxygenase 2, and is involved in regulation of both innate and adaptive immune system by MSCs [17]. Potent immunomodulatory cytokine TGF-β is continuously produced by MSCs, and its production can be enhanced by other anti-inflammatory factors such as IL-4 and IL-13 [18]. IL-10 is an anti-inflammatory cytokine, which can be produced either by MSCs themselves or by MSC-instructed immune cells [19]. Further soluble factors are also reported to be involved in MSC-mediated immunomodulation: human leukocyte antigen (HLA)-G5, galectins, hepatocyte growth factor, tumor necrosis factor α-stimulated gene 6 [20]. Direct cell-to-cell contact mediates immunosuppression effect of MSCs at least partially. This mechanism acts mainly through programmed death ligand 1 (PD-L1), which expression is upregulated by IFN-γ [21]. The membrane-bound HLA-G1 is another factor involved in direct interaction between MSCs and immune cells [21]. Summarizing, the mechanisms involved in MSC-mediated immunosuppression are complicated; they are specific for individual cell types and are largely determined by degree of inflammation and microenvironment (**Figure 1**).

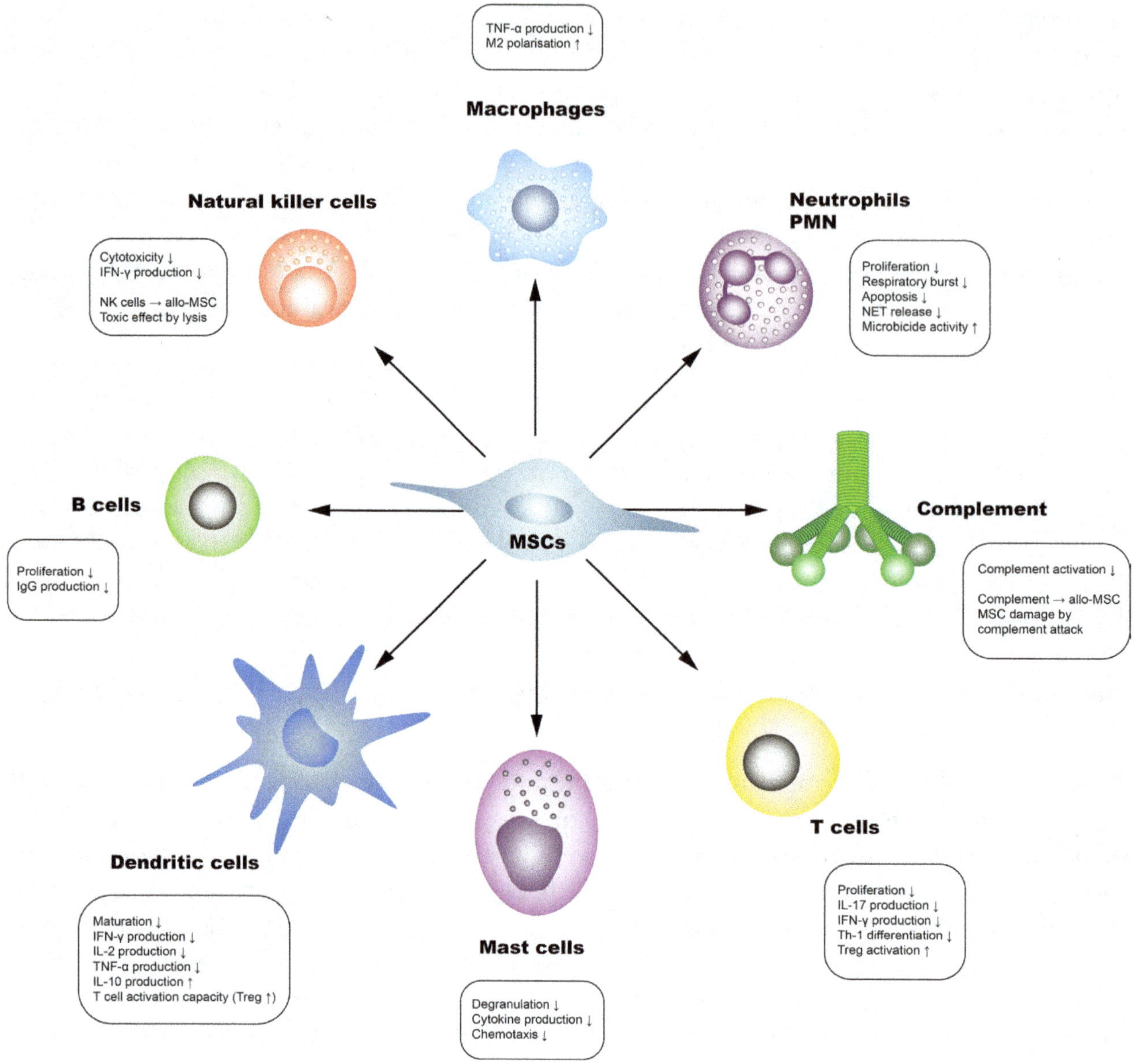

Figure 1. Immunomodulatory effects of MSCs on different components of innate and adaptive immunity.

2. Immunomodulatory effect of MSCs on different components of immune system and their role in dental tissues

2.1. T cells

T cells are one of the most important effector cells of the adaptive immune system, involved in the cell-mediated immune response. Antigen-specific activation of T cells via specialized antigen-presenting cells (APC) leads to clonal selection and differentiation of antigen-specific naïve T cells into different effector subtypes. Depending on which major histocompatibility complex (MHC) the antigen is presented, two different T cell subtypes evolve: CD4+ T-helper cell (MHC class II) with its different phenotypes (Th1/Th2/Th17/Treg) or CD8+ cytotoxic T cell

(MHC class I). The subtypes/phenotypes differ in their surface marker expression, their cytokine secretion profiles and their functions. CD8+ cytotoxic T cells are involved in destruction of virus-infected and tumor cells. Th1 cells are involved in eliminating pathogens, residing in vesicular compartments, whereas Th2 cells participate in B lymphocyte activation, leading to antibody producing plasma cells. In addition, Th17 cells detect extracellular pathogens, recruiting neutrophil granulocytes. Regulatory T cells exhibit a suppressive function, involved in the self-tolerance process and in diminishing inflammatory processes [22].

Although there are a lot of studies investigating the multiple roles of T lymphocytes in periodontitis, the function of T cells in the pathogenesis of periodontitis is still to be clarified [23]. Both Th1 and Th2 cells are detected concurrently in inflamed periodontal tissue [24] and seem to be directly involved in alveolar bone destruction, mainly by producing RANKL [25]. Recently discovered, Th17 cells play an essential role in periodontitis and are one of the primary sources of RANKL [23, 26]. Regulatory T cell-produced IL-10 inhibits RANKL expression of T cells [27]. Periodontitis is shown to be associated with both increased and decreased number of Treg cells [27, 28].

Among all immune cells, the effect of MSCs on T cells is studied at most [29]. It is already known that MSCs influence the activation, proliferation and differentiation of T cells, modulating T cell-mediated immune response [30]. MSCs are potent suppressors of T cell proliferation, including CD4+ T-helper and CD8+ cytotoxic T cells [29, 31]. This suppressive effect of MSCs is enhanced by priming with IFN-γ and TNF-α is mediated by IDO, PGE-2, HLA-G5 [32–34] as well as by cell-to-cell contact through PD-L1 and HLA-G1 [35, 36]. In addition, MSCs suppress proliferation of naïve but not maturated CD8+ T cells [37]. Furthermore, MSCs modulate CD4+ T-helper cell differentiation, their cytokine production and the balance between different CD4+ T-helper subtypes [38, 39]. The effect of MSCs on T cell polarization might depend on their activation state [40]. Interestingly, nonprimed MSCs stimulate proliferation of nonactivated T cells, but retain their ability to promote Treg formation [41].

MSCs from different dental tissues also show the ability to modulate T lymphocytes. T cell proliferation is inhibited by different IFN-γ primed dental MSCs, particularly DPSCs, PDLSCs, GMSC, and SCAP [8, 42–44]. DPSCs can also induce T cell apoptosis [45]. The inhibitory effect of dental MSCs on T cell proliferation is mediated mainly by IDO, hepatocyte growth factor (HGF), and TGF-β [29, 46]. Furthermore, DPSCs, PDLSCs, and SHED inhibit IL-17 production by T cells and stimulate formation of Treg cells, which might dampen periodontal inflammation [42, 44, 47]. Interestingly, immunomodulatory properties of PDLSCs on T cells are impaired under inflammatory conditions. PDLSCs isolated from inflamed tissue exhibit lower inhibitory effect on T cell proliferation, Th17 differentiation, and IL-17 production as well as induce lower number of regulatory Treg cells and IL-10 production [44]. Moreover, PDLSCs from inflamed tissue also inhibit IFN-γ production by T cells and Th1 cell differentiation, whereas PDLSCs from healthy tissue have no effect on these parameters [44].

2.2. Dendritic cells

Dendritic cells constitute a critical interface between innate and adaptive immune response and are responsible for initiating antigen-specific immune response [48]. The major function of classical dendritic cells is detection of invading pathogens and their presentation to the adaptive immune system, which results in initiation of long-lasting antigen-specific response. Besides antigen detection and presentation to T cells, classical DCs also produce pro-inflammatory cytokines, which plays a crucial role in T cell differentiation into different subsets. Classical DCs (cDCs) derive from bone marrow precursors and can be found in lymphoid tissue, bone marrow, and most nonlymphoid tissues. In the absence of pathogens, cDCs are immune tolerogenic and induce expansion of Treg [49]. Activation of cDCs by pattern recognition receptors induces their maturation, migration to lymph node and priming of T cells. Besides cDCs, there are several nonclassical DCs subsets: monocyte-derived DCs, plasmacytoid DCs and Langerhans cells [50].

In recent years, an importance of dendritic cells in both maintaining of periodontal health and progression of periodontal disease was recognized [51]. Under healthy conditions, immature DCs of periodontal tissue promote production of Treg cells and thus are involved in induction of immune tolerogenic state. Langerhans cells, which are present in sulcular and junctional epithelium, are also involved in maintenance of periodontal health homeostasis via induction of Treg cells [51]. Upon exposure to periodontal pathogens, DCs can contribute to different types of adaptive immune response. Activation of Th1, Th2, or Th17 response by DCs might be both beneficial and destructive for the host [52]. The activation and maturation of dendritic cells is influenced by periodontal pathogen *Porphyromonas gingivalis* [53], which is thought to lead to subversion of local immunity and alteration of host immune homeostasis.

The functional activity of dendritic cells is substantially affected by MSCs. Bone marrow MSCs inhibit differentiation of DCs from their precursors. This concerns both classical DCs and monocyte-derived DCs [54–56]. Furthermore, DCs differentiated in the presence of bone marrow MSCs exhibit impaired maturation upon stimulation with pattern recognition receptors and/or inflammatory cytokines [54, 57, 58]. Interestingly, no impaired maturation is observed when DCs are differentiated in the presence of MSCs isolated from inflamed tissue." ocktail [59]. In contrast to DCs differentiation, the effect of MSCs on the maturation of differentiated DCs is less obvious. On the one hand, some studies show that MSCs inhibit maturation of differentiated DCs [60, 61]. On the other hand, some studies show that MSCs have no effect on maturation of differentiated DCs [54] or even can potentiate this process [62, 63]. The process of DCs maturation is also stimulated by MSCs originating from inflamed tissue [59]. The effect of MSCs on DCs is often associated with production of IL-6 and PGE-2, which are known to inhibit DCs differentiation [64, 65] and stimulate their maturation [66]. Another important factor for interaction between MSCs and DCs is TNF-stimulated gene 6 protein (TSG-6), which is produced by MSCs and might inhibit DCs maturation [67].

MSCs derived from different dental tissues also exhibit an ability to modulate the function of DCs. Periodontal ligament STRO1+ CD146+ stem cells inhibit expression of nonclassical major histocompatibility complex-like glycoprotein CD1b, which results in inhibition of DC-mediated T cell proliferation [68]. Gingiva-derived MSCs are shown to inhibit maturation and activation of DCs resulting in attenuation of the inflammatory response, associated with PGE-2-dependent mechanisms [69]. MSCs derived from SHED are shown to influence differentiation, maturation, and T cell activation ability of monocyte-derived DCs [70]. Particularly, after exposure to SHED-derived MSC, DCs induce higher proportion of Treg cells, exhibit decreased production of pro-inflammatory cytokines IL-2, TNF-α, and IFN-γ and produce increased levels of anti-inflammatory IL-10 protein [70].

2.3. Natural killer cells

Natural killer cells (NK cells) are originally thought to be a component of innate immune system, but studies of last few years show that these cells have attributes of both innate and adaptive immune system [71]. NK cells can directly induce the death of tumor and virus-infected cells. Additionally, NK cells are considered as a major source of IFN-γ and also produce other cytokines. This makes them important players of immune system, regulating the function of other immune cells like DCs, macrophages, neutrophils, T cells and B cells [72–76]. Two major populations of NK cells are present in peripheral blood. Predominant population of NK cells is $CD56^{dim}CD16^{+}$ and exhibits moderate expression of CD56. Approximately 5% of all NK cells show $CD56^{bright}CD16^{-}$ phenotype and exhibit high expression of CD56 [77].

Although NK cells play an important role in both innate and adaptive immune response, their role in periodontal disease remains obscure [78]. Chronic periodontitis is associated with an increased number of NK cells in human gingiva [79, 80]. NK cells are considered as one of the major sources of IFN-γ [81], which can be associated with increased tissue destruction and periodontal disease severity [82, 83]. Besides, NK cells can directly interact with some periodontal pathogens. Interaction between *P. gingivalis* and NK cells leads to enhanced IFN-γ production and is involved in production of *P. gingivalis* specific IgG2 [84]. Another periodontal pathogen *A. actinomycetemcomitans* promotes IFN-γ production by NK cells either directly or mediated by DCs [85]. Direct recognition of *Fusobacterium nucleatum* by NK cells through their receptor NKp46 contributes to increased tissue destruction in experimental periodontitis [86].

NK cells and MSCs interact in a complex reciprocal manner. Cultured MSCs are recognized and lysed by NK cells that are activated by IL-2 or IL-15, which could be explained by low MHC class I expression on MSCs' surface. Interestingly, priming of MSCs by IFN-γ induces upregulation of MHC class I expression and prevents them from being killed by activated NK cells. The susceptibility of MSCs for NK cells mediated killing is also regulated by toll lile receptor (TLR) activation [87]. MSCs primed with TLR-3 are protected from being killed by activated NK cells, whereas priming with TLR-4 and TLR-7/-8 has no significant effect on MSCs susceptibility to NK cell mediated lysis [88]. In turn, MSCs also influence activity of NK cells. Particularly, MSCs suppress cytokine production and cytotoxicity of freshly isolated NK cells but not those of activated NK cells [37, 89, 90]. The effect of MSCs on NK cells is largely mediated by IDO and PGE-2 [89].

Information about interaction of dental MSCs and NK cells is rather limited. Similarly to bone marrow MSCs, dental pulp stem cells are susceptible to lysis by activated NK cells [91]. NK cells exert the strongest cytotoxic effect on undifferentiated DPSCs, whereas differentiated cells are less susceptible to lysis [92]. DPSCs could be protected from NK cell mediated cytotoxicity by co-culture with monocytes [92] or by overexpression of hypoxia-inducible factor 1 [93].

2.4. B cells

B cells are an indispensable component of the adaptive immune response, which is mainly involved in antibody production. B cells develop from hematopoietic progenitor cells in the fetal liver and in the bone marrow postnatal [94]. After exiting bone marrow, immature B cells migrate to secondary lymph organs like the spleen or lymph nodes, where they may encounter antigens through interaction with antigen-presenting cells like dendritic cells and macrophages. After interaction with antigen, B cells differentiate into short-lived antibody-producing plasma cells. Alternatively, B cells may enter a germinal center, where they undergo clonal expansion, class switch recombination and somatic hypermutation resulting in differentiation into high affinity antibody-producing plasma cells and memory B cells [95]. Recent studies revealed that beside antibody production, B cells are also involved in the processes of antigen presentation and cytokine production [96–98].

B cells and plasma cells are the major leukocytes in periodontal lesions and represent 18% and 50% of all infiltrating cells, respectively [99]. Despite this fact, the role of B cells in periodontitis is not characterized sufficiently. B cells comprise several functionally different subsets and their distribution is altered in patients with severe periodontitis [100]. The major function of B cells is producing specific antibodies against periodontal pathogens, which is an important step of bacteria elimination [101]. However, B cells are also considered as major source of deleterious effects of immune response. Particularly, B cells are known to be one of the major sources of RANKL, which plays a central role in bone resorption by osteoclasts [102]. Mice with B cells immunoglobulin D deficiency exhibit lower alveolar bone loss upon oral infection, suggesting an important role of B cells in tissue destruction [103]. Some B cells subsets are also involved in the autoimmune response in periodontitis [99].

The information about the effect of MSCs on B cells is rather controversial: it seems that this effect depends on several factors like B cells maturation state, stimuli used for B cells proliferation and differentiation and ratio between MSCs and B cells. Thus, MSCs inhibit B cell proliferation at MSC:B cell ratio 1:1 to 1:2 [104], but stimulate B cell proliferation at ratio 1:5 to 1:10 [104]. Interestingly, under highly proliferative conditions, MSCs inhibit B cell proliferation even at low MSC:B cells ratio [104]. MSCs stimulate proliferation of naïve and memory B cells [105]. MSCs enhance IgG production by B cells upon stimulation with lipopolysaccharide or cytomegalovirus [106], but inhibit production of IgG, IgA and IgM in mixed lymphocyte culture [107]. Pre-exposure of MSCs to IFN-γ enhances their inhibitory effect on B cell proliferation and IgG production [108, 109] but eliminate their ability to induce regulatory B cells [109]. The inhibitory effect of MSCs on B cells largely depends on cell-to-cell contact, in which interaction between programmed death-1 (PD-1) and its ligand PD-1 L takes place [108, 110].

The information about the effect of dental MSCs on functional activity of B cells is rather limited. The only one report shows that PDLSCs influence B cells both *in vitro* and *in vivo* [111]. Particularly, PDLSCs inhibit proliferation, differentiation and chemotaxis of B cells *in vitro* as well as fail to activate humoral immunity *in vivo* in miniature pig models [111]. This inhibitory effect of PDLSCs on B cells is achieved by interaction of PD-1 and its ligand PD-1 L [111].

2.5. Macrophages

Macrophages are phagocytic tissue resident cells of the innate immune system, which are generated from peripheral blood monocytes. Macrophages are found almost in all tissues and their differentiation is determined by specific tissue environments in physiological or inflammatory conditions [112]. The major function of macrophages is the elimination of pathogens by phagocytosis and antigen presentation to cells of the adaptive immune system [113]. In addition to pathogen elimination, macrophages are involved in regulation of immune response, inflammation resolution and immune suppression [114]. Besides their role in immunity, macrophages also play a central role in the clearance of apoptotic cells and damaged tissue [115]. In the early 1990s, a concept for classically activated pro-inflammatory M1 macrophages and alternatively activated anti-inflammatory M2 macrophages emerged. Nowadays, the M1-M2 concept of macrophages activation is extensively revisited since it became obvious that macrophages exhibit extremely high plasticity [116]. Upon activation, macrophages adapt an intermediate state which exhibits some features of both M1 and M2 types, which are considered as extreme states. The activation state of macrophages is driven by the environment and thereby, macrophages are thought to provide an optimal progression of the immune response.

Macrophages activation and polarization to M1-like or M2-like phenotypes play an essential role in the progression of periodontal disease. Upon infection, macrophages are polarized into M1-like phenotype, promote inflammatory response and are correlated with bone resorption [117]. These macrophages produce high amount of cytokines such as IL-1, TNF-α, IL-6, MMP-9, which are associated with periodontal tissue destruction. Moreover, M1 macrophages produce high amount of IL-12 and IL-23. These cytokines stimulate differentiation and proliferation of Th17 cells, which promote further tissue destruction [118]. In case of successful pathogen elimination, a switch into M2-like phenotype occurs. These macrophages play a crucial role in the clearance of apoptotic cells and damaged tissue as well as in wound healing promotion. The increased level of IL-10, which is produced by M2 macrophages, is associated with decreased severity of periodontitis. The ratio between M1 and M2 macrophages is increased in periodontal disease compared to the healthy state and gingivitis [119, 120]. Moreover, the enhanced levels of M1 macrophages correlate with the pocket depth and the levels of tissue destructive cytokines IL-1β and MMP-9 [120].

MSCs modulate the polarization of macrophages. Co-culture of macrophages with MSCs induces their polarization towards regulatory M2 phenotype and is characterized by decreased production of pro-inflammatory TNF-α and IL-12, increased production of IL-10, increased expression of M2 marker CD206 and enhanced phagocytic activity [121, 122]. The polarization of macrophages into M2 phenotype by MSCs is mediated mainly by PGE-2 and IDO [122, 123]. However, the contribution of direct cell-to-cell contact to MSC-mediated macrophage polarization cannot be excluded as well [124]. Induction of macrophages regulatory phenotype is also observed upon systemic or local MSCs administration [122, 125]. Macrophages co-cultured with MSCs are described as a novel type and called MSC-educated macrophages [121]. These macrophages are currently considered for potential clinical application in the treatment of myocardial infarction, graft rejection, diabetes mellitus, ischemic disease and so on [126].

Macrophages polarization is also influenced by different dental MSCs. Human gingiva-derived MSCs induce macrophages polarization into M2 phenotype, which can be associated with an acceleration of wound healing [127]. Human DPSCs isolated from both healthy and inflamed tissue markedly suppress LPS-induced TNF-α production by macrophages through IDO-dependent mechanism [128]. Transplantation of DPSCs into the unilateral hindlimb skeletal muscle suppresses inflammation of sciatic nerves by promoting macrophages M2 polarization [129]. Conditioned medium of periodontal ligament stem cells enhances periodontal regeneration, which was accompanied by alteration of macrophages activity [130]. Recently, SCAP is shown to attenuate neuro-inflammation, which was accompanied by regulation of macrophages activity [131].

2.6. Polymorphonuclear neutrophils

Polymorphonuclear neutrophils are the major fraction of leukocytes circulating in blood (50–70%) and form the first line of host defense against pathogens [132]. Under physiological conditions, up to 2×10^{11} neutrophils are generated from myeloid precursors in the bone marrow daily. To fulfill their key role in the innate immune response, neutrophils must be recruited from bloodstream to the sites of inflammation. Transendothelial migration of neutrophils is a complex process initiated upon activation of tissue-resident leukocytes by invading pathogens [133]. Neutrophils are rather short-lived cells and their lifespan in peripheral blood is thought to be up to 7 h and might be prolonged under inflammatory conditions [134]. Upon tissue migration, the lifespan of neutrophils might be extended up to 2 days [135]. Neutrophils possess several pathogen elimination mechanisms. First, pathogens can be phagocytized and exposed to reactive oxygen species or antibacterial proteins released from the neutrophils granules [136]. Another possibility is the elimination of pathogens via neutrophil extracellular traps (NETs), which consist mainly of DNA and are capable of direct degradation and elimination of bacteria [137]. Recently, a regulatory role of neutrophils in inflammatory response and inflammation resolution has been emerged [138].

Neutrophils play an important role in the homeostasis of periodontal tissue in both healthy and diseased conditions [139]. Neutrophils comprise more than 95% of all leukocytes recruited into the gingival sulcus by dental biofilm [140] and prevent potential bacterial invasion into gingival tissue under healthy conditions. Nevertheless, they are not sufficiently effective in control of dysbiotic microbiota [141]. In addition, keystone pathogen *P. gingivalis* can subvert neutrophil-mediated immunity and promote the conversion of symbiotic microbiota to dysbiotic one [142]. Congenital disorders associated with either neutrophil deficiency or impairment of their life cycle are characterized by the development of aggressive forms of periodontal disease [143]. The maintenance of periodontal health is critically dependent on number and distribution of neutrophils: both insufficient and unrestrained neutrophils recruitment is associated with periodontal inflammation [142].

The knowledge about the interaction of MSCs and neutrophils is rather limited. So far, MSCs were found to exhibit some modulating effects on polymorphonuclear neutrophils. Both resting and TLR-3 primed MSCs have been shown to exert antiapoptotic effects on neutrophils mediated by IL-6, IFN-β and granulocyte macrophage colony-stimulating factor (GM-CSF) [144].

These antiapoptotic effects have also been observed at very low MSC:neutrophil ratio of up to 1:500 in naïve and IL-8 activated neutrophils [145]. Additionally, MSCs dampened the N-formyl-l-methionin-l-leucyl-l-phenylalanine (f-MLP)-induced respiratory burst [145]. Furthermore, MSCs augment antibacterial activity of neutrophils [146]. Human MSCs from amniotic membrane inhibit NET release by neutrophils through a TSG-6 dependent mechanism [147]. The efficacy of MSCs to suppress neutrophils recruitment might also partially depend on MSCs' origin [148].

MSCs of dental origin were also shown to influence neutrophils' functional properties. Particularly, PDLSCs significantly reduce neutrophil apoptosis and enhance their antimicrobial function [149]. PDLSCs exhibit antiapoptotic and proliferation promoting effects on IL-8 activated neutrophils through IL-6 production [150]. The effect of PDLSCs on neutrophils seems to be independent on cell-to-cell contact. Human DFSCs infected with periodontal pathogens *P. intermedia* or *T. forsythia* reduce neutrophil chemotaxis, phagocytic activity and NET formation [151]. Further investigations are needed to clarify the interactions between MSCs of dental origin and polymorphonuclear neutrophils as well as their underlying mechanisms.

2.7. Mast cells

Mast cells are bone marrow-derived granule-containing immune cells, which are present in almost all tissues, including several dental tissues. Upon activation, mast cells release numerous inflammatory mediators from their granules, which are either preformed (histamine, TNF-α, cathepsin G, etc.) or synthesized de novo (interleukins, platelet activating factor, macrophage inhibitory factor 1α) [152]. Mast cells are recognized to be involved in allergic reaction and autoimmunity, but also play an important role in pathogenesis of some inflammatory diseases, particularly arthritis and multiple sclerosis [153, 154]. The functions of mast cells are phagocytosis, antigen presentation and regulation of other cells of the immune system, particularly monocytes, T cells and B cells [155]. Beside inflammatory mediators, mast cells also secrete different growth factors such as VEGF, FGF, TGF-β and PDGF [156].

The role of mast cells in periodontitis is investigated rather poorly and the existing data are sometimes controversial [157]. Two studies show that the density of mast cells is increased in patients with gingivitis and further increased in periodontitis patients suggesting a potential role of these cells in disease progression [158, 159]. In contrast, a decrease in mast cells density or even lack of these cells is reported for marginal chronic gingivitis and acute necrotizing gingivitis [160]. In human, degranulation of mast cells correlates with periodontal disease severity underlying the role of these cells in disease progression [161].

The effect of MSCs on mast cells function is investigated only by few studies. Bone marrow MSCs suppress mast cells degranulation, cytokine production and chemotaxis through production of PGE-2 by COX-2 [162, 163]. MSCs derived from human umbilical cord blood inhibit mast cells degranulation in pre-clinical model through PGE-2- and TGF-β1-dependent mechanisms [164]. The effect of dental MSCs on mast cells function is not investigated to date.

2.8. Complement

The complement system is a component of the innate immune system comprising more than 40 plasma proteins, which are primarily produced in the liver as inactive precursors [165]. The complement could be activated through three different pathways: classic, alternative and lectin pathway. All three pathways are converged at C3 complement component and lead to the generation of different effectors. Complement system components are involved in pathogen destruction, amplification of immune response through synergy with TLRs, mobilization of hematopoietic stem cells from the bone marrow and regulation of T cells subsets activation [166].

The complement system plays an important role in pathogenesis of periodontal disease [167, 168]. Component of complement system is present in the gingival crevice, and its concentration is increased in periodontitis. As the first defense line of immune system, complement system is involved in the control of oral microbiota and maintenance of host-microbial homeostasis in the oral cavity [169]. Exploitation of complement components by periodontal pathogens, particularly *P. gingivalis,* leads to dysregulation of host immune system, dysbiosis of oral microbiota and triggering destructive inflammatory processes [169, 170].

Interaction of MSCs with complement system is bilateral and not yet completely investigated. Upon intravenous injection, MSCs activate complement system, which leads to their damage by membrane attack complex [171]. However, MSCs might inhibit complement activation and associated damage by secreting factor H, which is increased by pro-inflammatory cytokines TNF-α and IFN-γ [172]. Bone marrow MSCs can also synthesize some components of complement system and thus influence some immune cells. Particularly, mycoplasma-induced production of C3 protein is shown to inhibit Ig production by B cells [173].

To date, only interaction of dental pulp cells with complement system was investigated. Upon stimulation with lipoteichoic acid, dental pulp progenitor cells produce almost all components required for activation of complement system [174]. Moreover, DPSCs express C3a- and C5a receptors, which are activated by complement system and induce cell proliferation and mobilization [174, 175].

3. Immunomodulatory effect of MSCs on different components of immune system and their role in dental tissues

Similarly to bone marrow MSCs, immunomodulatory properties of dental MSCs are not constitutive and are affected by surrounding microenvironment. Immunomodulation capacity of quiescent MSCs is usually low and can be drastically enhanced upon stimulation with inflammatory cytokines such as IFN-γ, TNF-α and IL-1β [176]. These cytokines are mainly produced by activated immune cells and thus MSCs and immune cells regulate each other reciprocally. This interaction plays an important role in tissue homeostasis as well as in the processes of inflammation and tissue repair. Upon activation with inflammatory cytokines, MSCs usually adapt an immunosuppressive phenotype and might dampen excessive inflammatory response [177]. However, under low levels of inflammation, MSCs might also stimulate immune response and promote inflammation [177]. In dental MSCs, inflammatory cytokines usually increase the expression of immunomodulatory proteins. Activated PBMCs enhances the expression of TGF-β1, hepatocyte growth factor and IDO-1 in PDLSCs, DPSCs, and gingival MSCs [178]. IDO expression is drastically upregulated by IFN-γ in different dental MSCs [16, 178].

The immunomodulatory capacity of MSCs is also influenced by different pathogen-associated molecular patterns through activation of TLRs, but the role of MSCs priming by TLR is rather controversial to date. In some cases, priming of MSCs by TLR-3 and TLR-4 ligands enhances their immunosuppressive effect [179]. Another report shows that TLR-3 and TLR-4 activation results in abolishment of MSCs ability to suppress T cells activation [180]. These differences could be explained by the fact that activation of TLRs in MSCs induces production of both anti-inflammatory and pro-inflammatory mediators. The role of TLRs in immunomodulatory capacity of dental MSCs is currently under investigation and might be tissue specific. TLR-3 agonist augments immunosuppressive potential of DPSCs and dental follicle stem cells, whereas TLR-4 agonist augments immunosuppressive properties of dental follicle stem cells but inhibits those of DPSCs [181]. Different bacterial lipopolysaccharides induce production of proinflammatory mediators IL-6, IL-8 or MCP-1 in PDLSCs and DPSCs [16, 182–184]. TLR-2 and TLR-4 agonists fail to induce the expression of IDO-1 on protein level in PDLSC, but TLR-2 agonist enhances IFN-γ-induced IDO-1 expression [16]. In turn, LPS also enhances production of anti-inflammatory PGE-2 by PDLSCs [184]. Thus, TLR agonist might activate both proinflammatory and anti-inflammatory properties of dental MSCs and their exact role in inflammatory response is determined by other factors, like degree of inflammation and microenvironment.

Dental MSCs are located in the region which is continuously exposed to different bacterial challenges. Inflammatory milieu has a substantial effect on immunomodulatory properties of dental MSCs. PDLSCs isolated from inflamed tissue exhibit higher migratory capacityas well as impaired ability to promote Treg induction and suppress Th17 differentiation compared to cells isolated from healthy tissue [44, 185]. Similarly, DPSCs derived from teeth with pulpitis fail to suppress proliferation of PBMCs, but this ability might be restored by IFN-γ [186]. In contrast to above data, one study found no difference between DPSCs isolated from normal and inflamed tissues in their ability to modulate macrophage function [128]. To summarize, the alteration of immunomodulatory properties of dental MSCs under inflammatory conditions might play an essential role in the progression of different inflammatory disease such as pulpitis, gingivitis and periodontitis.

4. Contribution of the immunomodulatory effects of MSCs in their tissue regenerative potential

Although the regenerative potential of MSCs is largely recognized, their application for tissue regeneration in clinic is still limited. The major hurdle for clinical application of MSCs is the fact that the mechanisms of their differentiation *in vivo* are largely unknown. Preclinical studies and clinical trials with MSCs transplantation show that the rate of MSCs engraftment is rather poor and does not correlate with the clinical outcome of MSC-based therapy. The lifetime of transplanted MSCs is rather short: for example, intravenously injected MSCs are accumulated in the lung, where they disappear within 24 h [187]. Although the exact mechanisms of MSCs differentiation *in vivo* are unknown, it is a fact that differentiation is regulated by the local microenvironment and interaction of transplanted MSCs with the hosts′ immune system is one of the key elements in this process [188]. The mechanisms underlying MSCs differentiation *in vivo* are also altered by diseased microenvironments [189]. Moreover, transplanted MSCs themselves contribute to the creation of the microenvironment through their immunomodulatory function and the production of different growth factors, which in turn promote activation of endogenous tissue repair mechanisms [190]. Immunomodulatory and tropic capacity of MSCs are now considered as the major mechanisms of their therapeutic effect *in vivo*. This statement is supported by the observations that the secretome of MSCs exert similar tissue regenerative effects as transplanted MSCs [191]. Furthermore, the secretome of MSCs possess also strong immunomodulatory effects [20, 192].

It is rather difficult to discriminate between the role of regenerative potential and immunomodulatory abilities in the output of MSC-based therapies. Tissue regeneration is a complex process, which consists of several timely overlapping phases and involves interaction between different cell types. The immune system plays an important role in the processes of tissue repair and regeneration. Different immune cells are involved in the different stages of tissue regeneration processes [193]. Neutrophils and macrophages are the major cells involved in the inflammatory phase and are responsible for bacteria phagocytosis and removal of tissue debris. Regenerative M2 macrophages and regulatory T cells secrete anti-inflammatory cytokines, which create microenvironments promoting tissue repair. Therefore, the modulation of the immune response by MSCs might be an important mechanism underlying their regenerative potential. Regenerative potential of MSCs and their immunomodulatory properties are tightly interconnected. Many factors mediating immunomodulatory effects of MSCs are also influencing their differentiation potential. Particularly, activation of IDO by IFN-γ alters osteogenic, adipogenic and neural differentiation of human MSCs [194]. TSG-6, another immunomodulatory factor produced by MSCs, plays a crucial role in their differentiation ability [195, 196]. TGF-β produced by MSCs is potentially involved in both regenerative and immunomodulatory function of these cells [197].

Immunomodulatory properties of dental MSCs also seem to play an important role in the regeneration of dental tissues [198]. The major information about the potential role of immunomodulatory properties in therapeutic efficacy of dental MSCs arise from animal studies. Most studies suggest that allogenic transplantation of dental MSCs is well tolerated by recipients' immune system and does not induce any immune rejection [199]. Systemic transplantation of SHED cells ameliorates ovariectomy-induced osteopenia presumably through induction of Treg cells and reducing Th1 and Th17 cells number [200]. Transplantation of allogenic bone marrow MSCs into periodontal defects suppressed local levels of pro-inflammatory cytokines IL-1β, TNF-α and IFN-γ, which indicates their immunomodulatory function *in vivo* [201]. An *in vitro* study shows that the differentiation potential of PDLSCs is influenced by inflammatory microenvironments and is largely determined by their immunomodulatory properties [202].

5. Conclusions

Dental MSCs, similarly to MSCs from other tissues, influence the properties of both the innate and the adaptive immune system. Particularly, dental MSCs change the functional activities of all components of the immune system: T cells, dendritic cells, natural killer cells, B cells, macrophages, neutrophils, mast cells and complement system. The effects of MSCs are mostly immunosuppressive, but in some cases, MSCs might also enhance the immune response. The immunomodulatory mechanisms of MSCs include both production of soluble mediators and cell-to-cell contact. The interaction between MSCs and the immune system is reciprocal: immunomodulatory ability of resting MSCs is rather low and is substantially enhanced by proinflammatory cytokines IFN-γ, TNF-α and IL-1β. This circumstance suggests a tight interaction between MSCs and the immune system, which plays an important role in the maintenance of local tissue homeostasis.

In some cases, dental MSCs isolated from inflamed tissues exhibit impaired immunomodulatory capacity. Furthermore, immunomodulatory properties of dental MSCs might also be influenced through activation of their TLRs by different pathogen-associated bacterial patterns. These observations suggest that dental MSCs might also play an important role in the pathogenesis of different inflammatory diseases and particularly periodontitis.

Although dental MSCs exhibit significant differentiation capacity *in vitro*, the mechanisms underlying their regenerative potential *in vivo* are still unclear. Since the immune system plays one of the key roles in tissue repair processes, immunomodulatory capacity of dental MSCs could be considered as one of the major mechanisms of their effects *in vivo*.

Acknowledgements

Supported by Austrian Science Foundation (Project 29440 to O.A.). The authors are thankful to Mrs. Cornelia Jungwirth (Medical University of Vienna) for help in drawing **Figure 1**.

Author details

Oleh Andrukhov*, Christian Behm, Alice Blufstein and Xiaohui Rausch-Fan

*Address all correspondence to: oleh.andrukhov@meduniwien.ac.at

Division of Conservative Dentistry and Periodontology, University Clinic of Dentistry, Medical University of Vienna, Austria

References

[1] Dominici M, Le Blanc K, Mueller I, Slaper-Cortenbach I, Marini F, Krause D, et al. Minimal criteria for defining multipotent mesenchymal stromal cells. The International Society for Cellular Therapy position statement. Cytotherapy. 2006;**8**:315-317

[2] Chamberlain G, Fox J, Ashton B, Middleton J. Concise review: Mesenchymal stem cells: Their phenotype, differentiation capacity, immunological features, and potential for homing. Stem Cells. 2007;**25**:2739-2749

[3] Gronthos S, Mankani M, Brahim J, Robey PG, Shi S. Postnatal human dental pulp stem cells (DPSCs) in vitro and in vivo. Proceedings of the National Academy of Sciences of the United States of America. 2000;**97**:13625-13630

[4] Miura M, Gronthos S, Zhao M, Lu B, Fisher LW, Robey PG, et al. SHED: Stem cells from human exfoliated deciduous teeth. Proceedings of the National Academy of Sciences of the United States of America. 2003;**100**:5807-5812

[5] Seo BM, Miura M, Gronthos S, Bartold PM, Batouli S, Brahim J, et al. Investigation of multipotent postnatal stem cells from human periodontal ligament. Lancet. 2004;**364**:149-155

[6] Sonoyama W, Liu Y, Yamaza T, Tuan RS, Wang S, Shi S, et al. Characterization of the apical papilla and its residing stem cells from human immature permanent teeth: A pilot study. Journal of Endodontics. 2008;**34**:166-171

[7] Morsczeck C, Gotz W, Schierholz J, Zeilhofer F, Kuhn U, Mohl C, et al. Isolation of precursor cells (PCs) from human dental follicle of wisdom teeth. Matrix Biology. 2005;**24**:155-165

[8] Zhang Q, Shi S, Liu Y, Uyanne J, Shi Y, Shi S, et al. Mesenchymal stem cells derived from human gingiva are capable of immunomodulatory functions and ameliorate inflammation-related tissue destruction in experimental colitis. Journal of Immunology. 2009;**183**:7787-7798

[9] Akintoye SO, Lam T, Shi S, Brahim J, Collins MT, Robey PG. Skeletal site-specific characterization of orofacial and iliac crest human bone marrow stromal cells in same individuals. Bone. 2006;**38**:758-768

[10] Sharpe PT. Dental mesenchymal stem cells. Development. 2016;**143**:2273-2280

[11] Bakopoulou A, About I. Stem cells of dental origin: Current research trends and key milestones towards clinical application. Stem Cells International. 2016;**2016**:4209891

[12] Shi S, Gronthos S. Perivascular niche of postnatal mesenchymal stem cells in human bone marrow and dental pulp. Journal of Bone and Mineral Research. 2003;**18**:696-704

[13] Mitsiadis TA, Feki A, Papaccio G, Caton J. Dental pulp stem cells, niches, and notch signaling in tooth injury. Advances in Dental Research. 2011;**23**:275-279

[14] Munn DH, Mellor AL. Indoleamine 2,3 dioxygenase and metabolic control of immune responses. Trends in Immunology. 2013;**34**:137-143

[15] Krampera M, Cosmi L, Angeli R, Pasini A, Liotta F, Andreini A, et al. Role for interferon-gamma in the immunomodulatory activity of human bone marrow mesenchymal stem cells. Stem Cells. 2006;**24**:386-398

[16] Andrukhov O, Hong JS, Andrukhova O, Blufstein A, Moritz A, Rausch-Fan X. Response of human periodontal ligament stem cells to IFN-gamma and TLR-agonists. Scientific Reports. 2017;**7**:12856

[17] Kalinski P. Regulation of immune responses by prostaglandin E2. Journal of Immunology. 2012;**188**:21-28

[18] Nemeth K, Keane-Myers A, Brown JM, Metcalfe DD, Gorham JD, Bundoc VG, et al. Bone marrow stromal cells use TGF-beta to suppress allergic responses in a mouse model of ragweed-induced asthma. Proceedings of the National Academy of Sciences of the United States of America. 2010;**107**:5652-5657

[19] Najar M, Raicevic G, Fayyad-Kazan H, De Bruyn C, Bron D, Toungouz M, et al. Bone marrow mesenchymal stromal cells induce proliferative, cytokinic and molecular changes during the T cell response: The importance of the IL-10/CD210 Axis. Stem Cell Reviews. 2015;**11**:442-452

[20] Fontaine MJ, Shih H, Schafer R, Pittenger MF. Unraveling the mesenchymal stromal cells' paracrine immunomodulatory effects. Transfusion Medicine Reviews. 2016;**30**:37-43

[21] Tipnis S, Viswanathan C, Majumdar AS. Immunosuppressive properties of human umbilical cord-derived mesenchymal stem cells: Role of B7-H1 and IDO. Immunology and Cell Biology. 2010;**88**:795-806

[22] Wan YY, Flavell RA. How diverse–CD4 effector T cells and their functions. Journal of Molecular Cell Biology. 2009;**1**:20-36

[23] Campbell L, Millhouse E, Malcolm J, Culshaw S. T cells, teeth and tissue destruction—What do T cells do in periodontal disease? Molecular Oral Microbiology. 2016;**31**:445-56

[24] Teng YT. The role of acquired immunity and periodontal disease progression. Critical Reviews in Oral Biology and Medicine. 2003;**14**:237-252

[25] Teng YT. Mixed periodontal Th1-Th2 cytokine profile in *Actinobacillus actinomycetemcomitans*-specific osteoprotegerin ligand (or RANK-L)-mediated alveolar bone destruction in vivo. Infection and Immunity. 2002;**70**:5269-5273

[26] Cardoso CR, Garlet GP, Crippa GE, Rosa AL, Junior WM, Rossi MA, et al. Evidence of the presence of T helper type 17 cells in chronic lesions of human periodontal disease. Oral Microbiology and Immunology. 2009;**24**:1-6

[27] Ernst CW, Lee JE, Nakanishi T, Karimbux NY, Rezende TM, Stashenko P, et al. Diminished forkhead box P3/CD25 double-positive T regulatory cells are associated with the increased nuclear factor-kappaB ligand (RANKL+) T cells in bone resorption lesion of periodontal disease. Clinical and Experimental Immunology. 2007;**148**:271-280

[28] Cardoso CR, Garlet GP, Moreira AP, Junior WM, Rossi MA, Silva JS. Characterization of CD4+CD25+ natural regulatory T cells in the inflammatory infiltrate of human chronic periodontitis. Journal of Leukocyte Biology. 2008;**84**:311-318

[29] Wada N, Gronthos S, Bartold PM. Immunomodulatory effects of stem cells. Periodontology 2000. 2013;**63**:198-216

[30] Castro-Manrreza ME, Montesinos JJ. Immunoregulation by mesenchymal stem cells: Biological aspects and clinical applications. Journal of Immunology Research. 2015;**2015**: 394917

[31] Duffy MM, Ritter T, Ceredig R, Griffin MD. Mesenchymal stem cell effects on T cell effector pathways. Stem Cell Research & Therapy. 2011;**2**:34

[32] Chen H, Min XH, Wang QY, Leung FW, Shi L, Zhou Y, et al. Pre-activation of mesenchymal stem cells with TNF-alpha, IL-1beta and nitric oxide enhances its paracrine effects on radiation-induced intestinal injury. Scientific Reports. 2015;**5**:8718

[33] Selmani Z, Naji A, Zidi I, Favier B, Gaiffe E, Obert L, et al. Human leukocyte antigen-G5 secretion by human mesenchymal stem cells is required to suppress T lymphocyte and natural killer function and to induce CD4+CD25highFOXP3+ regulatory T cells. Stem Cells. 2008;**26**:212-222

[34] Meisel R, Zibert A, Laryea M, Gobel U, Daubener W, Dilloo D. Human bone marrow stromal cells inhibit allogeneic T cell responses by indoleamine 2,3-dioxygenase-mediated tryptophan degradation. Blood. 2004;**103**:4619-4621

[35] Chinnadurai R, Copland IB, Patel SR, Galipeau J. IDO-independent suppression of T cell effector function by IFN-gamma-licensed human mesenchymal stromal cells. Journal of Immunology. 2014;**192**:1491-1501

[36] Giuliani M, Fleury M, Vernochet A, Ketroussi F, Clay D, Azzarone B, et al. Long-lasting inhibitory effects of fetal liver mesenchymal stem cells on T-lymphocyte proliferation. PLoS One. 2011;**6**:e19988

[37] Rasmusson I, Ringden O, Sundberg B, Le Blanc K. Mesenchymal stem cells inhibit the formation of cytotoxic T lymphocytes, but not activated cytotoxic T lymphocytes or natural killer cells. Transplantation. 2003;**76**:1208-1213

[38] Aggarwal S, Pittenger MF. Human mesenchymal stem cells modulate allogeneic immune cell responses. Blood. 2005;**105**:1815-1822

[39] Ghannam S, Pene J, Moquet-Torcy G, Jorgensen C, Yssel H. Mesenchymal stem cells inhibit human Th17 cell differentiation and function and induce a T regulatory cell phenotype. Journal of Immunology. 2010;**185**:302-312

[40] Carrion F, Nova E, Luz P, Apablaza F, Figueroa F. Opposing effect of mesenchymal stem cells on Th1 and Th17 cell polarization according to the state of CD4+ T cell activation. Immunology Letters. 2011;**135**:10-16

[41] Crop MJ, Baan CC, Korevaar SS, Ijzermans JN, Weimar W, Hoogduijn MJ. Human adipose tissue-derived mesenchymal stem cells induce explosive T cell proliferation. Stem Cells and Development. 2010;**19**:1843-1853

[42] Ozdemir AT, Ozgul Ozdemir RB, Kirmaz C, Sariboyaci AE, Unal Halbutogllari ZS, Ozel C, et al. The paracrine immunomodulatory interactions between the human dental

pulp derived mesenchymal stem cells and CD4 T cell subsets. Cellular Immunology. 2016;**310**:108-115

[43] Ding G, Liu Y, An Y, Zhang C, Shi S, Wang W, et al. Suppression of T cell proliferation by root apical papilla stem cells in vitro. Cells, Tissues, Organs. 2010;**191**:357-364

[44] Liu D, Xu J, Liu O, Fan Z, Liu Y, Wang F, et al. Mesenchymal stem cells derived from inflamed periodontal ligaments exhibit impaired immunomodulation. Journal of Clinical Periodontology. 2012;**39**:1174-1182

[45] Zhao Y, Wang L, Jin Y, Shi S. Fas ligand regulates the immunomodulatory properties of dental pulp stem cells. Journal of Dental Research. 2012;**91**:948-954

[46] Li Z, Jiang CM, An S, Cheng Q, Huang YF, Wang YT, et al. Immunomodulatory properties of dental tissue-derived mesenchymal stem cells. Oral Diseases. 2014;**20**:25-34

[47] Yamaza T, Kentaro A, Chen C, Liu Y, Shi Y, Gronthos S, et al. Immunomodulatory properties of stem cells from human exfoliated deciduous teeth. Stem Cell Research & Therapy. 2010;**1**:5

[48] Mildner A, Jung S. Development and function of dendritic cell subsets. Immunity. 2014;**40**:642-656

[49] Qu Y, Zhao Y. Regulatory CD4(+)CD25(+) T cells are controlled by multiple pathways at multiple levels. International Reviews of Immunology. 2007;**26**:145-160

[50] Collin M, McGovern N, Haniffa M. Human dendritic cell subsets. Immunology. 2013;**140**: 22-30

[51] Wilensky A, Segev H, Mizraji G, Shaul Y, Capucha T, Shacham M, et al. Dendritic cells and their role in periodontal disease. Oral Diseases. 2014;**20**:119-126

[52] Gaffen SL, Hajishengallis G. A new inflammatory cytokine on the block: Re-thinking periodontal disease and the Th1/Th2 paradigm in the context of Th17 cells and IL-17. Journal of Dental Research. 2008;**87**:817-828

[53] Zeituni AE, Jotwani R, Carrion J, Cutler CW. Targeting of DC-SIGN on human dendritic cells by minor fimbriated Porphyromonas gingivalis strains elicits a distinct effector T cell response. Journal of Immunology. 2009;**183**:5694-5704

[54] Li YP, Paczesny S, Lauret E, Poirault S, Bordigoni P, Mekhloufi F, et al. Human mesenchymal stem cells license adult CD34+ hemopoietic progenitor cells to differentiate into regulatory dendritic cells through activation of the Notch pathway. Journal of Immunology. 2008;**180**:1598-1608

[55] Nauta AJ, Kruisselbrink AB, Lurvink E, Willemze R, Fibbe WE. Mesenchymal stem cells inhibit generation and function of both CD34+-derived and monocyte-derived dendritic cells. Journal of Immunology. 2006;**177**:2080-2087

[56] Ramasamy R, Fazekasova H, Lam EW, Soeiro I, Lombardi G, Dazzi F. Mesenchymal stem cells inhibit dendritic cell differentiation and function by preventing entry into the cell cycle. Transplantation. 2007;**83**:71-76

[57] Jung JY, Yoo CI, Kim HT, Kwon CH, Park JY, Kim YK. Role of mitogen-activated protein kinase (MAPK) in troglitazone-induced osteoblastic cell death. Toxicology. 2007;**234**:73-82

[58] Zhang Y, Cai W, Huang Q, Gu Y, Shi Y, Huang J, et al. Mesenchymal stem cells alleviate bacteria-induced liver injury in mice by inducing regulatory dendritic cells. Hepatology. 2014;**59**:671-682

[59] Dokic J, Tomic S, Markovic M, Milosavljevic P, Colic M. Mesenchymal stem cells from periapical lesions modulate differentiation and functional properties of monocyte-derived dendritic cells. European Journal of Immunology. 2013;**43**:1862-1872

[60] Chiesa S, Morbelli S, Morando S, Massollo M, Marini C, Bertoni A, et al. Mesenchymal stem cells impair in vivo T cell priming by dendritic cells. Proceedings of the National Academy of Sciences of the United States of America. 2011;**108**:17384-17389

[61] Liu WH, Liu JJ, Wu J, Zhang LL, Liu F, Yin L, et al. Novel mechanism of inhibition of dendritic cells maturation by mesenchymal stem cells via interleukin-10 and the JAK1/STAT3 signaling pathway. PLoS One. 2013;**8**:e55487

[62] Spaggiari GM, Abdelrazik H, Becchetti F, Moretta L. MSCs inhibit monocyte-derived DC maturation and function by selectively interfering with the generation of immature DCs: Central role of MSC-derived prostaglandin E2. Blood. 2009;**113**:6576-6583

[63] van den Berk LC, Roelofs H, Huijs T, Siebers-Vermeulen KG, Raymakers RA, Kogler G, et al. Cord blood mesenchymal stem cells propel human dendritic cells to an intermediate maturation state and boost interleukin-12 production by mature dendritic cells. Immunology. 2009;**128**:564-572

[64] Chomarat P, Banchereau J, Davoust J, Palucka AK. IL-6 switches the differentiation of monocytes from dendritic cells to macrophages. Nature Immunology. 2000;**1**:510-514

[65] Obermajer N, Muthuswamy R, Lesnock J, Edwards RP, Kalinski P. Positive feedback between PGE2 and COX2 redirects the differentiation of human dendritic cells toward stable myeloid-derived suppressor cells. Blood. 2011;**118**:5498-5505

[66] Jonuleit H, Kuhn U, Muller G, Steinbrink K, Paragnik L, Schmitt E, et al. Pro-inflammatory cytokines and prostaglandins induce maturation of potent immunostimulatory dendritic cells under fetal calf serum-free conditions. European Journal of Immunology. 1997;**27**:3135-3142

[67] Liu Y, Yin Z, Zhang R, Yan K, Chen L, Chen F, et al. MSCs inhibit bone marrow-derived DC maturation and function through the release of TSG-6. Biochemical and Biophysical Research Communications. 2014;**450**:1409-1415

[68] Shin C, Kim M, Han JA, Choi B, Hwang D, Do Y, et al. Human periodontal ligament stem cells suppress T cell proliferation via down-regulation of non-classical major histocompatibility complex-like glycoprotein CD1b on dendritic cells. Journal of Periodontal Research. 2017;**52**:135-146

[69] Su WR, Zhang QZ, Shi SH, Nguyen AL, Le AD. Human gingiva-derived mesenchymal stromal cells attenuate contact hypersensitivity via prostaglandin E2-dependent mechanisms. Stem Cells. 2011;**29**:1849-1860

[70] Silva Fde S, Ramos RN, de Almeida DC, Bassi EJ, Gonzales RP, Miyagi SP, et al. Mesenchymal stem cells derived from human exfoliated deciduous teeth (SHEDs) induce immune modulatory profile in monocyte-derived dendritic cells. PLoS One. 2014;**9**:e98050

[71] Vivier E, Raulet DH, Moretta A, Caligiuri MA, Zitvogel L, Lanier LL, et al. Innate or adaptive immunity? The example of natural killer cells. Science (New York, NY). 2011;**331**:44-49

[72] Moretta A, Marcenaro E, Sivori S, Della Chiesa M, Vitale M, Moretta L. Early liaisons between cells of the innate immune system in inflamed peripheral tissues. Trends in Immunology. 2005;**26**:668-675

[73] Martin-Fontecha A, Thomsen LL, Brett S, Gerard C, Lipp M, Lanzavecchia A, et al. Induced recruitment of NK cells to lymph nodes provides IFN-gamma for T(H)1 priming. Nature Immunology. 2004;**5**:1260-1265

[74] Walzer T, Dalod M, Robbins SH, Zitvogel L, Vivier E. Natural-killer cells and dendritic cells: "l'union fait la force". Blood. 2005;**106**:2252-2258

[75] Robbins SH, Bessou G, Cornillon A, Zucchini N, Rupp B, Ruzsics Z, et al. Natural killer cells promote early CD8 T cell responses against cytomegalovirus. PLoS Pathogens. 2007;**3**:e123

[76] Ueda R, Narumi K, Hashimoto H, Miyakawa R, Okusaka T, Aoki K. Interaction of natural killer cells with neutrophils exerts a significant antitumor immunity in hematopoietic stem cell transplantation recipients. Cancer Medicine. 2016;**5**:49-60

[77] Parisi L, Bassani B, Tremolati M, Gini E, Farronato G, Bruno A. Natural killer cells in the orchestration of chronic inflammatory diseases. Journal of Immunology Research. 2017;**2017**:4218254

[78] Wilensky A, Chaushu S, Shapira L. The role of natural killer cells in periodontitis. Periodontology 2000. 2015;**69**:128-141

[79] Kopp W. Density and localization of lymphocytes with natural-killer (NK) cell activity in periodontal biopsy specimens from patients with severe periodontitis. Journal of Clinical Periodontology. 1988;**15**:595-600

[80] Wynne SE, Walsh LJ, Seymour GJ, Powell RN. In situ demonstration of natural killer (NK) cells in human gingival tissue. Journal of Periodontology. 1986;**57**:699-702

[81] Varma TK, Lin CY, Toliver-Kinsky TE, Sherwood ER. Endotoxin-induced gamma interferon production: Contributing cell types and key regulatory factors. Clinical and Diagnostic Laboratory Immunology. 2002;**9**:530-543

[82] Baker PJ, Dixon M, Evans RT, Dufour L, Johnson E, Roopenian DC. CD4(+) T cells and the proinflammatory cytokines gamma interferon and interleukin-6 contribute to alveolar bone loss in mice. Infection and Immunity. 1999;**67**:2804-2809

[83] Gorska R, Gregorek H, Kowalski J, Laskus-Perendyk A, Syczewska M, Madalinski K. Relationship between clinical parameters and cytokine profiles in inflamed gingival tissue and serum samples from patients with chronic periodontitis. Journal of Clinical Periodontology. 2003;**30**:1046-1052

[84] Kikuchi T, Willis DL, Liu M, Purkall DB, Sukumar S, Barbour SE, et al. Dendritic-NK cell interactions in *P. gingivalis*-specific responses. Journal of Dental Research. 2005;**84**:858-862

[85] Kikuchi T, Hahn CL, Tanaka S, Barbour SE, Schenkein HA, Tew JG. Dendritic cells stimulated with *Actinobacillus actinomycetemcomitans* elicit rapid gamma interferon responses by natural killer cells. Infection and Immunity. 2004;**72**:5089-5096

[86] Chaushu S, Wilensky A, Gur C, Shapira L, Elboim M, Halftek G, et al. Direct recognition of *Fusobacterium nucleatum* by the NK cell natural cytotoxicity receptor NKp46 aggravates periodontal disease. PLoS Pathogens. 2012;**8**:e1002601

[87] Delarosa O, Dalemans W, Lombardo E. Toll-like receptors as modulators of mesenchymal stem cells. Frontiers in Immunology. 2012;**3**:182

[88] Giuliani M, Bennaceur-Griscelli A, Nanbakhsh A, Oudrhiri N, Chouaib S, Azzarone B, et al. TLR ligands stimulation protects MSC from NK killing. Stem Cells. 2014;**32**:290-300

[89] Spaggiari GM, Capobianco A, Abdelrazik H, Becchetti F, Mingari MC, Moretta L. Mesenchymal stem cells inhibit natural killer-cell proliferation, cytotoxicity, and cytokine production: Role of indoleamine 2,3-dioxygenase and prostaglandin E2. Blood. 2008;**111**:1327-1333

[90] Sotiropoulou PA, Perez SA, Gritzapis AD, Baxevanis CN, Papamichail M. Interactions between human mesenchymal stem cells and natural killer cells. Stem Cells. 2006;**24**:74-85

[91] Jewett A, Man YG, Tseng HC. Dual functions of natural killer cells in selection and differentiation of stem cells; role in regulation of inflammation and regeneration of tissues. Journal of Cancer. 2013;**4**:12-24

[92] Tseng HC, Cacalano N, Jewett A. Split anergized natural killer cells halt inflammation by inducing stem cell differentiation, resistance to NK cell cytotoxicity and prevention of cytokine and chemokine secretion. Oncotarget. 2015;**6**:8947-8959

[93] Martinez VG, Ontoria-Oviedo I, Ricardo CP, Harding SE, Sacedon R, Varas A, et al. Overexpression of hypoxia-inducible factor 1 alpha improves immunomodulation by dental mesenchymal stem cells. Stem Cell Research & Therapy. 2017;**8**:208

[94] Hardy RR, Hayakawa K. B cell development pathways. Annual Review of Immunology. 2001;**19**:595-621

[95] Jacob J, Kelsoe G, Rajewsky K, Weiss U. Intraclonal generation of antibody mutants in germinal centres. Nature. 1991;**354**:389-392

[96] Lund FE. Cytokine-producing B lymphocytes-key regulators of immunity. Current Opinion in Immunology. 2008;**20**:332-338

[97] Bonilla FA, Oettgen HC. Adaptive immunity. The Journal of Allergy and Clinical Immunology. 2010;**125**:S33-S40

[98] Vazquez MI, Catalan-Dibene J, Zlotnik A. B cells responses and cytokine production are regulated by their immune microenvironment. Cytokine. 2015;**74**:318-326

[99] Berglundh T, Donati M. Aspects of adaptive host response in periodontitis. Journal of Clinical Periodontology. 2005;**32**(Suppl 6):87-107

[100] Demoersman J, Pochard P, Framery C, Simon Q, Boisrame S, Soueidan A, et al. B cell subset distribution is altered in patients with severe periodontitis. PLoS One. 2018;**13**:e0192986

[101] Ebersole JL. Humoral immune responses in gingival crevice fluid: Local and systemic implications. Periodontology 2000. 2003;**31**:135-166

[102] Kawai T, Matsuyama T, Hosokawa Y, Makihira S, Seki M, Karimbux NY, et al. B and T lymphocytes are the primary sources of RANKL in the bone resorptive lesion of periodontal disease. The American Journal of Pathology. 2006;**169**:987-998

[103] Baker PJ, Boutaugh NR, Tiffany M, Roopenian DC. B cell IgD deletion prevents alveolar bone loss following murine oral infection. Interdisciplinary Perspectives on Infectious Diseases. 2009;**2009**:864359

[104] Corcione A, Benvenuto F, Ferretti E, Giunti D, Cappiello V, Cazzanti F, et al. Human mesenchymal stem cells modulate B cell functions. Blood. 2006;**107**:367-372

[105] Traggiai E, Volpi S, Schena F, Gattorno M, Ferlito F, Moretta L, et al. Bone marrow-derived mesenchymal stem cells induce both polyclonal expansion and differentiation of B cells isolated from healthy donors and systemic lupus erythematosus patients. Stem Cells. 2008;**26**:562-569

[106] Rasmusson I, Le Blanc K, Sundberg B, Ringden O. Mesenchymal stem cells stimulate antibody secretion in human B cells. Scandinavian Journal of Immunology. 2007;**65**:336-343

[107] Comoli P, Ginevri F, Maccario R, Avanzini MA, Marconi M, Groff A, et al. Human mesenchymal stem cells inhibit antibody production induced in vitro by allostimulation. Nephrology, Dialysis, Transplantation: Official Publication of the European Dialysis and Transplant Association—European Renal Association. 2008;**23**:1196-1202

[108] Schena F, Gambini C, Gregorio A, Mosconi M, Reverberi D, Gattorno M, et al. Interferon-gamma-dependent inhibition of B cell activation by bone marrow-derived mesenchymal stem cells in a murine model of systemic lupus erythematosus. Arthritis and Rheumatism. 2010;**62**:2776-2786

[109] Luk F, Carreras-Planella L, Korevaar SS, de Witte SFH, Borras FE, Betjes MGH, et al. Inflammatory conditions dictate the effect of mesenchymal stem or stromal cells on B cell function. Frontiers in Immunology. 2017;**8**:1042

[110] Augello A, Tasso R, Negrini SM, Amateis A, Indiveri F, Cancedda R, et al. Bone marrow mesenchymal progenitor cells inhibit lymphocyte proliferation by activation of the programmed death 1 pathway. European Journal of Immunology. 2005;**35**:1482-1490

[111] Liu O, Xu J, Ding G, Liu D, Fan Z, Zhang C, et al. Periodontal ligament stem cells regulate B lymphocyte function via programmed cell death protein 1. Stem Cells. 2013;**31**:1371-1382

[112] Gordon S, Taylor PR. Monocyte and macrophage heterogeneity. Nature Reviews. 2005;**5**:953-964

[113] Shi C, Pamer EG. Monocyte recruitment during infection and inflammation. Nature Reviews. 2011;**11**:762-774

[114] Parihar A, Eubank TD, Doseff AI. Monocytes and macrophages regulate immunity through dynamic networks of survival and cell death. Journal of Innate Immunity. 2010;**2**:204-215

[115] Ogle ME, Segar CE, Sridhar S, Botchwey EA. Monocytes and macrophages in tissue repair: Implications for immunoregenerative biomaterial design. Experimental Biology and Medicine. 2016;**241**:1084-1097

[116] Martinez FO, Gordon S. The M1 and M2 paradigm of macrophage activation: Time for reassessment. F1000prime Reports. 2014;**6**:13

[117] Sima C, Glogauer M. Macrophage subsets and osteoimmunology: Tuning of the immunological recognition and effector systems that maintain alveolar bone. Periodontology 2000. 2013;**63**:80-101

[118] Allam JP, Duan Y, Heinemann F, Winter J, Gotz W, Deschner J, et al. IL-23-producing CD68(+) macrophage-like cells predominate within an IL-17-polarized infiltrate in chronic periodontitis lesions. Journal of Clinical Periodontology. 2011;**38**:879-886

[119] Yu T, Zhao L, Huang X, Ma C, Wang Y, Zhang J, et al. Enhanced activity of the macrophage M1/M2 phenotypes and phenotypic switch to M1 in periodontal infection. Journal of Periodontology. 2016;**87**:1092-1102

[120] Yang J, Zhu Y, Duan D, Wang P, Xin Y, Bai L, et al. Enhanced activity of macrophage M1/M2 phenotypes in periodontitis. Archives of Oral Biology. 2017. DOI: 0.1016/j.archoralbio.2017.03.006

[121] Kim J, Hematti P. Mesenchymal stem cell-educated macrophages: A novel type of alternatively activated macrophages. Experimental Hematology. 2009;**37**:1445-1453

[122] Nemeth K, Leelahavanichkul A, Yuen PS, Mayer B, Parmelee A, Doi K, et al. Bone marrow stromal cells attenuate sepsis via prostaglandin E(2)-dependent reprogramming of host macrophages to increase their interleukin-10 production. Nature Medicine. 2009;**15**:42-49

[123] Francois M, Romieu-Mourez R, Li M, Galipeau J. Human MSC suppression correlates with cytokine induction of indoleamine 2,3-dioxygenase and bystander M2 macrophage differentiation. Molecular Therapy: The Journal of the American Society of Gene Therapy. 2012;**20**:187-195

[124] Takizawa N, Okubo N, Kamo M, Chosa N, Mikami T, Suzuki K, et al. Bone marrow-derived mesenchymal stem cells propagate immunosuppressive/anti-inflammatory

macrophages in cell-to-cell contact-independent and -dependent manners under hypoxic culture. Experimental Cell Research. 2017;**358**:411-420

[125] Dayan V, Yannarelli G, Billia F, Filomeno P, Wang XH, Davies JE, et al. Mesenchymal stromal cells mediate a switch to alternatively activated monocytes/macrophages after acute myocardial infarction. Basic Research in Cardiology. 2011;**106**:1299-1310

[126] Eggenhofer E, Hoogduijn MJ. Mesenchymal stem cell-educated macrophages. Trans plantation Research. 2012;**1**:12

[127] Zhang QZ, Su WR, Shi SH, Wilder-Smith P, Xiang AP, Wong A, et al. Human gingiva-derived mesenchymal stem cells elicit polarization of m2 macrophages and enhance cutaneous wound healing. Stem Cells. 2010;**28**:1856-1868

[128] Lee S, Zhang QZ, Karabucak B, Le AD. DPSCs from inflamed pulp modulate macrophage function via the TNF-alpha/IDO Axis. Journal of Dental Research. 2016;**95**:1274-1281

[129] Omi M, Hata M, Nakamura N, Miyabe M, Kobayashi Y, Kamiya H, et al. Transplantation of dental pulp stem cells suppressed inflammation in sciatic nerves by promoting macrophage polarization towards anti-inflammation phenotypes and ameliorated diabetic polyneuropathy. Journal of Diabetes Investigation. 2016;**7**:485-496

[130] Nagata M, Iwasaki K, Akazawa K, Komaki M, Yokoyama N, Izumi Y, et al. Conditioned medium from periodontal ligament stem cells enhances periodontal regeneration. Tissue Engineering. Part A. 2017;**23**:367-377

[131] De Berdt P, Bottemanne P, Bianco J, Alhouayek M, Diogenes A, Llyod A, et al. Stem cells from human apical papilla decrease neuro-inflammation and stimulate oligodendrocyte progenitor differentiation via activin-A secretion. Cellular and Molecular Life Sciences. 2018

[132] Sadik CD, Kim ND, Luster AD. Neutrophils cascading their way to inflammation. Trends in Immunology. 2011;**32**:452-460

[133] Choi EY, Santoso S, Chavakis T. Mechanisms of neutrophil transendothelial migration. Frontiers in Bioscience. 2009;**14**:1596-1605

[134] Tak T, Tesselaar K, Pillay J, Borghans JA, Koenderman L. What's your age again? Determination of human neutrophil half-lives revisited. Journal of Leukocyte Biology. 2013;**94**:595-601

[135] Kennedy AD, DeLeo FR. Neutrophil apoptosis and the resolution of infection. Immunologic Research. 2009;**43**:25-61

[136] Borregaard N. Neutrophils, from marrow to microbes. Immunity. 2010;**33**:657-670

[137] Brinkmann V, Reichard U, Goosmann C, Fauler B, Uhlemann Y, Weiss DS, et al. Neutrophil extracellular traps kill bacteria. Science (New York, NY). 2004;**303**:1532-1535

[138] Selders GS, Fetz AE, Radic MZ, Bowlin GL. An overview of the role of neutrophils in innate immunity, inflammation and host-biomaterial integration. Regenerative Biomaterials. 2017;**4**:55-68

[139] Hajishengallis G, Chavakis T, Hajishengallis E, Lambris JD. Neutrophil homeostasis and inflammation: Novel paradigms from studying periodontitis. Journal of Leukocyte Biology. 2015;**98**:539-548

[140] Delima AJ, Van Dyke TE. Origin and function of the cellular components in gingival crevice fluid. Periodontology 2000. 2003;**31**:55-76

[141] Ryder MI. Comparison of neutrophil functions in aggressive and chronic periodontitis. Periodontology 2000. 2010;**53**:124-137

[142] Hajishengallis G. Periodontitis: From microbial immune subversion to systemic inflammation. Nature Reviews. 2015;**15**:30-44

[143] Hajishengallis E, Hajishengallis G. Neutrophil homeostasis and periodontal health in children and adults. Journal of Dental Research. 2014;**93**:231-237

[144] Cassatella MA, Mosna F, Micheletti A, Lisi V, Tamassia N, Cont C, et al. Toll-like receptor-3-activated human mesenchymal stromal cells significantly prolong the survival and function of neutrophils. Stem Cells. 2011;**29**:1001-1011

[145] Raffaghello L, Bianchi G, Bertolotto M, Montecucco F, Busca A, Dallegri F, et al. Human mesenchymal stem cells inhibit neutrophil apoptosis: A model for neutrophil preservation in the bone marrow niche. Stem Cells. 2008;**26**:151-162

[146] Brandau S, Jakob M, Bruderek K, Bootz F, Giebel B, Radtke S, et al. Mesenchymal stem cells augment the anti-bacterial activity of neutrophil granulocytes. PLoS One. 2014;**9**:e106903

[147] Magana-Guerrero FS, Dominguez-Lopez A, Martinez-Aboytes P, Buentello-Volante B, Garfias Y. Human amniotic membrane mesenchymal stem cells inhibit neutrophil extracellular traps through TSG-6. Scientific Reports. 2017;**7**:12426

[148] Munir H, Luu NT, Clarke LS, Nash GB, McGettrick HM. Comparative ability of mesenchymal stromal cells from different tissues to limit neutrophil recruitment to inflamed endothelium. PLoS One. 2016;**11**:e0155161

[149] Cianci E, Recchiuti A, Trubiani O, Diomede F, Marchisio M, Miscia S, et al. Human periodontal stem cells release specialized proresolving mediators and carry immunomodulatory and prohealing properties regulated by lipoxins. Stem Cells Translational Medicine. 2016;**5**:20-32

[150] Wang Q, Ding G, Xu X. Periodontal ligament stem cells regulate apoptosis of neutrophils. Open Medicine. 2017;**12**:19-23

[151] Hieke C, Kriebel K, Engelmann R, Muller-Hilke B, Lang H, Kreikemeyer B. Human dental stem cells suppress PMN activity after infection with the periodontopathogens *Prevotella intermedia* and *Tannerella forsythia*. Scientific Reports. 2016;**6**:39096

[152] Walsh LJ. Mast cells and oral inflammation. Critical Reviews in Oral Biology and Medicine. 2003;**14**:188-198

[153] Theoharides TC, Cochrane DE. Critical role of mast cells in inflammatory diseases and the effect of acute stress. Journal of Neuroimmunology. 2004;**146**:1-12

[154] Woolley DE. The mast cell in inflammatory arthritis. The New England Journal of Medicine. 2003;**348**:1709-1711

[155] Steinsvoll S, Helgeland K, Schenck K. Mast cells—A role in periodontal diseases? Journal of Clinical Periodontology. 2004;**31**:413-419

[156] Artuc M, Steckelings UM, Henz BM. Mast cell-fibroblast interactions: Human mast cells as source and inducers of fibroblast and epithelial growth factors. The Journal of Investigative Dermatology. 2002;**118**:391-395

[157] Gaje PN, Amalia Ceausu R, Jitariu A, Stratul SI, Rusu LC, Popovici RA, et al. Mast cells: Key players in the shadow in oral inflammation and in squamous cell carcinoma of the oral cavity. BioMed Research International. 2016;**2016**:9235080

[158] Agrawal R, Gupta J, Gupta KK, Kumar V. Correlation of mast cells in different stages of human periodontal diseases: Pilot study. Journal of Oral and Maxillofacial Pathology: JOMFP. 2016;**20**:91-95

[159] Lagdive SS, Lagdive SB, Mani A, Anarthe R, Pendyala G, Pawar B, et al. Correlation of mast cells in periodontal diseases. Journal of Indian Society of Periodontology. 2013;**17**:63-67

[160] Natah SS, Hayrinen-Immonen R, Hietanen J, Malmstrom M, Konttinen YT. Quantitative assessment of mast cells in recurrent aphthous ulcers (RAU). Journal of Oral Pathology & Medicine. 1998;**27**:124-129

[161] Huang S, Lu F, Chen Y, Huang B, Liu M. Mast cell degranulation in human periodontitis. Journal of Periodontology. 2013;**84**:248-255

[162] Liu J, Kuwabara A, Kamio Y, Hu S, Park J, Hashimoto T, et al. Human mesenchymal stem cell-derived microvesicles prevent the rupture of intracranial aneurysm in part by suppression of mast cell activation via a PGE2-dependent mechanism. Stem Cells. 2016;**34**:2943-2955

[163] Brown JM, Nemeth K, Kushnir-Sukhov NM, Metcalfe DD, Mezey E. Bone marrow stromal cells inhibit mast cell function via a COX2-dependent mechanism. Clinical and Experimental Allergy: Journal of the British Society for Allergy and Clinical Immunology. 2011;**41**:526-534

[164] Kim HS, Yun JW, Shin TH, Lee SH, Lee BC, Yu KR, et al. Human umbilical cord blood mesenchymal stem cell-derived PGE2 and TGF-beta1 alleviate atopic dermatitis by reducing mast cell degranulation. Stem Cells. 2015;**33**:1254-1266

[165] Kohl J. Self, non-self, and danger: A complementary view. Advances in Experimental Medicine and Biology. 2006;**586**:71-94

[166] Merle NS, Church SE, Fremeaux-Bacchi V, Roumenina LT. Complement system part I—Molecular mechanisms of activation and regulation. Frontiers in Immunology. 2015;**6**:262

[167] Damgaard C, Holmstrup P, Van Dyke TE, Nielsen CH. The complement system and its role in the pathogenesis of periodontitis: Current concepts. Journal of Periodontal Research. 2015;**50**:283-293

[168] Hajishengallis G, Maekawa T, Abe T, Hajishengallis E, Lambris JD. Complement involvement in periodontitis: Molecular mechanisms and rational therapeutic approaches. Advances in Experimental Medicine and Biology. 2015;**865**:57-74

[169] Hajishengallis G, Abe T, Maekawa T, Hajishengallis E, Lambris JD. Role of complement in host-microbe homeostasis of the periodontium. Seminars in Immunology. 2013;**25**:65-72

[170] Wang M, Krauss JL, Domon H, Hosur KB, Liang S, Magotti P, et al. Microbial hijacking of complement-toll-like receptor crosstalk. Science Signaling. 2010;**3**:ra11

[171] Li Y, Lin F. Mesenchymal stem cells are injured by complement after their contact with serum. Blood. 2012;**120**:3436-3443

[172] Tu Z, Li Q, Bu H, Lin F. Mesenchymal stem cells inhibit complement activation by secreting factor H. Stem Cells and Development. 2010;**19**:1803-1809

[173] Lee DS, Yi TG, Lee HJ, Kim SN, Park S, Jeon MS, et al. Mesenchymal stem cells infected with *Mycoplasma arginini* secrete complement C3 to regulate immunoglobulin production in B lymphocytes. Cell Death & Disease. 2014;**5**:e1192

[174] Chmilewsky F, Jeanneau C, Laurent P, About I. Pulp fibroblasts synthesize functional complement proteins involved in initiating dentin-pulp regeneration. The American Journal of Pathology. 2014;**184**:1991-2000

[175] Rufas P, Jeanneau C, Rombouts C, Laurent P, About I. Complement C3a mobilizes dental pulp stem cells and specifically guides pulp fibroblast recruitment. Journal of Endodontics. 2016;**42**:1377-1384

[176] Krampera M. Mesenchymal stromal cell 'licensing': A multistep process. Leukemia. 2011;**25**:1408-1414

[177] Bernardo ME, Fibbe WE. Mesenchymal stromal cells: Sensors and switchers of inflammation. Cell Stem Cell. 2013;**13**:392-402

[178] Wada N, Menicanin D, Shi S, Bartold PM, Gronthos S. Immunomodulatory properties of human periodontal ligament stem cells. Journal of Cellular Physiology. 2009;**219**:667-676

[179] Rashedi I, Gomez-Aristizabal A, Wang XH, Viswanathan S, Keating A. TLR3 or TLR4 activation enhances mesenchymal stromal cell-mediated Treg induction via notch Signaling. Stem Cells. 2017;**35**:265-275

[180] Liotta F, Angeli R, Cosmi L, Fili L, Manuelli C, Frosali F, et al. Toll-like receptors 3 and 4 are expressed by human bone marrow-derived mesenchymal stem cells and can inhibit their T cell modulatory activity by impairing Notch signaling. Stem Cells. 2008;**26**:279-289

[181] Tomic S, Djokic J, Vasilijic S, Vucevic D, Todorovic V, Supic G, et al. Immunomodulatory properties of mesenchymal stem cells derived from dental pulp and dental follicle are susceptible to activation by toll-like receptor agonists. Stem Cells and Development. 2011;**20**:695-708

[182] Bindal P, Ramasamy TS, Kasim NHA, Gnanasegaran N, Lin CW. Immune responses of human dental pulp stem cells in lipopolysaccharide induced microenvironment. Cell Biology International. 2018. DOI: 10.1002/cbin.10938

[183] Chang J, Zhang C, Tani-Ishii N, Shi S, Wang CY. NF-kappaB activation in human dental pulp stem cells by TNF and LPS. Journal of Dental Research. 2005;**84**:994-998

[184] Kukolj T, Trivanovic D, Djordjevic IO, Mojsilovic S, Krstic J, Obradovic H, et al. Lipopolysaccharide can modify differentiation and immunomodulatory potential of periodontal ligament stem cells via ERK1,2 signaling. Journal of Cellular Physiology. 2018;**233**:447-462

[185] Park JC, Kim JM, Jung IH, Kim JC, Choi SH, Cho KS, et al. Isolation and characterization of human periodontal ligament (PDL) stem cells (PDLSCs) from the inflamed PDL tissue: In vitro and in vivo evaluations. Journal of Clinical Periodontology. 2011;**38**:721-731

[186] Sonoda S, Yamaza H, Ma L, Tanaka Y, Tomoda E, Aijima R, et al. Interferon-gamma improves impaired dentinogenic and immunosuppressive functions of irreversible pulpitis-derived human dental pulp stem cells. Scientific Reports. 2016;**6**:19286

[187] Eggenhofer E, Luk F, Dahlke MH, Hoogduijn MJ. The life and fate of mesenchymal stem cells. Frontiers in Immunology. 2014;**5**:148

[188] Liu Y, Wang L, Kikuiri T, Akiyama K, Chen C, Xu X, et al. Mesenchymal stem cell-based tissue regeneration is governed by recipient T lymphocytes via IFN-gamma and TNF-alpha. Nature Medicine. 2011;**17**:1594-1601

[189] Sui BD, Hu CH, Liu AQ, Zheng CX, Xuan K, Jin Y. Stem cell-based bone regeneration in diseased microenvironments: Challenges and solutions. Biomaterials. 2017. DOI: 10.1016/j.biomaterials.2017.10.046

[190] Wang Y, Chen X, Cao W, Shi Y. Plasticity of mesenchymal stem cells in immunomodulation: Pathological and therapeutic implications. Nature Immunology. 2014;**15**:1009-1016

[191] Vizoso FJ, Eiro N, Cid S, Schneider J, Perez-Fernandez R. Mesenchymal stem cell secretome: Toward cell-free therapeutic strategies in regenerative medicine. International Journal of Molecular Sciences. 2017;**18**(9):1852

[192] Bruno S, Deregibus MC, Camussi G. The secretome of mesenchymal stromal cells: Role of extracellular vesicles in immunomodulation. Immunology Letters. 2015;**168**:154-158

[193] Julier Z, Park AJ, Briquez PS, Martino MM. Promoting tissue regeneration by modulating the immune system. Acta Biomaterialia. 2017;**53**:13-28

[194] Croitoru-Lamoury J, Lamoury FM, Caristo M, Suzuki K, Walker D, Takikawa O, et al. Interferon-gamma regulates the proliferation and differentiation of mesenchymal stem cells via activation of indoleamine 2,3 dioxygenase (IDO). PLoS One. 2011;**6**:e14698

[195] Lee RH, Yu JM, Foskett AM, Peltier G, Reneau JC, Bazhanov N, et al. TSG-6 as a biomarker to predict efficacy of human mesenchymal stem/progenitor cells (hMSCs) in modulating sterile inflammation in vivo. Proceedings of the National Academy of Sciences of the United States of America 2014;**111**:16766-71

[196] Qi Y, Jiang D, Sindrilaru A, Stegemann A, Schatz S, Treiber N, et al. TSG-6 released from intradermally injected mesenchymal stem cells accelerates wound healing and reduces tissue fibrosis in murine full-thickness skin wounds. The Journal of Investigative Dermatology. 2014;**134**:526-537

[197] Ng F, Boucher S, Koh S, Sastry KS, Chase L, Lakshmipathy U, et al. PDGF, TGF-beta, and FGF signaling is important for differentiation and growth of mesenchymal stem cells (MSCs): Transcriptional profiling can identify markers and signaling pathways important in differentiation of MSCs into adipogenic, chondrogenic, and osteogenic lineages. Blood. 2008;**112**:295-307

[198] Wada N, Tomokiyo A, Gronthos S, Bartold PM. Immunomodulatory properties of PDLSC and relevance to periodontal regeneration. Current Oral Health Reports. 2015;**2**:245-251

[199] Li C, Wang X, Tan J, Wang T, Wang Q. The immunomodulatory properties of periodontal ligament stem cells isolated from inflamed periodontal granulation. Cells, Tissues, Organs. 2014;**199**:256-265

[200] Liu Y, Wang L, Liu S, Liu D, Chen C, Xu X, et al. Transplantation of SHED prevents bone loss in the early phase of ovariectomy-induced osteoporosis. Journal of Dental Research. 2014;**93**:1124-1132

[201] Du J, Shan Z, Ma P, Wang S, Fan Z. Allogeneic bone marrow mesenchymal stem cell transplantation for periodontal regeneration. Journal of Dental Research. 2014;**93**:183-188

[202] Zhang J, Li ZG, Si YM, Chen B, Meng J. The difference on the osteogenic differentiation between periodontal ligament stem cells and bone marrow mesenchymal stem cells under inflammatory microenviroments. Differentiation; Research in Biological Diversity. 2014;**88**:97-105

6

Periodontal Diseases in Patients with Special Health Care Needs

Mônica Fernandes Gomes,
Andrea Carvalho De Marco,
Lilian Chrystiane Giannasi and
Miguel Angel Castillo Salgado

Abstract

A wide variation of people with an impairment or disability requires a "special care dentistry" once their general manifestations directly act in the oral cavity. This target public is inserted into the following categories: neuromotor disability, sensory disability, mental disorder, infecto-contagious diseases, chronic systemic diseases, and systemic conditions. Among the several oral illnesses found in these groups, periodontal diseases have been the most frequent, becoming a major challenge for the dental practitioners. Thus, we described the microbiological, histopathological, and clinical features of periodontal diseases in each "special health care needs" group. Advances in "Omic" technologies have suggested the application of molecular biology methods to assess the genomics (genes), proteomics (proteins), transcriptomics (mRNA), and metabolomics (metabolites) aspects of periodontal diseases. These researches aim to promote a better understanding of the mechanisms involved in the pathogenesis and in the identification of new bio markers of periodontal diseases that help in diagnosis of periodontal diseases and in tissue responses after treatments of gingivitis and periodontitis. As an alternative therapy, some bioactive materials and photobiomodulation may be indicated once they strongly stimulate the periodontal tissue regeneration, attenuate the inflammatory processes, and/or promote the reconstruction of the microstructure of the periodontium.

Keywords: periodontal diseases, special health care needs, "Omic" technologies, bioactive materials, photobiomodulation

1. Introduction

The World Health Organization (WHO) estimates that there are more than one billion people in the world living with some form of impairment or disability, of whom nearly 200 million have considerable difficulties in functioning [1]. There is a growing proportion of *people* with disabili ties worldwide, and these are vulnerable groups in both developed and developing countries.

Currently, the National Organization on Disability (NOD), a private and nonprofit organization, estimates that 54 million children and adults in the United States have one or more disabilities, with 35 million Americans being severely disabled [2–4]. The proportion of children with disabilities is estimated to be 12.5 million or around 18% [3–5]. According to the estimated data by National Health and National Health and Nutrition Examination Survey (NHANES), 46% of adults in the United States have periodontitis, and 8.9% have severe periodontitis [6].

The geopolitical and social plurality of states and regions in Brazil have shown the emerging need for effective public policies to meet the specific needs of this diversity. According to the *Brazilian Institute of Geography and Statistics*, 45.6 million Brazilian citizens (equivalent to 23.9% of the population) have some type of neuropsychomotor impairment as physical, sensory—visual and auditory—and intellectual disabilities. Among these, 17.7 million people (6.7% of the population) have severe disability. The majority of this target public is found in urban areas and is aged between 15 and 64 years; further, the northeastern areas have a higher number of cities with at least one person with disability [7]. Hence, oral health care needs should be emphasized mainly for this target public due to high susceptibility to infection risks and great vulnerability to develop illnesses. Mental disorders associated or not with disabilities must also be considered in these individuals. In this condition, the familiar influence shall be taken into account for these groups once their human development directly depends on the good relationship among them.

Regarding children with developmental disorders, especially the autism spectrum disorder (ASD), attention-deficit/hyperactivity disorder (AD/HD), or specific learning disorder (LD), the field of "special care dentistry" is rapidly gaining recognition as a necessary service once they require oral health care needs at all times [8]. According to American Psychiatric Association (APA) [9], these disorders have relatively been growing due to the increase in birth rates and life expectancy of these individuals. Another relevant factor would be the ability or difficulty to perform their self-care, in particular, in the mouth, resulting in a negative impact of precarious oral conditions. The main oral signs and symptoms found in this target public include poor oral hygiene, dental caries, and severity of periodontal diseases (PD). High incidence of dental hypoplasia, traumatic lesion (factitious, iatrogenic, and accidental), drug-induced gingival overgrowth, dental malocclusion, and tooth missing are also evidenced [8, 10]. It is important to highlight that the large dental loss of intact teeth is caused by the destruction of the collagen fibers of the periodontal ligament (PDL) and severe resorption of alveolar bone tissue from the persistent supra and subgingival and periopathogenic microbiota, recognized as periodontal disease [11]. Therefore, this disease is one of the most common oral chronic infections in people with special health care needs (SHCN), becoming an important dental public health problem.

Based on combined data from the literature and our scientific experiences, we discussed the microbiological, histopathological, and clinical features of PD in each "special care needs" group. Furthermore, we reported some advances in "Omic" technologies which are molecular biology methods used to assess the genomics (genes), proteomics (proteins), transcriptomics (mRNA), and metabolomics (metabolites) aspects of PD. These methods promote a better *understanding* of the mechanisms involved in the *etiopathogenesis* and in the identification of new biomarkers of PD that help in the diagnosis of PD and in tissue responses after treatments of gingivitis and periodontitis. In addition, alternative therapies to PD in patients with SHCN were recommended in order to aggregate new scientific knowledge, some of them being investigated at the Center of Biosciences Applied to Persons with Special Care Needs (CEBAPE) of the Institute of Science and Technology of the São Paulo State University (UNESP).

2. Special Health Care Needs (SHCN) in dentistry

The field of "special care dentistry" is rapidly gaining recognition as a service that should be provided to persons with physical, mental, or intellectual disabilities by general physicians, pediatric physicians, geriatric physicians, dental practitioners, and dental hygienists. Considering the limited opening of the oral cavity and the great difficulty of clinical procedure handling, the special needs patients may be treated under applying of psychological, physical, or pharmacological techniques in order to control their behavior and the voluntary or involuntary body movements. These patients may be affected by several comorbid physical illnesses including diabetes mellitus, cardiovascular diseases, respiratory illnesses as aspiration pneumonia, sleep disturbance as obstructive sleep apnea, malignant neoplasms, and so on.

Extrinsic and intrinsic factors may corroborate to the installation and perpetuation of PD, as well as increase the susceptibility to supra and subgingival periopathogens in these individuals, even after oral hygiene promotion and/or intensive conventional mechanical treatment, combined or not with a supportive therapy. Concerning the main extrinsic factors, previous studies have considered oral mucositis-inducing chemotherapy drugs, saliva flow-reducing medications, respiratory disturbances as mouth breathing leading to oral hyperventilation and, as a consequence, dry mouth, motor deficit, cognitive impairment, learning difficulty and disability, crowded teeth, and inappropriate diet. The intrinsic factors include immune response deficiency, a high amount of periopathogens, sleep disorders such as obstructive sleep apnea, dysfunction of the oropharyngeal muscles resulting in severe dysphagia, and the risk of occurrence for aspiration pneumonia. Previous studies confirm the presence of respiratory pathogens in the oral cavity which may be aspirated into the lung alveoli due to severe dysphagia, developing aspiration pneumonia [12, 13]. This comorbidity may negatively influence the oral health homeostasis, aggravating the preexistent inflammatory processes, in particular, the PD.

Current researches confirm that the therapy applying neuromuscular electrical stimulation on the masticatory muscles was effective in adults with cerebral palsy. This *biostimulating effect* also reflected in the electrical activity of the oropharyngeal muscles, favoring their functional performance; then, a positive effect on the apnea and hypopnea index was found. These episode cascades reduced the number of pathological respiratory events, promoting improvements in the quality of life for these patients [12–14].

Regarding the oral health status of these populations, the main oral manifestations are dental caries, dental hypoplasia, dental agenesis, orofacial traumas, drug-induced gingival overgrowth, and, in particular, PD [8]. Recent studies have shown that the presence of periodontopathic microbiota at the oral biofilm and/or spread throughout the saliva may explain the higher susceptibility to PD in this target public [15, 16].

According to the Joint Advisory Committee for Special Care Dentistry (JACSD), "special care dentistry" provides oral services for people with an impairment or disability including physical, sensory, intellectual, mental, medical, social, or a combination of one or more of these [17]. Several conditions, disorders, and/or disabilities lead these patients to the need of specialized oral assistance. In Brazil, the Federal Council of Dentistry has recognized the specialty of Dentistry for Patients with Special Health Care Needs as a dental service which has been assisting people with simple or complex disabilities, of acute or chronic nature, and temporary or permanent conditions or disorders. This target public is inserted into the following categories: neuromotor disability (1), sensory disability (2), mental disorder (3), infecto-contagious diseases (4), chronic systemic diseases (5), and systemic conditions (6).

The neuromotor disorders (1) include people with physical and intellectual disabilities which are from an unknown, environmental, and a genetic origin. These disorders consist of cerebral palsy, cerebrovascular disturbances (e.g., ischemic and hemorrhagic cerebral strokes), spinal cord injury, myelomeningocele, infectious disease (e.g., poliomyelitis or infantile paralysis), autoimmune diseases (e.g., myasthenia gravis and multiple sclerosis), muscular dystrophy resulting in muscle weakness and cellular degeneration, metabolic bone diseases (e.g., rachitis or osteomalacia caused by genetic, nutritional and/or hormonal abnormalities affecting bone growth and remodeling), and bone genetic disorder (e.g., dysostosis, osteopetrosis and imperfect osteogenesis). The congenital and acquired abnormalities, resulting in craniomaxillofacial deformities, complex malformations, and syndromes are also included in the neuromotor disorders. It is important to emphasize that the intellectual disabilities may be associated with these conditions.

The sensory disorders (2) include the hearing and visual disabilities, generating immediate harmful effects as depression, isolation, dementia, and decrease of quality of life [18]. The severity of these impairments may result in the disruption of interpersonal relations and decrease of self-sufficiency in daily living activities, both of which are critical to the well-being of a person [19]. Hearing disability, with its resultant difficulties in communication function, pervades multiple domains of function in the individuals, decreasing activity, increasing depressive symptoms, and confounding assessment of cognitive ability. Although it is not curable, this impairment is often remediable with appropriate audiologic evaluation and the prescription of amplification devices. Visual disability also affects multiple domains of function, limiting the individuals' ability and increasing the risk of falls, fractures, and morbidity. In order to attenuate the consequences of visual disability, the cause must be identified to obtain an effective treatment [20].

Conforming to the fifth edition of the Diagnostic and Statistical Manual of Mental Disorders (DSM-5) published by the American Psychiatric Association (APA) under coordination of the Division of Mental Health of the World Health Organization (WHO) and the National

Institute of Mental Health (NIMH), a mental disorder (3) is a syndrome characterized by clinically significant disturbances in an individual's cognition, emotion regulation, or behavior which reflects a dysfunction in psychological, biological, or developmental processes underlying mental functioning [9]. Thus, mental disorders are usually associated with significant distress or disability in social, occupational, or other important activities. An expectable or culturally approved response to a common stressor or loss (e.g., the death of a loved one) is not considered a mental disorder [9]. For a better elucidation, the new North American classification of mental disorders is briefly mentioned in **Figure 1**.

Among the different groups of psychopathologies, it is worth mentioning the neurodevelopmental disorders which include intellectual disabilities (mild, moderate, and severe levels), autism spectrum disorder (ASD), attention deficit and hyperactivity disorder (ADHD), communication disorders (speech and language impairments), specific learning disorder, motor disorders (e.g., stereotyped movement disorder and tic disorders), and so on [9]. Children with neurodevelopmental disorders may experience difficulties with language and speech, motor skills, behavior, memory, learning, or other neurological functions [14]. While the symptoms and behaviors of neurodevelopmental disabilities often change or evolve as a child grows older, some disabilities are permanent. Diagnosis and treatment of these disorders may be difficult, frequently involving a combination of professional therapy, pharmaceuticals, and home- and school-based programs.

Considering the most common mental disorders including dementia, depression, generalized anxiety disorder, panic disorder, obsessive–compulsive disorder, posttraumatic stress, and phobias, the psychiatric patients have presented high susceptibility to PD. These illnesses have been caused by a set of processes such as the presence of oral microbial biofilm due to poor oral hygiene, psychotropic medication-induced dry mouth, and gingival hyperplasia [15, 21]. Mental health clinicians should also be aware of the oral consequences of prescribed medications, especially the antipsychotic drugs [15]. About this, the depression may dysregulate regulatory mechanisms within the brain involved in immune regulation, alter the immune system responses, and thereby influence the development and progression of infections and inflammatory diseases, including periodontitis [22]. As a support therapy, antidepressant drugs, such as fluoxetine, tianeptine (selective serotonin reuptake inhibitor), and venlafaxine (serotonin-norepinephrine reuptake inhibitor) are used; however, the side effects could affect the periodontal tissue health [23]. Current studies using animal models showed that the fluoxetine reduced the alveolar bone loss due to suppression of inflammatory response and protection against periodontal bone resorption and collagen fibers destruction of the periodontal ligament (PDL), while the tianeptine influenced the immune system, enhancing the plasma concentrations of pro-inflammatory and T regulatory cytokines and interleukins in response to the gram-negative bacterial lipopolysaccharide (LPS) antigen. As a consequence of these processes, there is an inhibition of the periodontal disease progression [24, 25]. On the other hand, the venlafaxine influenced the increase of alveolar bone loss, most likely due to its anti-inflammatory and immunoregulatory effects on the periodontitis once it is considered an inflammatory disorder and an immunologically compromised disease [22].

Therefore, an increased focus on the physical health of psychiatric patients should encompass oral health including closer collaboration between the dental practitioners and clinicians. Possible interventions must include the following approaches: to apply the best

CATEGORIES OF MENTAL DISORDERS	
1. **Neurodevelopmental Disorders:** disabilities associated primarily with the functioning of the neurological system and brain (e.g. Autism Spectrum Disorder).	12. **Sleep-Wake Disorders:** insomnia, hypersomnia, and arousal disorder
2. **Schizophrenia Spectrum and Other Psychotic Disorders**	13. **Sexual Dysfunction**
3. **Bipolar and Other Related Disorders:** a psychological illness that causes severe changes in mood, energy, behavior and thoughts. People who suffer from this disease oscillate between periods of depression and periods of exacerbated mood and euphoria.	14. **Paraphilic Disorders** (i.e. feel personal distress about their interest, not merely distress resulting from society's disapproval; or have a sexual desire or behavior that involves another person's psychological distress, injury, or death, or a desire for sexual behaviors involving unwilling persons or persons unable to give legal consent).
4. **Depressive Disorders** (i.e. characterized by sadness severe enough or persistent enough to interfere with function and often by decreased interest or pleasure in activities).	15. **Gender Dysphoria** (i.e. very discomfort with the gender identity and, as a consequence, non-acceptance with the body which was assigned).
5. **Anxiety Disorders** (i.e. defined as "a state of intense apprehension, uncertainty, and fear resulting from the anticipation of a threatening event or situation, often to a degree that normal physical and psychological functioning is disrupted"): separation anxiety disorder, selective mutism, specific phobia, social disorder, panic disorders, agoraphobia, generalized anxiety disorder, and substance-induced anxiety disorder.	16. **Disruptive, Impulse-Control, and Conduct Disorders** (i.e. Disruptive, impulse-control, and conduct disorders (i.e. characterized by a recurrent pattern of negativistic, hostile behavior and disobedience toward the societal standards and authority figures, and violation to the rights of others by physical and verbal aggression and destruction of property).
6. **Obsessive-Compulsive and Other Related Disorders** (i.e. characterized by obsessions and compulsions that require a considerable amount of time, getting in the way of social activities and personal values; other relates disorders are body dysmorphic disorder, trichotillomania or hair-pulling disorder, hoarding disorder, and excoriation disorder or skin-picking disorder.	17. **Substance-Related and Addictive Disorders** (i.e. marked by physiological dependence to substances, including alcohol, caffeine, cannabis, hallucinogens, inhalants, opioids, sedatives, stimulants, tobacco, and other, and, as a consequence, leading to a drug-seeking behavior, tolerance, and/or withdrawal).
7. **Trauma and Stress-Related Disorders** (i.e. outcomes of exposure to potentially traumatic stressful life events): reactive attachment disorder, disinhibited social engagement disorder, posttraumatic stress disorder, acute stress disorder, and adjustment disorders.	18. **Neurocognitive Disorders:** dementia as Alzheimer's disease, vascular dementia, and others.
8. **Dissociative Disorders** (i.e. disruptions or discontinuity of consciousness, memory, identity, emotion, perception, body representation, motor control, and behavior).	19. **Personality Disorders** (i.e. an enduring pattern that deviates from the expectations of the individual's culture in two or more of the following areas: cognition; affectivity; interpersonal functioning; impulse control; the enduring pattern is inflexible and pervasive across a broad range of situations; and the enduring pattern leads to clinically significant distress or impairment).
9. **Somatic Symptoms and Other Related Disorders** (i.e. preoccupation with one or more distressing physical symptoms, resulting in disruption of daily life.)	20. **Drugs-induced movement disorders**
10. **Feeding and Eating Disorders** (e.g. anorexia nervosa and bulimia nervosa)	21. **Other Adverse Effects of Drugs**
11. **Elimination Disorders** (i.e. involuntary elimination of urine, enuresis, or defecation, encopresis, in inappropriate places or at inappropriate times by childhood or adolescence)	22. **Other Conditions that may *be a* focus of Clinical Attention** (i.e. affective problems including feelings of sadness, apathy, or anger about the other individual in the relationship).

Figure 1. Different condition groups of mental disorders described in the fifth edition of the diagnostic and statistical manual of mental disorders published by the American Psychiatric Association [9].

practices in health care focusing the transdisciplinary, to remove first the infectious foci as oral microbial biofilm and dental calculus through dental scaling and root planning for an appropriate teeth cleaning and reduction or inactivation of periodontal pockets, to guide the regular use of dental floss or interdental brushes and tooth brushing, to insert monitoring processes on oral self-care such as to create a strategic planning on interdental cleaning behaviors according to the difficulty levels of learning and the motor and cognitive dysfunction of each individual, and to perform periodic oral appraisals for necessary methodological adjustments in order to ensure the maintenance and the preservation of good oral health. Before introducing these procedures, the dental practitioner must comprehend the profile of each patient with SHCN, so as to know the physical and intellectual limitations, to identify the presence of comorbid diseases which may affect the overall health, and to assess the psychiatric behavior related to oral self-care. Surely, this systemic overview may favor the homeostasis of the stomatognathic system and improve the general health conditions, once these approaches can prevent the development of extensive and severe PD avoiding dental mobilities and/or loss.

The infecto-contagious diseases (4) is a subset category of highly dangerous transmissible diseases which include mainly infected patients with human immunodeficiency virus (HIV) infection and acquired immune deficiency syndrome (AIDS), patients with active tuberculosis disease, patients with viral hepatitis, and other such patients.

The chronic systemic diseases (5) are illnesses that spread throughout the body, affecting multiple organs and body systems, which may evolve into comorbidities, complicating the diagnosis and, consequently, influencing the prognosis. Considering this concept, the diseases imply juvenile rheumatoid arthritis, diabetes mellitus, congenital and acquired heart diseases, hematological diseases or disorders, chronic renal failure, autoimmune diseases (lichen planus, pemphigoid, pemphigus vulgar, erythema multiforme, lupus erythematosus, epidermolysis bullosa, etc.), vesiculobullous diseases, and so on.

The systemic conditions (6) are recognized as secondary factors that may modulate the disease initiation or progression rather than acting as primary etiological factors. These circumstances may affect the onset, progression, and treatment of such disease. Several patient types are included in these conditions, such as patients submitted to radiotherapy and chemotherapy in the head and neck regions, patients who received an organ transplant, patients with medication-induced immunosuppression, and similar others that may affect the general health conditions of the individual.

To better comprehend the relation among the environmental, genetic, and social effects and a person, a diagram was elaborated showing the occurrence of diseases, conditions, and/or disorders which may manifest during the life course of an individual. It is important to emphasize that these etiopathological factors may contribute to the development of one or more disabilities, leading to an acquired or congenital disability. On the other hand, an individual may be born with one or more disabilitiy and, concomitantly, develop diseases or disorders due to the high susceptibility to the environment and the different levels of disability complexity, characterizing the person with SHCN. It is noteworthy that the social impact resulting from precarious conditions of survival on the people with SHCN could explain the causes of health disparities or high occurrence of oral diseases (**Figure 2**). Socially disadvantaged groups have demonstrated poorer overall and oral health than the general population, becoming an aggravating factor, especially, in groups with SHCN. Therefore, a better attention to the public services in oral health for this population should be one of the main goals in government plans.

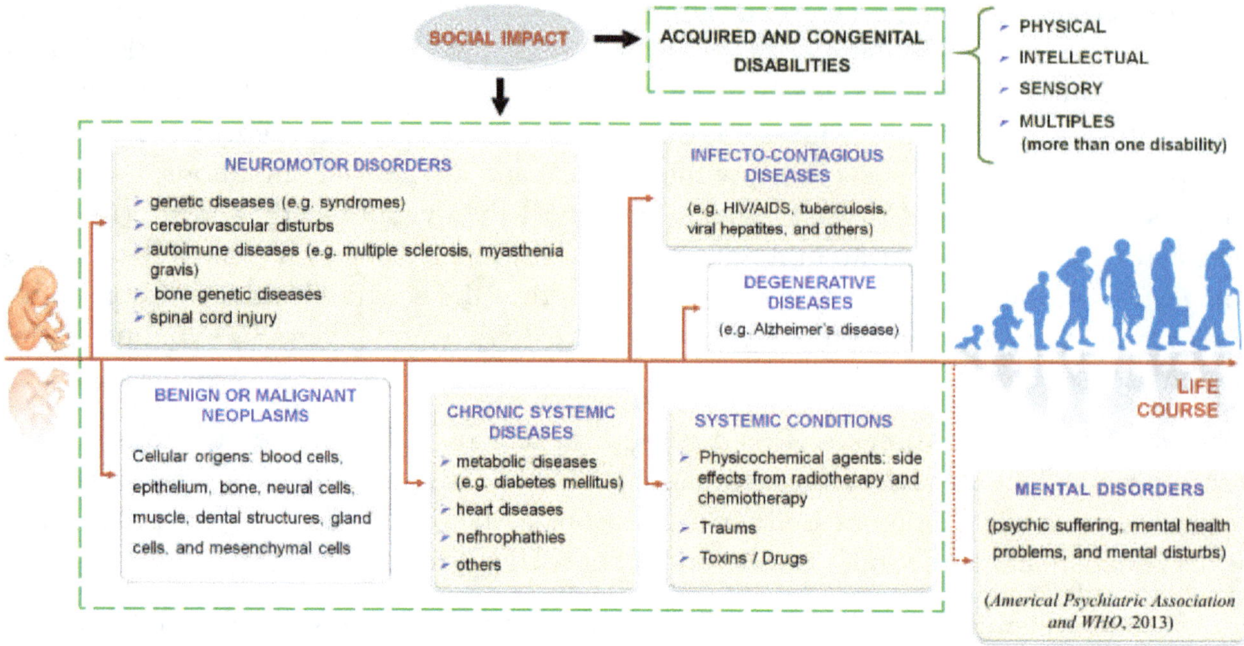

Figure 2. Diagram showing the life course of a susceptible individual to several extrinsic and intrinsic factors which may lead him/her to a disorder, disease, and/or a disability.

2.1. Types of periodontal diseases in patients with SHCN

Some case reports of patients with SHCN were briefly described in relation to their clinical, radiographic, histopathological, and laboratorial characteristics together with the oral manifestations, clinical procedures, and transdisciplinary approaches; then, we correlate them with the findings found in the literature. Furthermore, we mainly discuss the clinical management related to the PD. The additional commentaries are aimed to reinforce the importance of the early diagnosis and an appropriate dental treatment for each complexity of disability. Types of PD that were correlated with some categories of people with SHCN are depicted in the following section.

2.1.1. Case 1: chronic periodontitis associated with genetic disorder

A 14-year-old adolescent girl with Robinow syndrome had low stature, mild exophthalmos, hyperthyroidism, frequent thrombocytopenia, splenomegaly, and genital abnormality such as hypoplastic clitoris and small lips (a). Esophageal reflux was reported in the initial years of life. Using the Nicodemo et al. [26] and Grenlieh-Pyle [27] methods, dental and bone ages were 11.4 and 12, respectively. The intraoral examination showed mouth respiration, angular cheilitis, dental malocclusion, and ulcerated gingival surface (b and c) and accentuated alveolar bone loss (d), especially, at the region of mandibular incisors. Histologically, gingival tissues showed intense infiltration of mononuclear inflammatory cells diffusely spread throughout the connective tissue. Junctional epithelium hyperplasia with intense exocytosis (e) and extensive areas with no epithelium cover associated with infiltration of polymorphonuclear inflammatory cells into the lamina propria were also evidenced. In addition, presence of bacterial colonies (black arrows) and necrotic alveolar bone tissue fragments (blue arrows) was found (f and g). The diagnosis was chronic periodontitis with ulceration areas (**Image 1**).

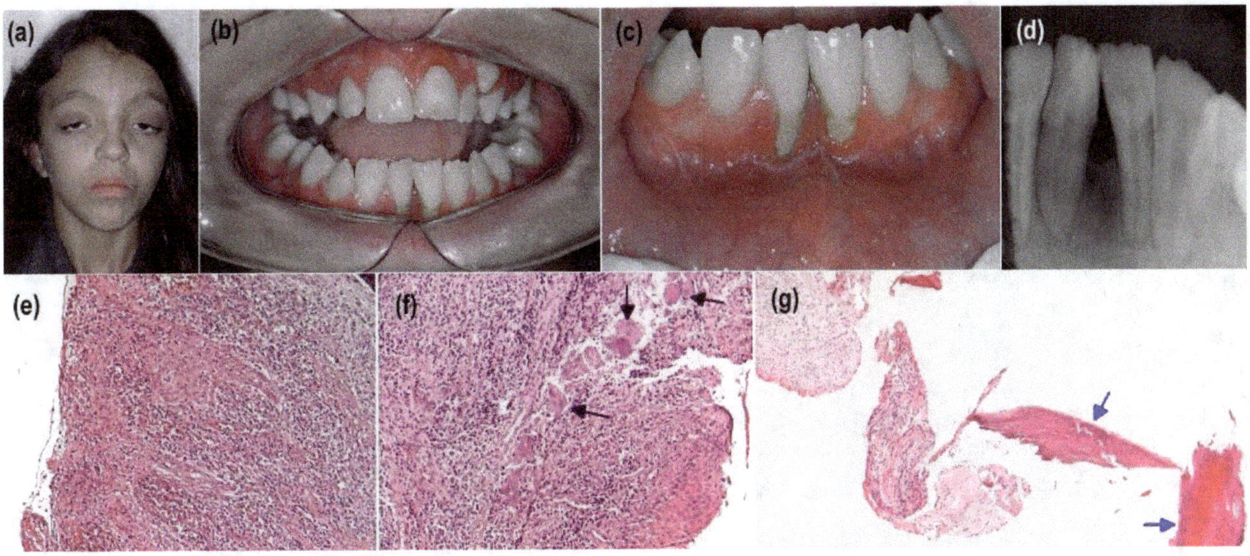

Image 1. Chronic periodontitis associated with genetic disorder (hematoxylin–eosin; original magnifications 100 and 50×).

2.1.2. Case 2: chronic gingivitis associated with genetic disorders plus uncommon abnormalities

A 19-year-old young man with Down syndrome associated with ectodermal anomalies. The extraoral features displayed dry skin and alopecia of eyelashes, eyebrows, and hair (a) while, the intraoral features showed dry mouth due to the severe reduction of saliva flow and mouth breathing, frequent angular cheilitis resulting from immune system deficiency, bilateral absence of the inner and upper third molars, presence of left upper and right lower deciduous canines, upper lateral incisors with microdontia, unerupted left upper permanent canine, generalized chronic gingivitis (a–d), and absence of caries. The recommended dental treatment was periodontal prophylaxis through the use of disclosing agents such as the scaling and root planning (e–g). It is important to point out that oral hygiene orientation and diet control must be continuously performed because of the neuromotor dysfunction of these patients, resulting in great understanding difficulties and difficulties in handling of cleaning devices and leading to a poor oral hygiene. Concerning dental education, we consider that the learning for repetition and use of ludic techniques or resources are effective strategies which must be implemented by dental practitioners. We also suggest the saliva analysis to assess their physicochemical properties, to determine the susceptibility to stress measuring the concentrations levels of salivary amylase or cortisol, and to identify the occurrence risk for aspiration pneumonia using as a biomarker the *Pseudomonas aeruginosa*. It is important to highlight that patients with Down syndrome present immune system disorders; therefore, oral infections must be avoided for general health balance and maintenance (**Image 2**).

2.1.3. Case 3: severe medications-induced gingival overgrowth

A 11-year-old female child with West syndrome had multiple epileptic spasms and, as a consequence, a severe neuropsychomotor impairment. The electroencephalography showed a hypsarrhythmia pattern confirming the diagnosis. The recommended treatment to this

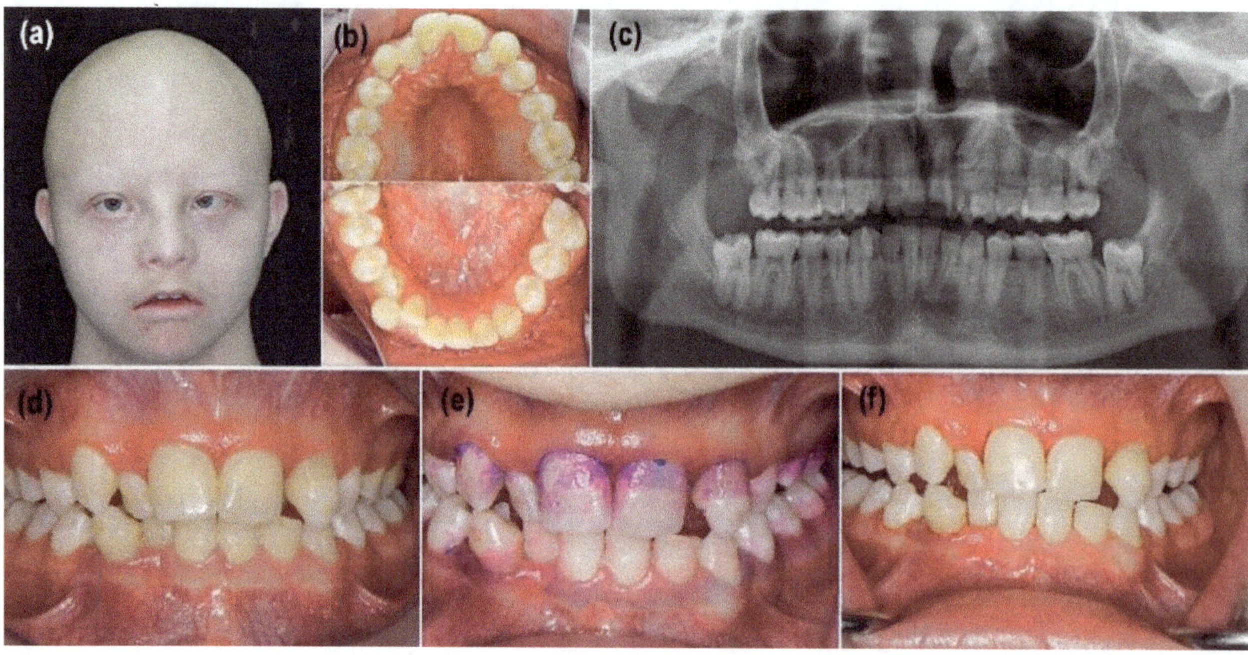

Image 2. Chronic gingivitis associated with genetic disorders plus ectodermal anomalies.

condition has been the use of phenobarbital and/or valproic acid since birth. The intraoral features were drug-induced generalized gingival proliferative lesion with partial covering of the posterior teeth and gingival bleeding. Some permanent teeth were still impacted due to the presence of gingival fibrosis (a–c). The recommended dental therapy was the prophylactic periodontal treatment and gingivectomy (**Image 3**).

To illustrate this case, histopathological features were depicted in order to show the medication effects on the oral mucosa, in particular, on the gingival tissues (epithelium and connective tissue) (**Figure 3**).

2.1.4. Case 4: discreet chronic gingivitis associated with severe bruxism

A 7-year-old male child with spastic quadriplegic cerebral palsy, caused by hypoxic–ischemic brain damage, exhibited poor cognitive function and has been feeding on semi-solid food since 3 years of age. Ranitidine hydrochloride was used to treat gastroesophageal reflux, and botulinum toxin was never used to decrease the severity of the sleep bruxism. As a consequence, severe upper and lower teeth wear reaching the region of the dental pulp were evidenced (a).

This child was in primary dentition phase and exhibited discreet chronic gingivitis, mouth-breathing pattern, severe dysphagia, and involuntary tongue movements. First, oral hygiene orientation and diet control under supervision were done due to his severe neuromotor dysfunction. Posteriorly, we used a masticatory device denominated "hyperbola" to attenuate the sleep bruxism and, consequently, to improve the quality of his life. After the proposed therapy, we obtained satisfactory results, including reduction of the sleep bruxism and improvements of sucking-swallowing movements at meals. (Source: Giannasi, et al. [14]) (**Image 4**).

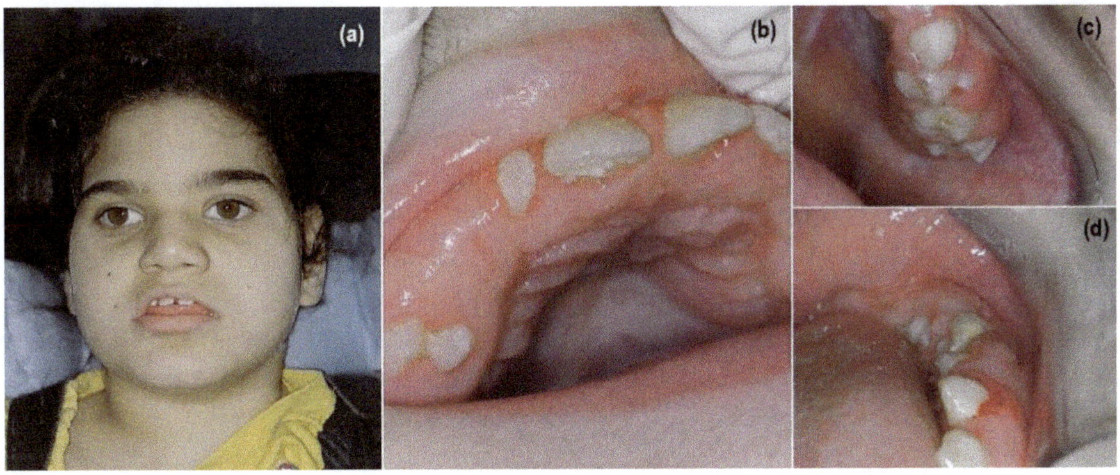

Image 3. Severe medications-induced gingival overgrowth.

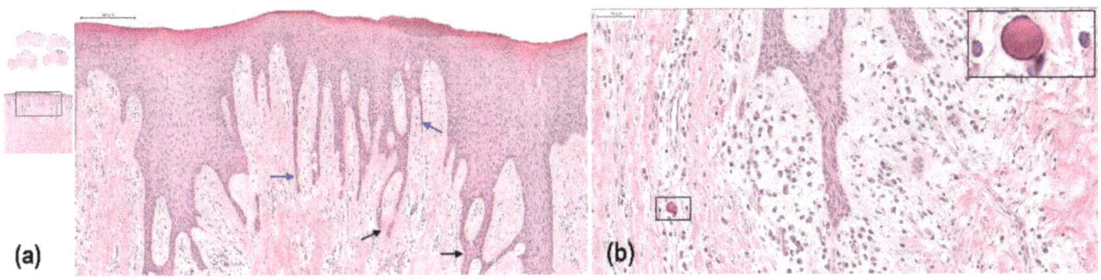

Figure 3. Medication-related gingival hyperplasia. Photomicrography showing gingival hyperplasia characterized by the epithelium hyperplasia and proliferation of dense connective tissue. Epithelial crest projections were thin and long (blue arrows), interconnecting them (black arrows) (a). A lamina propria exhibited infiltration of mononuclear inflammatory cells, especially lymphocytes, plasma cells, and macrophages. Furthermore, scattered eosinophilic globules of gamma globulin, known as Russell bodies (b; square), were also seen (hematoxylin–eosin; bars = 200 and 50 μm).

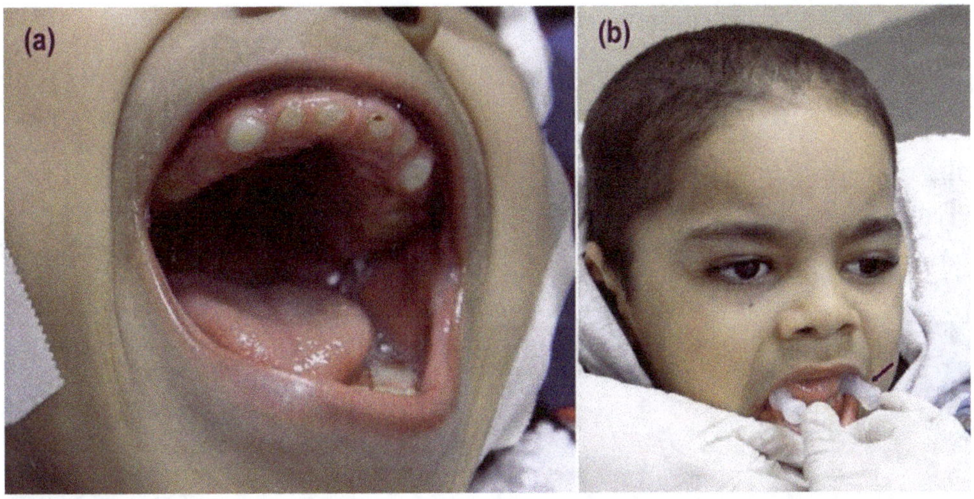

Image 4. Discreet chronic gingivitis associated with severe bruxism. (Source: Giannasi, et al. [14]).

2.1.5. Case 5: chronic gingivitis associated with sensory disabilities and metabolic disease

A 9-year-old male child with visual disability resulting from the intracranial hypertension and/ or alterations in the vascularization of the optical nerves which were caused by the cystic craniopharyngioma. Diabetes insipidus was developed as a complication of this disease, whereas, the motor functions, learning ability, memory, and mental health were preserved. The intraoral features showed generalized chronic gingivitis and deep caries, in particular, in the molar regions, resulting from poor oral hygiene. Considering that the periodontal disease is one of the main oral complications of diabetes, the oral health balance must be a major goal of the dentists once hyperglycemic control in a diabetic child becomes is a great challenge for parents and doctor (**Image 5**).

2.1.6. Case 6: necrotizing periodontal disease associated with AIDS and metabolic disorder

A 59-year-old man with diagnosis of active positive-HIV had squamous cell carcinoma in the vestibular fornix region. In the clinical history, the patient was a smoker since the age 13 and had arterial hypertension, saphenous bridge, and type 2 diabetes mellitus. The diagnosis of positive-HIV was confirmed when the patient was 36 years old. To treat the malignant neoplasm, chemotherapy and radiotherapy were indicated by the oncologists; however, no emergency dental treatment was done before the recommended therapies in order to first eliminate the dentoalveolar infection foci. We imply that the severe periodontitis combined with periapical lesion caused by the presence of residual root, quickly evolves into an abscess with spontaneous extraoral suppurative drainage. The neoplasm overgrowth and the indicated therapies with no support dental treatment surely influenced this infectious process (a and b). Severe candidiasis was spread on the hard palate and, in particular, superior alveolar ridge (c). The exfoliative cytology confirmed the diagnosis, showing a great amount of *Candida albicans* hyphae (d) and indicating a highly immunocompromised patient. As a consequence of the oral condition, this patient was with a severe malnutrition and cachexia resulting in hypoglycemic shock and, then, progressing to his death in 15 days. Most likely, there was no favorable response to the medical therapeutic protocols due to the severity of the immunosuppression and the presence of generalized acute oropharyngeal infections (**Image 6**).

2.1.7. Case 7: generalized chronic periodontitis associated with heart and metabolic diseases

A 61-year-old man had uncontrolled and insulin-dependent type 2-diabetes mellitus, arterial hypertension, ankylosing spondylitis, and hepatitis C. Regarding the diabetes control, the patient was treated with sinvastatina (10 mg), galvus (100 mg) and lantus (44 mL). The

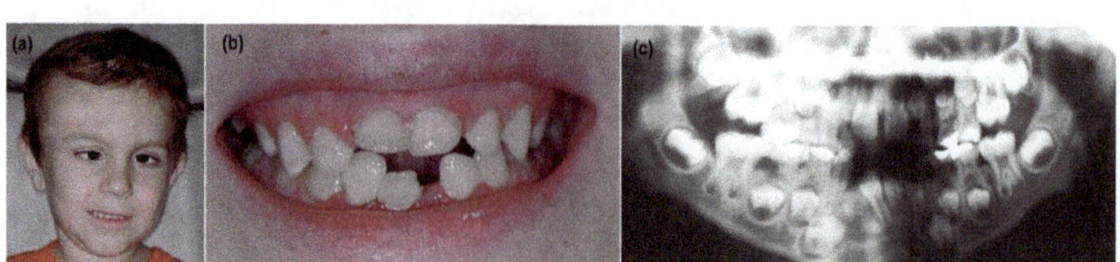

Image 5. Chronic gingivitis associated with visual disability and metabolic disease.

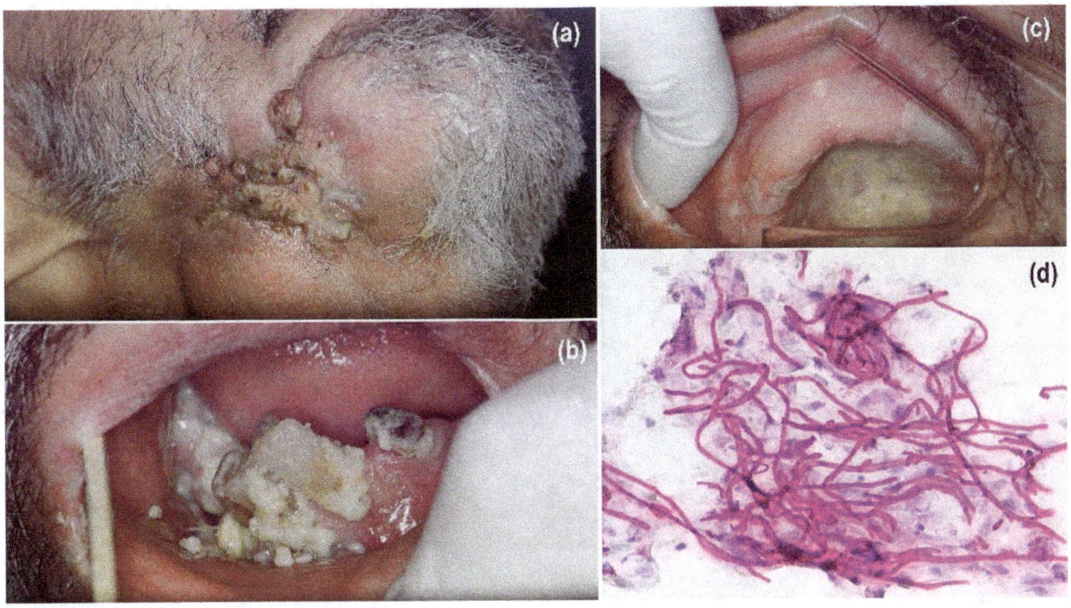

Image 6. Necrotizing periodontal disease in combination with AIDS and metabolic disorder (Papanicolaou stain, original magnification 400×).

glycated hemoglobin (HbA1c) value was 9.1% (Reference values: normal: ≤5,6%, *prediabetes:* 5,7–6,4%, and diabetes mellitus: ≥6,5%, in accordance with the American Diabetes Association) [28]. In the intraoral features, generalized chronic periodontitis characterized by the clinical attachment loss and the periodontal abscess with suppurative drainage placed, in particular, at the right canine region were evidenced (a, b, c, and d). Oral hygiene was unsatisfactory, most likely because of the pain and the gingival bleeding stimulated by the use of cleaning devices. The periodontal treatment was done associated with prophylactic drugs as antibiotics. No local vasoconstrictive anesthetic agent was administered during the clinical procedures. (Courtesy: Professor Doctor Ana Cristina Solis) (**Image 7**).

Concerning the etiology of PD in patients with uncontrolled diabetes, the progressive attachment loss was detected due to the function and reduction of polymorphonuclear leukocyte chemotaxis leading to an increase in infection susceptibility, collagen synthesis and maturation reduction, increased collagenase activity, and the formation of advanced glycation end products (AGEs) that bind to the receptor for advanced glycation end products (RAGEs) in macrophages and monocytes. The effects of AGE accumulation increase tissue oxidant stress, alter the endothelial cell functions, elevate the activity of matrix metalloproteinases leading to the production of free radicals, and promote vascular dysfunction and cellular death. These factors may directly affect the migration and activity of inflammatory cells, impairing the mechanisms of defense against microorganisms and delaying the periodontal tissue repair processes, resulting in great losses of support structures [11].

To clarify these clinical findings, periodontal tissue alterations resulting from oral complications of diabetes were depicted, including intense alveolar bone resorption at the furcation region, proliferation of junctional epithelium (hyperplasia) toward the furcation, diffuse infiltration of mononuclear inflammatory cells which consisted of macrophages, lymphocytes,

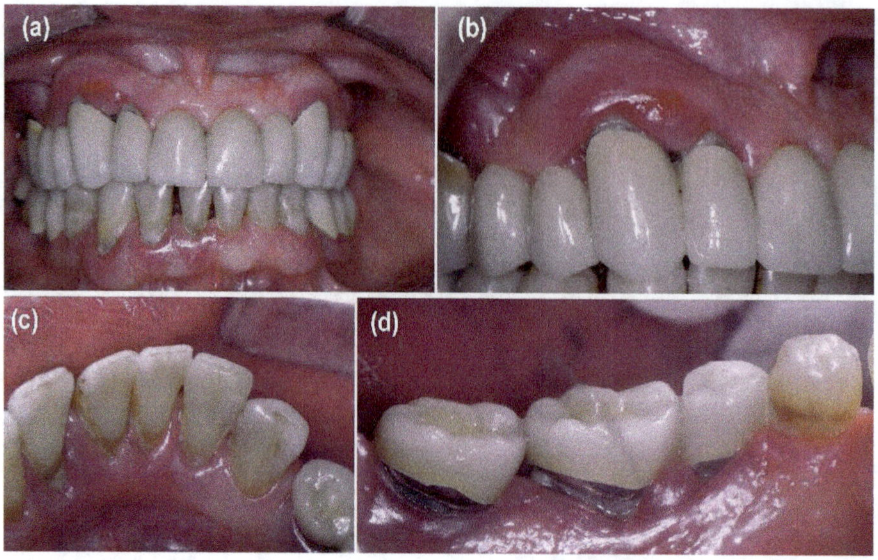

Image 7. Generalized chronic periodontitis associated with heart and metabolic diseases. (Courtesy: Doctor Professor Ana Cristina Solis).

and especially plasma cells. Numerous blood vessels were congested and the diapedesis mechanism (leukocyte extravasation into connective tissue) were well evidenced, justifying the great amount of inflammatory cells at the lamina propria (**Figure 4**).

2.1.8. Case 8: autoimmune disease associated gingivitis (desquamative gingivitis)

A 33-year-old woman with chronic mucocutaneous inflammatory disorder of immunological background showing aggressive and extensive oral lesions with erythematous, erosive and extensive areas, especially in the marginal and attached gingivae (a and b). Histopathological features showing a band of infiltration of lymphocytic inflammatory cells under the surface epithelium extending throughout the gingiva (c), besides hydropic degeneration and sharpness loss of the basal layer (d) (hematoxylin and eosin, 50× and 100×). The diagnosis was lichen planus. (Source: Gomes et al. [29]) (**Image 8**).

2.1.9. Case 9: gingivitis associated with hematological disorders

A 23-year-old young woman with Fanconi's anemia had severe pancytopenia and a prolonged, long-term immunosuppression which resulted in the development of an abscess on the infra-orbicular region. This process progressed to phlegmon causing tissue necrosis of the nostrils, nasal septum, nasal fossa, and posterior orbit region of the right side (a). The etiologic agent of the phlegmon was *Streptococcus parasanguinis*. The myelogram shows moderately hypocellular bone marrow with cellular dysplasia involving the granulocytic, erythrocytic, and megakaryocytic (arrow) series (b). The intrabuccal examination showed abundant and spontaneous gingival bleeding, edema on the interdental papillae, hematomas on the superior and inferior lips, and inadequate oral hygiene (c and d). No caries, alveolar bone loss, and periodontal pockets were evidenced. No bone marrow transplant was performed due to incompatibility of donors; thus, the only available option was an alternative treatment through the erythrocytes and platelets-concentrated transfusion to prevent

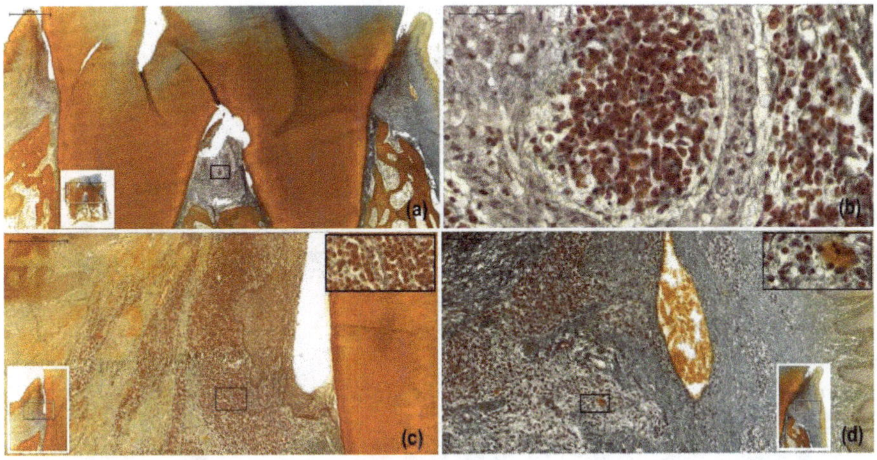

Figure 4. Photomicrography showing chronic periodontitis related to Case 7 (Masson's trichrome; bars = 1000, 200, 100, and 50 μm).

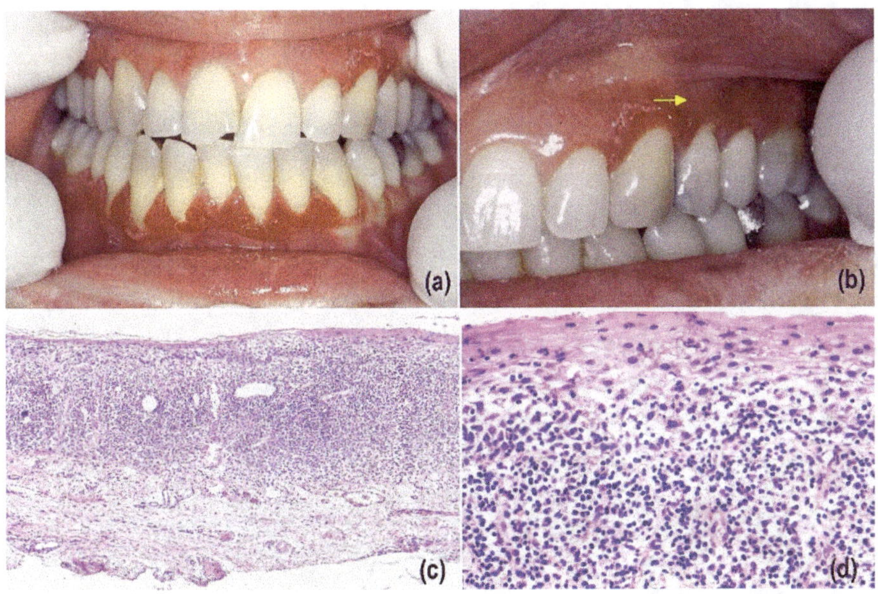

Image 8. Gingivitis associated with autoimmune disease (desquamative gingivitis) (Source: Gomes et al. [29]).

spontaneous hemorrhages and severe anemia. Oral exfoliative cytology was performed, showing superficial epithelial cells with nuclear and cytoplasmic alterations, erythrocytes, bacterial colonies (cocci), and numerous hyphae and spores of *Candida albicans* (e). Based on this, drug administrations, as antifungal medication and antibiotics, were also indicated to treat the oral acute inflammatory processes caused by bacterial and fungal infections. It is important to emphasize that the dental interventions were done together to the recommended medical therapy until the disease remission period. Initially, the periodontal prophylaxis was carried out by dentist and, posteriorly, the orientation and control of oral hygiene and diet accomplished by nurses and caregivers after adequate training in oral health. The health multiprofessional team, who may participate in this treatment process, corroborated in favor of supportive health care, leading to a quick recovery time of the patient (Source: Gomes et al. [30]) (**Image 9**).

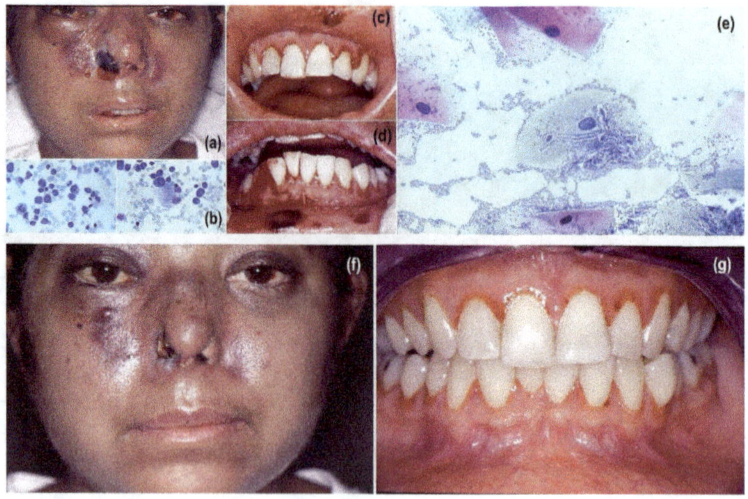

Image 9. Gingivitis associated with hematological disorders (Leishmann stain, 600×; Papanicolaou stain, 400×) (Source: Gomes et al. [30]).

2.1.10. Case 10: necrotizing ulcerative gingivitis associated with hematological disorder plus chemical and physical agents

A 14-year-old adolescent boy with Acute Lymphoblastic Leukemia (ALL) underwent the chemotherapy and radiotherapy on the region of the central nervous system for relapse prophylaxis of the primary disease (a). The myelogram before the medical therapies displayed hypercellular bone marrow composed exclusively by lymphoblastic cells with numerous atypical mitoses (square) (b and c). Extra and intraoral features of the patient, before the recommended dental treatment, were acute necrotizing ulcerative gingivitis, severe oral mucositis with areas necrosis associated to pseudomembranes, and facial asymmetry with signs of

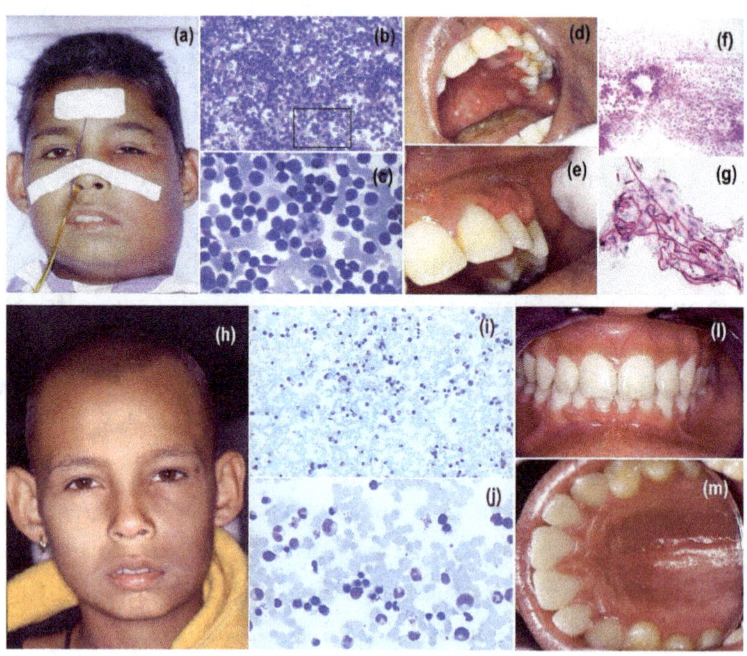

Image 10. Necrotizing ulcerative gingivitis associated with hematological disorder plus chemical and physical agents (Leishmann stain, 600×; Papanicolaou stain, 400×) (Source: Gomes et al. [31]).

phlogistic processes (d and e). The exfoliative cytology of the hard palate and attached and free gingivae shows a great number of inflammatory polymorphonuclear and mononuclear cells, besides a great amount of *Candida albicans* hyphae confirming the diagnosis of candidiasis (f and g). The dental treatment protocol, inserted together to the medical therapies until the primary disease remission period, corroborated in favor of the patient's general recovery time and of the elimination of the oral acute inflammatory process (h). The myelogram after the remission phase of the disease showed normal bone marrow (i and j). In extra- and intraoral features, the patient showed discreet facial asymmetry, discreet chronic gingivitis, and palate mucosae with normal features (l and m). Considering these clinical and histological findings, we dare reinforce that the insertion of a dental practitioner into the hospital transdisciplinary team is crucial to the medical therapy success and to the good quality of health services, in particular, for systemically highly compromised patients. (Source: Gomes et al. [31]) (**Image 10**).

3. "Omic" technologies applied in periodontal diseases

With advances in genomic (genes), transcriptomic (mRNA), proteomic (proteins), and metabolomic (metabolites) capabilities, an increased interest has emerged in the biologic system to define the complex regulatory networks that result in health or disease [32]. This implies a greater understanding of the data related to the etiopathogenesis of PD. These diseases are a multifactorial, highly complex disease involving some factors as host, environment, and microbiota. However, it is the host inflammatory response which may lead to the soft and hard tissue destruction. In severe diseases, this can lead to tooth loss [33].The host response to the infections draws upon the innate, inflammatory, and adaptive immune systems which provide an appropriate response to the aggressive microorganisms. In some individuals and with some bacteria, this phenomenon will be an innate-only response, others will need to invoke the inflammatory response, and yet others will require the adaptive immune response (cellular, humoral, or both) in order to reduce the microbial activities [33, 34].

Although much of what Page and Schroeder proposed in 1976 has stood the test of time, advances in the fields of basic and periodontal immunology need a reassessment of their work, as well as their integration with emerging new concepts [35]. Major advances have been made regarding the cellular and molecular mechanisms underlying the induction, regulation, and effector functions of immune and inflammatory responses. Likewise, Kornman [36] described a new look of the PD pathogenesis when he reported the specific bacteria and immunoinflammatory mechanisms related to innate differences among individuals and changes in environmental factors. This fact may accelerate or attenuate these biochemical changes [37].

With emerging genomic, proteomic, and metabolomic data and tools of biology systems for interpreting data, it is now possible to start describing the basic elements of a new model of pathogenesis [36]. Stunning new findings have begun to clarify several complexities of the host-pathogen interaction of PD, pointing to key roles for microbial dysboisis and immune imbalance in the pathogenesis of disease [34].

Regarding the genomic knowledge, inflammation, cellular infiltration, and expression of a complex array of cytokines, chemokines, and lipid mediators are key characteristics of PD. In

PD, the presence of elevated inflammatory cytokines, including tumor necrosis factor (TNF)-α, interleukin (IL)-1, IL-6, interferon (IFN)-γ, and IL-12, is considered a central force when coupled with cell activation and RANKL (receptor activator of nuclear factor kappa-B ligand) activation in driving pathogen elicited bone loss [38, 39]. In addition to pro-inflammatory cytokines, an array of chemokines including IL-8 and monocyte chemotactic protein (MCP)-1 and others are frequently elevated in PD [40]. Some examples of this type of interaction are described in the literature, for example, studies that reported a positive association between polymorphism of the IL-1 and PD [41, 42]. In addition, the presence of antiinflammatory and regulatory cytokines, such as transforming growth factor-beta (TGF-β), IL-10 and IL-4, has been reported [43, 44].

T lymphocyte cells (T cells) are well known as key regulating cells which orchestrate the host immune response. Considering the cells arise from the $CD4^+$ population and are based on cytokine profiling, early studies showed that these cells were segregated into Th1 and Th2 populations. Modern cytokine profiling and transcription factor analysis have led to a much more detailed classification of Th cells and the emergence of the Th17, Treg, TFH, Th9, and Th22 subsets [45, 46]. More advances have been recognized in what concerns the Toll-like receptors (TLRs) and TLR signaling; TIR-domain-containing adapter-inducing interferon-β (TRIF), interferon regulatory factors and type 1 interferon, and other pattern recognition receptors and PD, including scavenger receptors (SRs) and *nucleotide-binding-oligomerization-domain (NOD)-like receptors* (NLRs) [34].

With a similar importance, the transcriptomics aspects are defined as gene expression profile and when altered may influence the microbiota composition of periodontal pocket, as observed by Papapanou et al. [47]. In the same way, recent studies started to use proteomic techniques, promoting high resolution in the evaluation of proteins and molecular pathways involved in gingival inflammation [48, 49].

The gingival fluid composition of inflamed sites of patients with generalized aggressive periodontitis was evaluated by Bostanci et al. [50], demonstrating the proportion of enzymes associated with neutrophils, metalloproteinase of matrix-8, catepsin G, mieloperoxidase in addition to bacterial, viral, and yeast proteins that were increased in aggressive periodontitis when compared to healthy sites of individuals without periodontitis. Cystatin B and defensins, defense proteins, were detected only in healthy individuals.

Proteins involved in immune response and antimicrobial function, such as α-amylases, calgranulin A, cystatin, C-lysozyme, and cathepsin G were regulated positively in the induction phase of gingivitis. In the resolution phase, several histones and neutrophilic proteins, including cathepsin G, myeloperoxidase, and defensin-1 had their production decreased [49].

Concerning metabolomic aspects, among the earliest host-response molecules found in response to infection are lipid mediators [51]. Resolution of inflammation involves the production of lipid mediators named immunoresolvents and includes the resolvins, protectins, lipoxins, and maresins [51, 52]. Functionally, resolvins limit inflammation in part through prevention of neutrophil penetration, limiting inflammation at the local level, and promote tissue regeneration. The reduction of inflammation, through the use of resolvin-based approaches, may represent a novel strategy to potentially augment PD treatment approaches [53].

New models in the next few years will be merely frameworks for integrating key knowledge as it becomes available from the "Omic" technologies for diagnosis, providing by identifying one or more biomarkers the detection of active disease, predict future progression, and evaluate the response to periodontal therapy, thereby improving clinical management through early diagnosis and intervention, especially in case of patients with SHCN.

4. Alternative therapy for periodontics

As an alternative treatment to obtain the regeneration of the periodontium, the photobiomodulation (PBM) and some bioactive materials may be indicated, once they strongly stimulate the periodontal tissue response, attenuate the inflammatory processes, and/or promote the microstructural reconstruction of the periodontium. However, in the indication of these therapies, PBM must be carefully studied, since it depends exclusively on the general and oral health status of each patient.

Concerning the patients with SHCN associated to immune system deficiency, the PBM, also known as low-level laser therapy (LLLT), has been largely used to promote therapeutic and biostimulating effects, such as analgesia, antiinflammatory action, angiogenesis, and mitogenesis [11]. Gomes et al. [11] assessed the impact of the GaAlAs diode laser on the periodontal tissues and investigated its effects on the alveolar bone remodeling process during orthodontic tooth movement in normoglycemic and diabetic rats. The authors demonstrated that the PMB strongly stimulated the alveolar bone remodeling and favored the continuous reorganization of the soft periodontal tissues, leading to the maintenance and the integrity of periodontal microstructures under orthodontic force, especially in uncontrolled diabetic rats (**Figure 5**).

Several bioactive materials have been used in the regenerative medicine, especially in patients with complex metabolic and cellular disorders. Among them, we highlighted homogenous demineralized dentin matrix (HDDM), amniotic membrane (AM) used as a biological dressing, and different types of platelet concentrates such as platelet-rich plasma (PRP) and platelet-rich fibrin (PRF). These biomaterials were applied in the craniomaxillofacial complex resulting in tissue regeneration and microstructural reconstruction due to their effective inductive and conductive properties. The HDDM, PRP, and AM in implantation sites may initiate an inductive cascade as chemotaxis

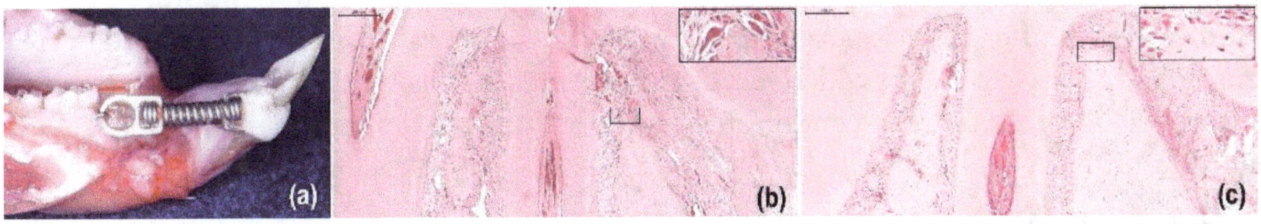

Figure 5. Low-level laser therapy applied on the periodontal tissues under orthodontic force (a) in a period of 21 days. Photomicrographs showing furcation region of the right mandibular first molar in diabetic rats: (b) diabetic rats with no laser irradiation displaying alveolar bone loss due to intense osteoclastic activity (square); and (c) diabetic rats with laser irradiation exhibiting suitable alveolar bone formation because of the intense osteoblastic activities (square) and the integrity of the periodontal ligament fibers (Source: Gomes et al. [11]).

of progenitor cells, mitogenesis, angiogenesis, and differentiation into a wide variety of cells. The cell recruitment, division rate, and differentiation of cell lines are under the direct control of several growth factors and stem cells which are found in these biomaterials [54–56].

In particular, the AM is a huge source for multipotent mesenchymal stem cells (MSCs) with the ability to differentiate into a wide variety of cells, such as chondroblasts, osteoblasts, adipocytes and fibroblasts, myocytes, endothelial cells, neuronal cells, and hepatocytes, leading to formation of cartilage, bone, connective tissue, muscle, blood vessel, nerve, and liver tissue, respectively [56–58]. This membrane acts as a barrier, preventing the entry of pathogens and toxins, preserving the tissue structures, and, consequently, reducing the levels of local pro-inflammatory cytokines [58, 59]. Thus, it could be largely used to selectively guide the tissue regeneration in the periodontium following destructive PD.

Regarding the second-generation platelet concentrate, the PRF clot forms a strong and dense natural fibrin mesh full of growth factors that can stimulate proliferation of PDL cells and osteoblasts; besides, it favors various cytokine entrapment and preserves the growth factors from proteolysis [60]. This concentrate is characterized by a high content of platelets and leukocytes that release an array of growth factors such as platelet-derived growth factor (PDGF), *transforming growth factor-beta 1 (TGF*-β1), insulin-like growth factor (IGF), vascular endothelial growth factor (*VEGF),* and the antiinflammatory cytokines [61].

Although the use of autologous platelet concentrates is not new to periodontics, current researches are strongly encouraging the combination of platelet concentrates, such as PRP, PRF, and concentrated growth factors, with bone graft materials, membranes for guided tissue regeneration and MSCs to stimulate the periodontal regeneration. Most likely, this pool has synergistic effects, favoring the environment and the development of desirable periodontal tissues which were seriously compromised by the periodontal disease.

5. Considerations

Considering the high susceptibility to PD in people with SHCN, it is important that the dental practitioners know the different levels of disability complexity and how the undesirable environment may impair the human and physical development, leading to temporary or permanent disorders and/or diseases. Among the most common oral diseases, periodontal disease is an inflammatory condition which has been identified as a potential risk factor for systemic diseases. Therefore, it must be continuously controlled by the dentists to maintain the general health status of this individual.

In addition, other treatments for oral rehabilitation may be indicated when the periodontium is healthy, such as orthodontics, dental implants and/or the use of dental prostheses, contributing to the balance of the stomatognathic system, the preservation of the general health, a better quality of life, and, consequently, social inclusion.

In search of alternative therapies for this target public, the photobiomodulation for periodontal tissue biostimulation and the reconstructive surgeries using bioactive materials may be recommended in order to favor the periodontal regeneration, to protect the periodontium under daily actions of physicochemical agents and psychic conditions, and to restore lost periodontal microstructures.

Despite the entire scientific and technological development for people with SHCN, we may presume that the major challenges for health multiprofessionals are to promote the best transdisciplinary practices in oral healthcare on dental services and hospitals due to the high complexity of disabilities, conditions, disorders and diseases of these individuals; to perform people management focusing on the good interpersonal relationship among the health multiprofessionals, patient, family and caregivers; and to combat the several environmental and social factors that may strongly affect the decision-making power of the patient to carry out a satisfactory self-care.

Acknowledgements

This book chapter was supported by the São Paulo State Secretariat for the Rights of the Person with Disability (SEDPcD) and State of São Paulo Research Foundation (FAPESP; grant number: 2017/06835-8), in Brazil. The authors would like to thank the Associate Professor Sergio Lúcio Pereira de Castro Lopes, the Associate Professor Maria Aparecida Neves Jardini, the Doctor Professor Ana Cristina Solis, and the dentist Mario Augusto Gomes by the technical support and radiographic and clinical assistances.

List of abbreviations

ADHD	attention-deficit and hyperactivity disorder
AGEs	advanced glycation end products
AIDS	acquired immune deficiency syndrome
AM	amniotic membrane
ALL	Acute Lymphoblastic Leukemia
APA	American Psychiatric Association
ASD	autism spectrum disorder
DSM	Diagnostic and Statistical Manual of Mental Disorders
GaAlAs	gallium-aluminum-arsenide
HbA1c	glycated hemoglobin
HDDM	homogenous demineralized dentin matrix
HIV	human immunodeficiency virus

IFN	interferon
IFN-γ	interferon-gamma
IGF	insulin-like growth factor
IL	interleukin
IL-1	interleukin-1
IL-10	interleukin-10
IL-12	interleukin-12
IL-4	interleukin-4
IL-6	interleukin-6
IL-8	interleukin-8
JACSD	Joint Advisory Committee for Special Care Dentistry
LLLT	low-level laser therapy
LPS	bacterial lipopolysaccharide
MCP-1	monocyte chemotactic protein-1
mRNA	messenger ribonucleic acid
MSCs	mesenchymal stem cells
NHANES	National Health and Nutrition Examination Survey
NIMH	National Institute of Mental Health
NLRs	nucleotide-binding-oligomerization-domain (NOD)-like receptors
PBM	photobiomodulation
PD	periodontal diseases
PDGF	platelet-derived growth factor
PDL	periodontal ligament
PRF	platelet-rich fibrin
PRP	platelet-rich plasma
RAGEs	*r*eceptor for advanced glycation end products
RANKL	receptor activator of nuclear factor kappa-B ligand
SHCN	special health care needs
SRs	scavenger receptors
T cells	T lymphocyte

TFH	T-follicular helper cell
TGF	transforming growth factor
Th cells	T helper cells
Th1	T helper cell 1
Th17	T helper cell 17
Th2	T helper cell 2
Th22	T helper cell 22
Th9	T helper cell 9
TLRs	Toll-like receptors
TNF	tumor necrosis factor
TNF-α	tumor necrosis factor-alpha
Treg	regulatory T cell
TRIF	TIR-domain-containing adapter-inducing interferon-β
VEGF	vascular endothelial growth factor
WHO	World Health Organization

Author details

Mônica Fernandes Gomes[1]*, Andrea Carvalho De Marco[1], Lilian Chrystiane Giannasi[1,2,3] and Miguel Angel Castillo Salgado[1]

*Address all correspondence to: mfgomes@ict.unesp.br

1 Center of Biosciences Applied to Patients with Special Health Care Needs (CEBAPE), Institute of Science and Technology, UNESP, São José dos Campos, São Paulo, Brazil

2 Metropolitan University of Santos, UNIMES, Santos, São Paulo, Brazil

3 Universitary Center of Anápolis, UniEVANGÉLICA, Anápolis, Goiás, Brazil

References

[1] Hosseinpoor AR, Williams JAS, Gautam J, Posarac A, Officer A, Verdes E, Kostanjsek N, Chatterji S. Socioeconomic inequality in disability among adults: A multicountry study using the world health survey. American Journal of Public Health. 2013;**103**:1278-1286

[2] American Academy on Pediatric Dentistry. Council on Clinical Affairs. Guideline on management of dental patients with special health care needs. Pediatric Dentistry. 2008-2009;**30**(7Suppl):107-111

[3] Dolan TA. Professional education to meet the oral health needs of older adults and persons with disabilities. Special Care Dentist. 2013;**33**:190-197

[4] Douglass CW, Glassman P. The oral health of vulnerable older adults and persons with disabilities. Special Care Dentist. 2013;**33**:156-163

[5] American Academy of Pediatric Dentistry. Council on Clinical Affairs. Guideline on management of dental patients with special health care needs. Pediatric Dentistry. 2012-2013;**34**:152-157

[6] Eke PI, Dye BA, Wei L, Slade GD, Thornton-Evans GO, Borgnakke WS, Taylor GW, Page RC, Beck JD, Genco RJ. Update on prevalence of periodontitis in adults in the United States: NHANES 2009 to 2012. Journal of Periodontology. 2015;**86**(5):611-622

[7] Instituto Brasileiro de Geografia e Estatística (IBGE). Censo Demográfico 2010 [Internet]. Rio de Janeiro (RJ): Ministério do Planejamento, Orçamento e Gestão. [acesso em 31 Jul 2013]. Disponível em: ftp://ftp.ibge.gov.br/Censos/Censo_Demografico_2010/Caracteristicas_Gerais_Religiao_Deficiencia/caracteristicas_religiao_deficiencia.pdf

[8] Morisaki I. Oral healthcare for the persons with special needs. Clinical Calcium. 2017; **27**(10):1417-1425

[9] Diagnostic and Statistical Manual of Mental Disorders: DSM-5. 5th ed. Arlington, VA: American Psychiatric Association, 2013. 947 p

[10] Leroy R, Declerck D. Oral health-care utilization in adults with disabilities in Belgium. European Journal of Oral Sciences. 2013;**121**:36-42

[11] Gomes MF, Da Graças Vilela Goulart M, Giannasi LC, Hiraoka CM, De Fátima Santana Melo G, De Sousa AGV, Nóbrega CJP, Zangaro RA, Salgado MAC. Effects of the GaAlAs diode laser (780 nm) on the periodontal tissues during orthodontic tooth movement in diabetes rats: Histomorphological and immunohistochemical analysis. Lasers in Medical Science. 2017;**32**(7):1479-1487

[12] Giannasi LC, Matsui MY, Freitas SR, Caldas BF, Grossmann E, Amorim JB, dos Santos Idos R, Oliveira LV, Oliveira CS, Gomes MF. Effects of neuromuscular electrical stimulation on the masticatory muscles and physiologic sleep variables in adults with cerebral palsy: A novel therapeutic approach. PLoS One. 2015;**10**(8):e0128959

[13] Matsui MY, Giannasi LC, Batista SR, Amorim JB, Oliveira CS, Oliveira LV, Gomes MF. Differences between the activity of the masticatory muscles of adults with cerebral palsy and healthy individuals while at rest and in function. Archives of Oral Biology. 2017;**73**:16-20

[14] Giannasi LC, Freitas Batista SR, Matsui MY, Hardt CT, Gomes CP, Oliveira Amorim JB, Oliveira CS, de Oliveira LV, Gomes MF. Effect of a hyperbolide mastication apparatus for the treatment of severe sleep bruxism in a child with cerebral palsy: Long-term follow-up. Journal of Bodywork and Movement Therapies. 2014;**18**(1):62-67

[15] Brown LF, Ford PJ, Symons AL. Periodontal disease and the special needs patient. Periodontology 2000. 2017;**74**(1):182-193

[16] Gomes MF, Sichi LGB, Giannasi LC, Amorim JBO, Rocha JC, Koga-Ito CY, Salgado MAC. Phenotypic features and salivary parameters in patients with ectodermal dysplasia: Report of three cases. Case Reports in Dentistry. 2018. ID 2409212

[17] Woof M. Specialisation in special care dentistry—Where from, where now, where to? Journal of Disability and Oral Health. 2000;**1**(1):34-38

[18] Keller BK, Morton JL, Thomas VS, Potter JF. The effect of visual and hearing impairments on functional status. Journal of the American Geriatrics Society. 1999 Nov;**47**(11): 1319-1325

[19] Wallhagen MI, Strawbridge WJ, Shema SJ, Kurata J, Kaplan GA. Comparative impact of hearing and vision impairment on subsequent functioning. Journal of the American Geriatrics Society. 2001;**49**(8):1086-1092

[20] Lichtenstein MJ. Hearing and visual impairments. Clinics in Geriatric Medicine. 1992;**8**(1): 173-182

[21] Kisely S, Sawyer E, Siskind D, Lalloo R. The oral health of people with anxiety and depressive disorders—A systematic review and meta-analysis. Journal of Affective Disorders. 2016;**200**:119-132

[22] Carvalho RS, de Souza CM, Neves JC, Holanda-Pinto SA, Pinto LM, Brito GA, de Andrade GM. Effect of venlafaxine on bone loss associated with ligature-induced periodontitis in Wistar rats. Journal of Negative Results in Biomedicine. 2010;**9**:3

[23] Oliveira-Solis AC, Araújo ÁC, Corchs F, Bernik M, Duran ÉP, Silva C, Lotufo-Neto F. Impact of post-traumatic stress disorder on oral health. Journal of Affective Disorders. 2017;**219**:126-132

[24] Breivik T, Gundersen Y, Osmundsen H, Fonnum F, Opstad PK. Neonatal dexamethasone and chronic tianeptine treatment inhibit ligature-induced periodontitis in adult rats. Journal of Periodontal Research. 2006;**41**(1):23-32

[25] Branco-de-Almeida LS, Franco GC, Castro ML, Dos Santos JG, Anbinder AL, Cortelli SC, Kajiya M, Kawai T, Rosalen PL. Fluoxetine inhibits inflammatory response and bone loss in a rat model of ligature-induced periodontitis. Journal of Periodontology. 2012;**83**(5):664-671

[26] Moraes ME, Bastos MS, Santos LR, Castilho JC, Moraes LC, Medici Filho E. Dental age in patients with Down syndrome. Brazilian Oral Research. 2007;**21**(3):259-264

[27] Greulich WW, Pyle SI. Radiographic Atlas of Skeletal Development of the Hand and Wrist. 2nd ed. California: Stanford University Press; 1959

[28] American Diabetes Association. Standards of Medical Care in Diabetes—2017. Diabetes Care. 2017;**40**(1):S1-S135

[29] Gomes MF, Werbicky V, Nogueira TO. Lyophilized human amniotic membrane over wounds in areas of oral biopsy. Revista da Associação Paulista de Cirurgiões Dentistas. 2001;**55**(5):327-331

[30] Gomes MF, Teixeira RT, Plens G, Silva MM, Pontes EM, da Rocha JC. Naso-orbicular tissue necrosis by *Streptococcus parasanguis* in a patient with Fanconi's anemia: Clinical and laboratory aspects. Quintessence International. 2004;**35**(7):572-576

[31] Gomes MF, Kohlemann KR, Plens G, Silva MM, Pontes EM, da Rocha JC. Oral manifestations during chemotherapy for acute lymphoblastic leukemia: A case report. Quintessence International. 2005;**36**(4):307-313

[32] Horgan RP, Kenny LC. 'Omic' technologies: Genomics, transcriptomics, proteomics and metabolomics. The Obstetrician & Gynaecologist. 2011;**13**:189-195

[33] Benakanakere M, Kinane DF. Innate cellular responses to the periodontal biofilm. Frontiers of Oral Biology. 2012;**15**:41-55

[34] Huang N, Gibson FC 3rd. Immuno-pathogenesis of periodontal disease: Current and emerging paradigms. Current Oral Health Reports. 2014;**1**(2):124-132

[35] Page RC, Schroeder HE. Pathogenesis of inflammatory periodontal disease. A summary of current work. Laboratory Investigations. 1976;**34**(3):235-249

[36] Kornman KS. Mapping the pathogenesis of periodontitis: A new look. Journal of Periodontology. 2008;**79**(8 Suppl):1560-1568

[37] Hajishengallis G, Korostoff JM. Revisiting the Page & Schroeder model: The good, the bad and the unknowns in the periodontal host response 40 years later. Periodontology 2000. 2017;**75**(1):116-151

[38] Cochran DL. Inflammation and bone loss in periodontal disease. Journal of Periodontology. 2008;**79**(8 Suppl):1569-1576

[39] Yuan H, Gupte R, Zelkha S, Amar S. Receptor activator of nuclear factor kappa B ligand antagonists inhibit tissue inflammation and bone loss in experimental periodontitis. Journal of Clinical Periodontology. 2011;**38**(11):1029-1036

[40] Tonetti MS, Imboden MA, Gerber L, Lang NP, Laissue J, Mueller C. Localized expression of mRNA for phagocyte-specific chemotactic cytokines in human periodontal infections. Infection and Immunity. 1994;**62**(9):4005-4014

[41] Meisel P, Siegemund A, Dombrowa S, Sawaf H, Fanghaenel J, Kocher T. Smoking and polymorphisms of the interleukin-1 gene cluster (IL-1alpha, IL-1beta, and IL-1RN) in patients with periodontal disease. Journal of Periodontology. 2002;**73**(1):27-32

[42] Schäefer AS, Richter GM, Nothnagel M, Manke T, Dommisch H, Jacobs G, Arlt A, Rosenstiel P, Noack B, Groessner-Schreiber B, Jepsen S, Loos BG, Schreiber S. A genome-wide association study identifies GLT6D1 as a susceptibility locus for periodontitis. Human Molecular Genetics. 2010;**19**(3):553-562

[43] Gamonal J, Acevedo A, Bascones A, Jorge O, Silva A. Levels of interleukin-1 beta, −8, and −10 and RANTES in gingival crevicular fluid and cell populations in adult periodontitis patients and the effect of periodontal treatment. Journal of Periodontology. 2000;**71**(10):1535-1545

[44] Salvi GE, Brown CE, Fujihashi K, Kiyono H, Smith FW, Beck JD, Offenbacher S. Inflammatory mediators of the terminal dentition in adult and early onset periodontitis. Journal of Periodontal Research. 1998;**33**(4):212-225

[45] Nakajima T, Ueki-Maruyama K, Oda T, Ohsawa Y, Ito H, Seymour GJ, Yamazaki K. Regulatory T-cells infiltrate periodontal disease tissues. Journal of Dental Research. 2005;**84**(7):639-643

[46] Aranha AM, Repeke CE, Garlet TP, Vieira AE, Campanelli AP, Trombone AP, Letra A, Silva RM, Garlet GP. Evidence supporting a protective role for Th9 and Th22 cytokines in human and experimental periapical lesions. Journal of Endodontics. 2013;**39**(1):83-87

[47] Papapanou PN, Behle JH, Kebschull M, Celenti R, Wolf DL, Handfield M, Pavlidis P, Demmer RT. Subgingival bacterial colonization profiles correlate with gingival tissue gene expression. BMC Microbiology. 2009;**9**:221

[48] Grant MM, Creese AJ, Barr G, Ling MR, Scott AE, Matthews JB, Griffiths HR, Cooper HJ, Chapple IL. Proteomic analysis of a noninvasive human model of acute inflammation and its resolution: The twenty-one day gingivitis model. Journal of Proteome Research. 2010;**9**(9):4732-4744

[49] Bostanci N, Ramberg P, Wahlander Å, Grossman J, Jönsson D, Barnes VM, Papapanou PN. Label-free quantitative proteomics reveals differentially regulated proteins in experimental gingivitis. Journal of Proteome Research. 2013;**12**(2):657-678

[50] Bostanci N, Heywood W, Mills K, Parkar M, Nibali L, Donos N. Application of label-free absolute quantitative proteomics in human gingival crevicular fluid by LC/MS E (gingival exudatome). Journal of Proteome Research. 2010;**9**(5):2191-2199

[51] Bannenberg G, Serhan CN. Specialized pro-resolving lipid mediators in the inflammatory response: An update. Biochimica et Biophysica Acta. 2010;**1801**(12):1260-1273

[52] Freire MO, Van Dyke TE. Natural resolution of inflammation. Periodontology 2000. 2013;**63**(1):149-164

[53] Hasturk H, Kantarci A, Goguet-Surmenian E, Blackwood A, Andry C, Serhan CN, Van Dyke TE. Resolvin E1 regulates inflammation at the cellular and tissue level and restores tissue homeostasis in vivo. Journal of Immunology. 2007;**179**(10):7021-7029

[54] Gomes MF, Banzi EC, Destro MF, Lavinicki V, Goulart M. Homogenous demineralized dentin matrix for application in cranioplasty of rabbits with alloxan-induced diabetes: Histomorphometric analysis. The International Journal of Oral & Maxillofacial Implants. 2007;**22**(6):939-947

[55] Gomes MF, Valva VN, Vieira EM, Giannasi LC, Salgado MA, Vilela-Goulart MG. Homogenous demineralized dentin matrix and platelet-rich plasma for bone tissue engineering in cranioplasty of diabetic rabbits: Biochemical, radiographic, and histological analysis. International Journal of Oral and Maxillofacial Surgery. 2016;**45**(2):255-266

[56] Gomes MF, Amorim JB, Giannase LC, Salgado MAC. Biomaterials for tissue engineering applications in diabetes mellitus. In: Dobrzanski LA, editor. Biomaterials in Regenerative Medicine [e-book]. Rijeka: InTech Open; 2018. pp. 410-435

[57] Vilela-Goulart M, Teixeira RT, Rangel DC, Niccoli-Filho W, Gomes MF. Homogenous amniotic membrane as a biological dressing for oral mucositis in rats: Histomorphometric analysis. Archives of Oral Biology. 2008;**53**(12):1163-1171

[58] Lima GMG, Severo MC, Santana-Melo GF, Cardoso MA, Vilela-Goulart MG, Salgado MAC, Gomes MF. Amniotic membrane as a biological dressing for 5-fluoruracil-induced oral mucositis in rats. International Journal of Oral and Maxillofacial Surgery. 2015;**44**:845-851

[59] Gomes MF, dos Anjos MJ, Nogueira TO, Guimarães SA. Histologic evaluation of the osteoinductive property of autogenous demineralized dentin matrix on surgical bone defects in rabbit skulls using human amniotic membrane for guided bone regeneration. The International Journal of Oral & Maxillofacial Implants. 2001;**16**(4):563-571

[60] Moradian H, Rafiee A, Ayatollahi M. Design and fabrication of a novel transplant combined with human bone marrow mesenchymal stem cells and platelet-rich fibrin: New horizons for periodontal tissue regeneration after dental trauma. Iranian Journal of Pharmaceutical Research. 2017;**16**(4):1370-1378

[61] Panda S, Sankari M, Satpathy A, Jayakumar D, Mozzati M, Mortellaro C, Gallesio G, Taschieri S, Del Fabbro M. Adjunctive effect of autologus platelet-rich fibrin to barrier membrane in the treatment of periodontal intrabony defects. Journal of Craniofacial Surgery. 2016;**27**(3):691-696

7

Desquamative Gingivitis: Early Sign of Mucous Membrane Pemphigoid and Pemphigus Vulgaris

Hiroyasu Endo, Terry D. Rees, Hideo Niwa, Kayo Kuyama, Maya Oshima, Tae Serizawa, Shigeo Tanaka, Morio Iijima, Masamichi Komiya and Takanori Ito

Abstract

Early signs and symptoms of autoimmune bullous diseases such as mucous membrane pemphigoid (MMP) or pemphigus vulgaris (PV) develop in the oral cavity in almost all cases. Desquamative gingivitis (DG) is a clinical manifestation common to several diseases or disorders and is frequently associated with autoimmune bullous diseases. This is a retrospective study of 37 patients with MMP (24 cases) or PV (13 cases) including 10 males and 27 females with a mean age of 58.4 years. The study indicates that DG is an early sign of autoimmune bullous diseases such as MMP or PV. About 70.3% of the oral lesions were confined only to the gingiva, and DG was the only manifestation of the diseases. Since some lesions remain limited to the oral cavity for a long period of time, patients diagnosed with MMP or PV should be closely followed because they must be immediately referred to other experts when they develop lesions on parts of their body other than the oral cavity. The oral healthcare provider should collaborate with other healthcare experts including dermatologists, ophthalmologists, and otolaryngologists to evaluate and manage patients with autoimmune bullous diseases in the oral cavity.

Keywords: gingival diseases/pemphigus/pemphigoid, benign mucous membrane/autoimmune diseases/mouth diseases

1. Introduction

Early signs and symptoms of autoimmune bullous diseases such as mucous membrane pemphigoid (MMP) or pemphigus vulgaris (PV) develop in the oral cavity in almost all cases. MMP is the most commonly recognized, followed by PV [1]. MMP is one of a group of autoimmune, subepithelial blistering diseases that predominantly affect the mucous membranes. MMP is considered to be a disease phenotype related to one or more different anti-basement membrane zone (BMZ) autoantibodies. Various components in the hemidesmosomes have been recognized as the target antigens of MMP, including bullous pemphigoid antigen 2 (BP180), bullous pemphigoid antigen 1 (BP230), laminin 332, type VII collagen, and β4 or α6 integrin subunits [2–5]. Most MMP patients are in the fifth or sixth decade of life, and the majority of them are women [6–8]. Oral lesions are observed in almost all cases, and the primary lesion often appears in the oral cavity [6–10]. PV is an autoimmune bullous disease characterized by acantholysis and suprabasilar separation in the epithelium of skin and/or mucous membranes. The main target antigen of PV is desmoglein (Dsg) 3, which is a constituent of desmosomes on the keratinocyte [11, 12]. Almost all PV patients with lesions limited to the oral mucosa have circulating autoantibodies to Dsg3 [12–15]. PV patients with lesions in the oral mucosa and skin also have Dsg1 autoantibodies, the main antigen of pemphigus foliaceus [12, 14, 15]. PV can develop at any age, but is most commonly observed in middle-aged and elderly individuals [16–19]. Early signs and symptoms of PV develop in the oral cavity in about 80% of patients [19].

Since patients with MMP or PV frequently experience only oral symptoms of pain and discomfort, they often visit the dentist or periodontist before other health care workers [20–22]. Desquamative gingivitis (DG) is a condition characterized by painful erythematous gingiva not resulting from dental plaque, sloughing of gingival tissues, erosions and ulcerations of the gingival epithelium and bulla formation on the gingiva [23–26]. It is a clinical manifestation common to several diseases or disorders [23–26]. Most DG patients are caused by mucocutaneous diseases. The differential diagnoses include oral lichen planus, MMP, and PV [24]. MMP is responsible for 35–48% and PV for 3–15% of DG [26]. Contact allergic reactions to various oral hygiene products, dental materials, or food flavoring and preservatives have also been reported in the differential diagnosis of DG [23, 24]. Gingival desquamation is a prominent clinical feature, and Nikolsky's sign often shows a positive reaction in DG caused by autoimmune bullous diseases [21]. This sign involves the application of a firm sliding or rubbing force on normal-appearing gingiva, inducing epithelial desquamation [21, 27].

Although an accurate diagnosis of oral mucosal disease or disorder causing DG is required to provide proper treatment, it is almost impossible to do so based solely on clinical appearance. Therefore, histopathological examination and direct immunofluorescence (DIF) testing are often required to establish the final diagnosis [24]. The specific disease or disorder causing DG, the severity of the DG lesions, the presence or absence of extraoral lesions, and the medical history of the patient are the key factors in determining the selection of a topical or systemic treatment [10, 23, 24]. In some patients, DG can be successfully managed with moderate to very high-potency topical corticosteroids combined with effective plaque control. Patients with severe and/or multiple oral lesions, or recalcitrant lesions, may need aggressive systemic treatment. The presence of extraoral lesions also may require systemic treatment for effective management. Although scarring with MMP is rarely a feature of the oral mucosa, conjunctival scarring may lead to blindness if not treated aggressively [28, 29]. Airway obstruction due to laryngeal scarring is a rare condition, but it may occasionally be a fatal complication [30, 31]. PV is a life-threatening condition if left untreated [32], so it is important to diagnose and treat it in its early stages. This study describes in detail the clinical and diagnostic findings of MMP or PV as a common oral manifestation of autoimmune bullous diseases.

2. Materials and methods

This is a retrospective study of 37 patients with MMP (24 cases) or PV (13 cases) who were seen by the authors at Nihon University, School of Dentistry at Matsudo between 2001 and 2017. Patients participating in the study included 10 males and 27 females, aged 24–83 years, with a mean age of 58.4 years. The medical records included information on each patient's clinical features, intraoral site involvement, presence or absence of extraoral lesions, duration from the onset of symptoms until presentation for diagnosis, and diagnostic information provided to the patient. A biopsy was obtained that included perilesional tissue and was then submitted for routine histopathology and DIF study for each of the 37 patients. DIF study was performed using conjugates for immunoglobulin (Ig) G, IgA, IgM, complement C3, and fibrinogen. Patients were diagnosed with MMP or PV through clinical examination supported by histologic diagnosis and DIF testing [24, 25, 33]. Some of the 37 patients presented in this study have been previously reported [9, 13, 14, 21, 34]. The current study was approved by the institutional review board (Ethics Committee Approval no. EC14-011-1).

3. Results

The results summarizing the intraoral involvement in 37 patients are shown in **Table 1**. All 37 patients described DG lesions including erythema, erosions, ulcerations, and epithelial desquamation (**Figures 1–4**). The oral lesions were confined to gingiva in 70.3% of patients. In a small number of patients, ulcers and erosions were also observed in the buccal mucosa, soft palate or tongue (**Figures 5–7**). **Table 2** summarizes the diagnostic pattern in the 37 patients. Diagnosis delays of more than 6 months were experienced by 30.8% of the PV patients and 54.2% of the MMP patients. 16.7% of patients with MMP were delayed for more than 12 months from onset to diagnosis. The results summarizing the characteristics of the biopsy

Site	MMP (n = 24)	PV (n = 13)	Total (n = 37)
Gingiva only	17 (70.8%)	9 (69.2%)	26 (70.3%)
Gingiva + buccal mucosa + tongue	1 (4.2%)	2 (15.4%)	3 (8.1%)
Gingiva + buccal mucosa + soft palate	0 (0%)	1 (7.7%)	1 (2.7%)
Gingiva + buccal mucosa	2 (8.3%)	1 (7.7%)	3 (8.1%)
Gingiva + soft palate	3 (12.5%)	0 (0%)	3 (8.1%)
Gingiva + tongue	1 (4.2%)	0 (0%)	1 (2.7%)

Table 1. Intraoral site involvement in 37 patients.

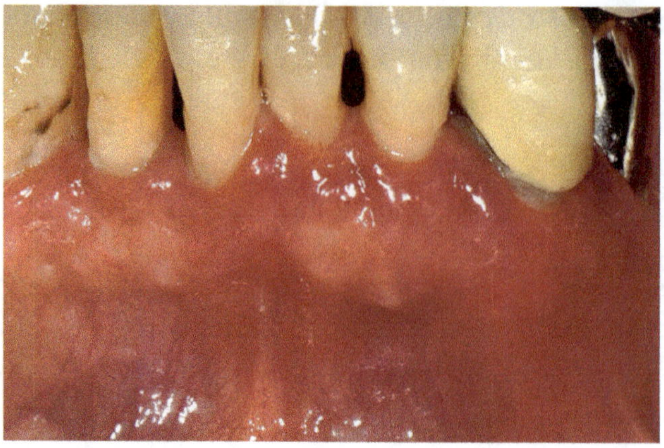

Figure 1. Desquamative gingivitis associated with mucous membrane pemphigoid. Diffuse erythematous lesions on the gingiva.

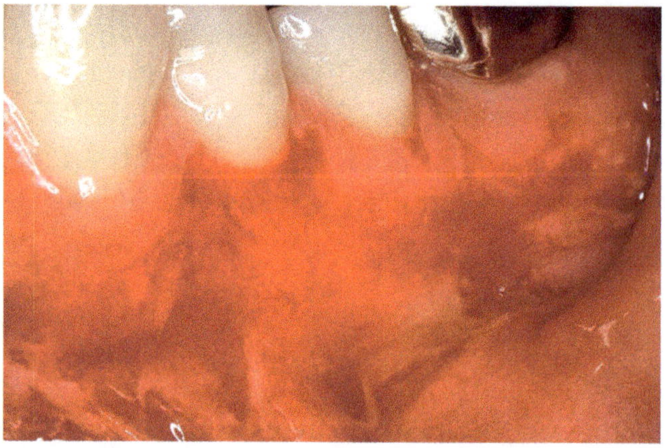

Figure 2. Desquamative gingivitis associated with pemphigus vulgaris. Patchy erythematous lesions were found on the gingiva.

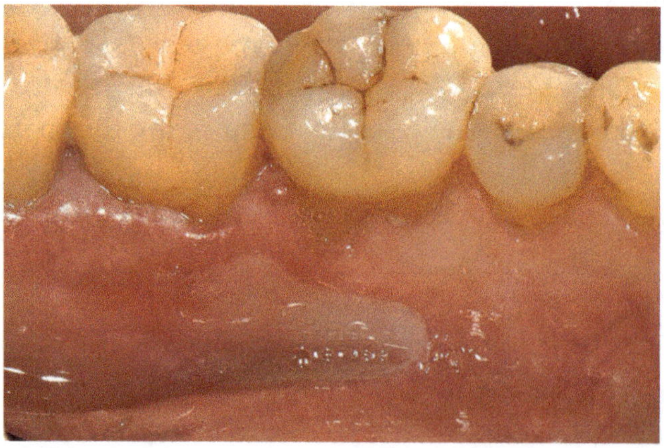

Figure 3. Pseudomembrane-covered erosion of the gingiva associated with mucous membrane pemphigoid.

findings in these 37 patients are shown in **Table 3**. Subepithelial separation was observed in the H&E-stained section in 20 patients with MMP (**Figure 8**). Three MMP samples showed nonspecific inflammation, and one MMP sample was nondiagnostic because of a total lack

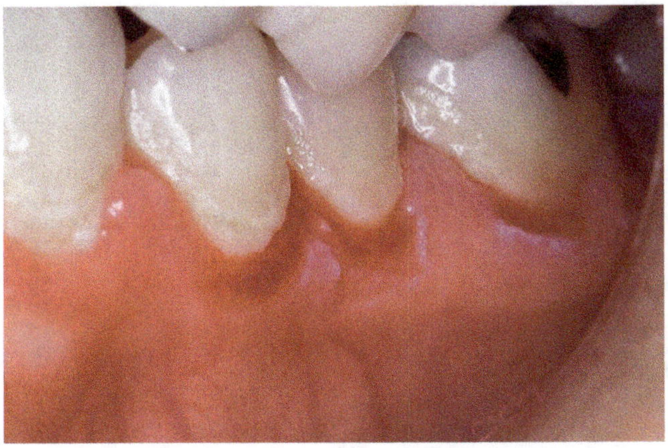

Figure 4. Localized erosions of the gingiva associated with pemphigus vulgaris.

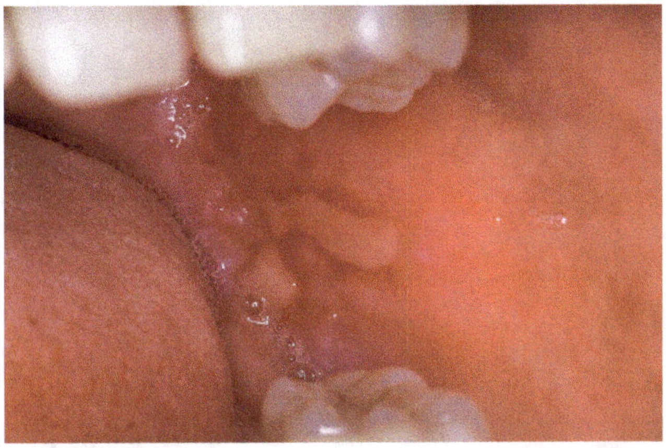

Figure 5. Pseudomembrane-covered erosion of the buccal mucosa associated with mucous membrane pemphigoid.

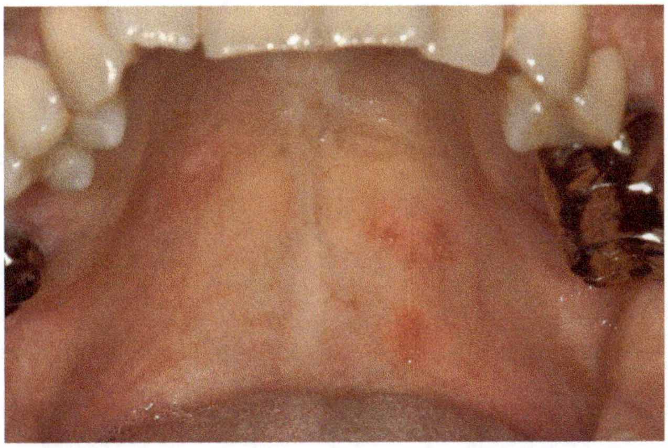

Figure 6. Localized erosions of the palatal mucosa associated with pemphigus vulgaris.

of the epithelium in the H&E-stained section. In contrast, acantholysis and a suprabasilar separation in the epithelium were observed in the H&E-stained section in all 13 PV patients (**Figure 9**). In the DIF testing, all 37 samples showed positive staining at the BMZ (MMP **Figure 10**) or at the intercellular space (PV **Figure 11**).

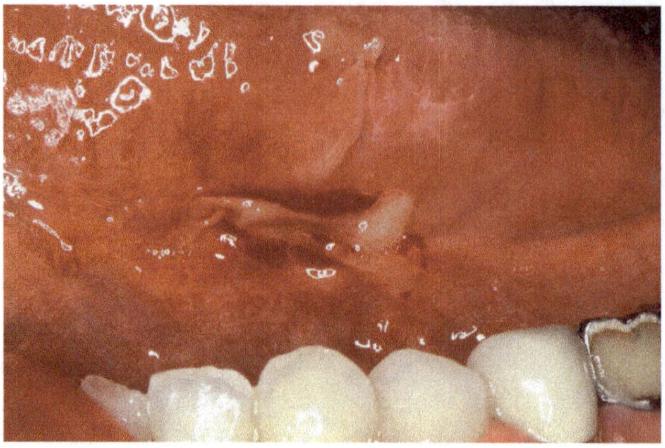

Figure 7. Desquamative lesion of the tongue associated with pemphigus vulgaris.

Diagnostic delay	Diagnosis		
	MMP (n = 24)	PV (n = 13)	Total (n = 37)
≤6 months	11 (45.8%)	9 (69.2%)	20 (54.1%)
7–12 months	9 (37.5%)	4 (30.8%)	13 (35.1%)
>12 months	4 (16.7%)	0 (0%)	4 (10.8%)

Table 2. Diagnostic pattern in 37 patients.

	MMP (n = 24)	PV (n = 13)
Histopathology		
Subepithelial separation	20	0
Acantholysis and suprabasilar separation	0	13
Non-specific	3	0
Non-diagnostic	1	0
Direct immunofluorescence		
Positive	24*	13**
Negative	0	0

*A linear BMZ deposition of varying combinations of IgG, IgA, fibrinorgen and complement C3.
**An epithelial intercellular deposition of IgG and complement C3.

Table 3. Biopsy findings in 37 patients.

After a diagnosis of MMP or PV, patients were advised to confirm the presence or absence of extraoral lesions by a dermatologist, otorhinolaryngologist, and ophthalmologist. Eleven (eight patients with MMP and three patients with PV) of the 37 patients (29.7%) confirmed the presence of extraoral lesions. The sites where clinical involvement was found were skin (5 patients), upper airway (10 patients), and eye (2 patients). Multiple extraoral mucosal involvements were

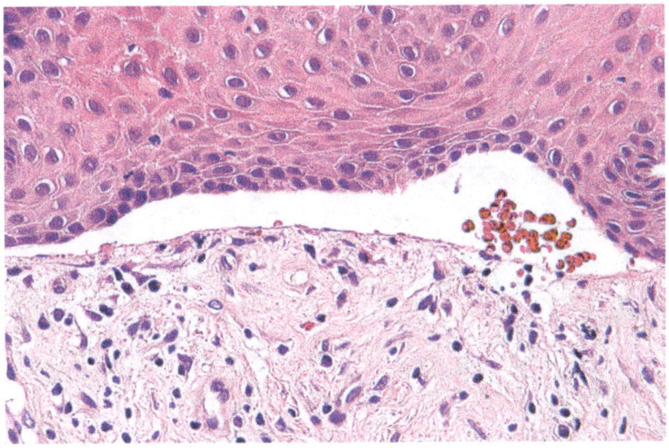

Figure 8. Hematoxylin-eosin-stained section of mucous membrane pemphigoid. A subepithelial separation was found.

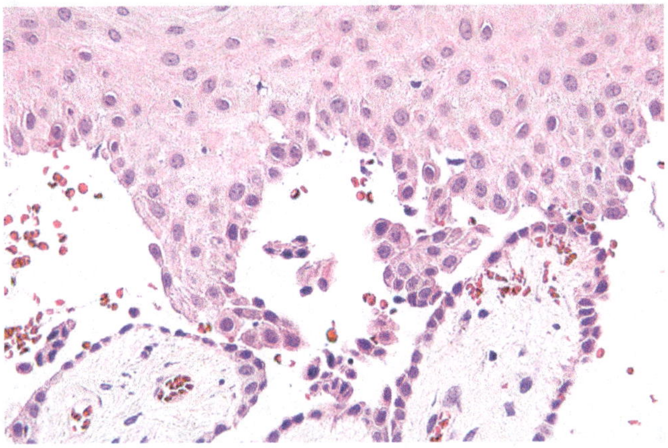

Figure 9. Hematoxylin-eosin-stained section of pemphigus vulgaris. Acantholysis and a suprabasilar separation in the epithelium were observed.

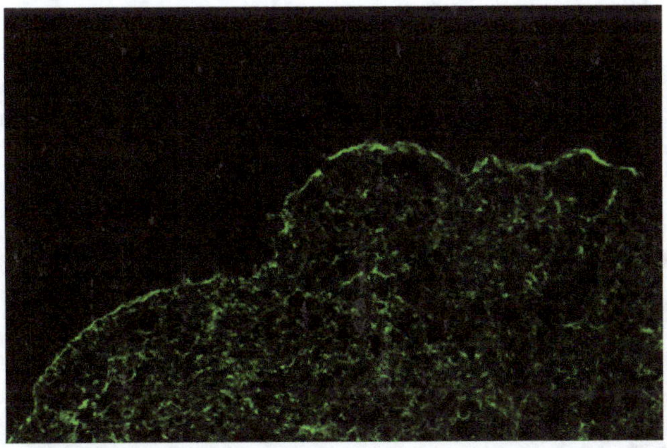

Figure 10. Direct immunofluorescence of the mucous membrane pemphigoid. A linear deposition of IgG at the basement membrane zone was recognized.

found in four patients with MMP and two patients with PV. All patients with extraoral involvement were managed by medical specialists with systemic treatment with or without hospitalization (**Figure 12a** and **b**). Patients with exclusively oral lesions were managed at the authors' hospital using a topical corticosteroid combined with effective plaque control. Patients were carefully monitored at 2–3 week intervals, and complete remission or minimalization of symptoms was achieved (**Figure 13a** and **b**).

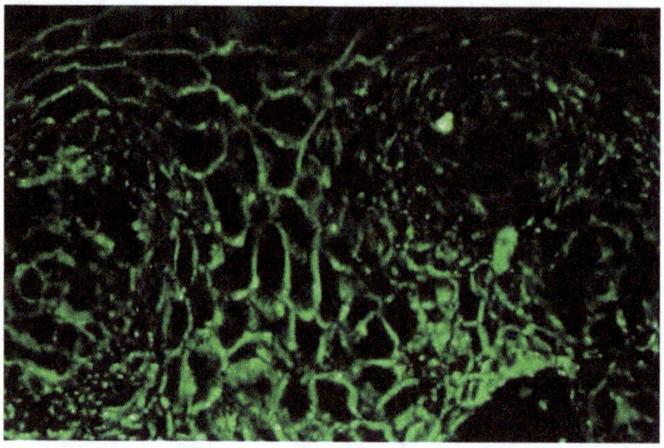

Figure 11. Direct immunofluorescence of pemphigus vulgaris. An intercellular deposition of IgG was evident.

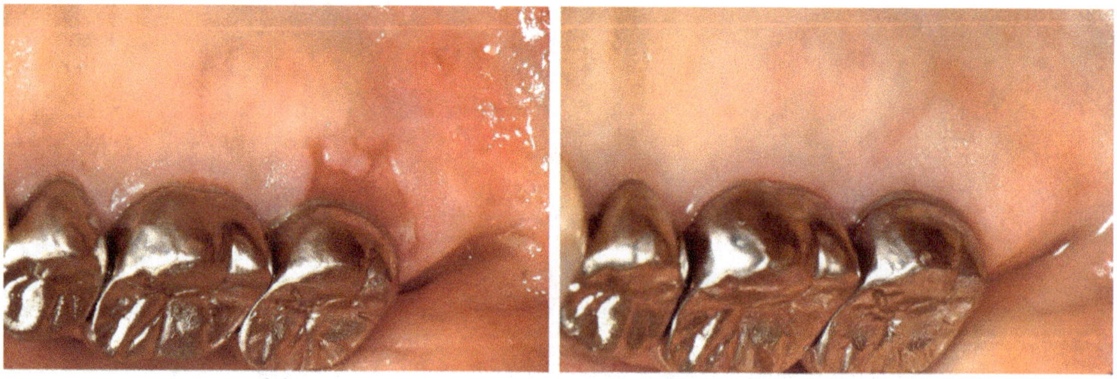

(a) (b)

Figure 12. (a) Desquamative gingivitis associated with pemphigus vulgaris. Localized erosion was observed on the palatal mucosa. Lesions were also found on the skin and upper airway. (b) Treatment response. The patient was managed by dermatologists with systemic treatment with hospitalization.

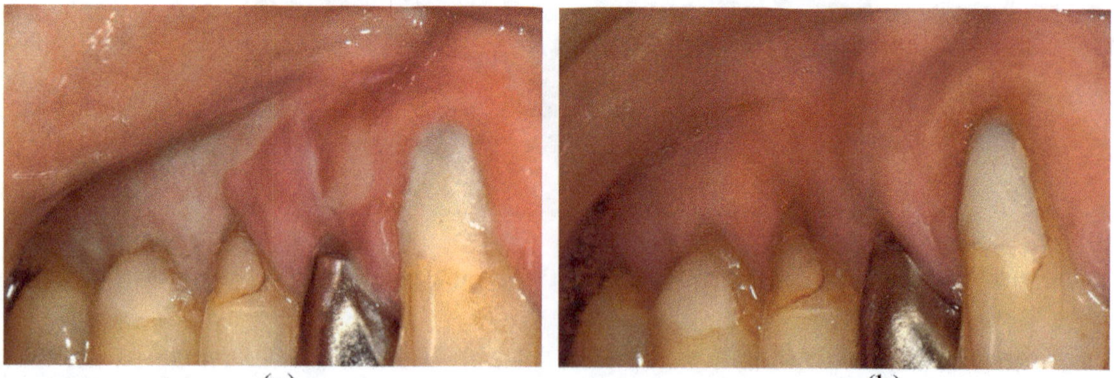

(a) (b)

Figure 13. (a) Desquamative gingivitis associated with mucous membrane pemphigoid. (b) Treatment response. Desquamative gingivitis was successfully managed using a topical corticosteroid combined with effective plaque control.

4. Discussion

The results of this study indicate that DG is an early sign of autoimmune bullous diseases such as MMP or PV. Although multiple oral sites were affected in some patients, 70.3% of the oral lesions were confined only to the gingiva, and DG was the only manifestation of the diseases. Data from this study indicate 70.8% of MMP patients had oral lesions confined only to the gingiva. This figure agrees with other reports [8, 25]. In contrast, in the present study, the frequency of oral lesions limited to the gingiva in PV patients is higher (69.2%) than previous reports (3–30%) [17–19, 25, 35]. The oral lesions of PV are usually multiple, typically in the buccal mucosa and soft palate [17, 18]. This disparity may be due to the selected bias due to an author's speciality (periodontist), as the patients may have been presenting for treatment of gingival lesions. Another limitation is that the number of PV cases is limited.

Nearly half (45.9%) of the patients in this study had experienced diagnostic delays longer than 6 months, indicating that early diagnosis of autoimmune bullous diseases in the oral cavity was still difficult. According to the survey of Sirois et al. [19] diagnostic delays greater than 6 months were common in oral PV, but 100% of cutaneous PV patients were correctly diagnosed within 6 months. Mobini et al. [36] reported that the mean period from onset of the disease until diagnosis was 7.57 months in patients with MMP. In this study, diagnosis was delayed more than 1 year for 16.7% of the MMP patients. This may be related to the characteristics of MMP. The initial symptoms of MMP often tend to undergo repeated episodes of onset and remission, and spontaneous remission was also observed in a few MMP patients. Furthermore, obtaining diagnostic biopsies from MMP patients is technically challenging. An inadequate surgical technique or surgical site selection, or improper tissue handling may easily lead to the loss of the gingival epithelium [25, 34, 37]. Four of the patients diagnosed with MMP at the author's clinic were previously biopsied at other facilities, but diagnosis was not rendered. This may be because the intact epithelium was not retained in those specimens. To avoid this problem, the authors reported a stab-and-roll biopsy technique designed to maintain the gingival epithelium for patients with DG [25, 34]. In this technique, more than 90% of biopsies were obtained exhibiting successful retention of intact epithelium, and all biopsies offered diagnostic support [34]. This biopsy technique may facilitate early diagnosis and treatment of diseases causing DG.

To establish a correct diagnosis of DG-associated diseases, conventional microscopic examination and DIF testing are essential. In particular, DIF testing is the gold standard used to diagnose autoimmune bullous diseases and is required for a definitive diagnosis [25, 33, 38]. In this study, all 37 autoimmune bullous diseases showed positive DIF staining. In H&E findings, acantholysis and a suprabasilar separation in the epithelium was observed in all 13 patients with PV. In contrast, a subepithelial separation was observed in 20 patients with MMP (83.3%). Since epithelial acantholysis is quite distinctive, it may be possible that correct diagnosis to be rendered based on H&E findings alone [38]. In contrast, the subepithelial separation, which is a characteristic of MMP patients, is a nondiagnostic finding as it is also found in other vesiculobullous diseases. Therefore, the international expert consensus on MMP does not consider results from conventional microscopic studies as an absolute criterion for the diagnosis [2].

In this study, extraoral lesions were confirmed in 11 of the 37 cases (29.7%) at the time of diagnosis. Since the oral cavity is the site of most problematic lesions, the patients came to the author's hospital first. Concomitant extraoral lesions were more common in MMP, and the patients tended to be affected in multiple mucosal sites or skin. Multiple target antigens of MMP were identified in BMZ components by the appearance of circulating autoantibodies in the patients' serum [2–5]. Therefore, it is currently believed that MMP is not a single entity but has distinct clinical subsets. For example, some MMP patients have involvement limited to the conjunctiva. They are referred to as having ocular cicatricial pemphigoid [39, 40]. Similarly, Mobini et al. [36] proposed that the MMP lesions confined only to the oral cavity are called "oral pemphigoid." In these clinical subsets, other mucous membranes and/or skin are not involved at long-term follow-up [4, 36, 41]. Di Zenzo et al. [42] pointed out in their review that it is important to know whether the exclusive oral lesion is only a stage of the course of MMP or if it represents the phenotype of a distinct clinical entity. In some long-term studies, MMP patients with exclusively oral lesions show that lesions do not develop in other mucous membranes and/or skin during follow-up [4, 36, 41]. In contrast, other studies indicate that MMP patients with initial oral lesions have a risk of developing ocular involvement with a calculated incidence rate from 0.03 to 0.05 persons per year [28, 29]. Several authorities suggest that early diagnosis of ocular MMP lesions is essential to successful management yet early signs of MMP may not be readily evident to other healthcare workers. Consequently, it may be advisable to refer any MMP patient to an ophthalmologist for immediate and long-term follow-up. Although there is a possibility that the clinical subset of MMP is classified based on the antibody profiles in their serum [3], at present, there is no known correlation between antigen-specific autoantibodies and the prognosis of disease [2].

PV frequently begins with oral lesions and later progresses to skin lesions [19]. Patients with PV with exclusively oral lesions should be followed closely and referred to other experts immediately if they develop signs or symptoms of lesions elsewhere on the body. Although the necessity of systemic therapy is decided with reference to the circulating anti-Dsg antibody titer in some cases, the therapeutic approach to PV is largely based on expert opinion rather than empirical evidence [43–46]. The monitoring of PV disease activity is mainly based on clinical findings at the present moment [43, 45, 46]. In any case, PV limited to oral cavity should be followed for a long period of time and perhaps indefinitely.

5. Conclusion

DG is an early sign of autoimmune bullous diseases such as MMP or PV in the oral cavity. In this study, about 70% of the oral lesions are confined to the gingiva, and DG was the only manifestation of the diseases. To establish a correct diagnosis of DG caused by autoimmune bullous diseases, conventional microscopic examination and DIF testing are essential. In particular, DIF testing is the gold standard used to diagnose of MMP or PV. Since some lesions remain limited to the oral cavity for a long period of time, patients diagnosed with MMP or PV should be closely followed because they must be immediately referred to other experts when they develop lesions on parts of their body other than the oral cavity. The oral healthcare provider should collaborate with other healthcare experts including dermatologists, ophthalmologists, and otolaryngologists to evaluate and manage patients with autoimmune bullous diseases in the oral cavity.

Acknowledgements

This study was supported by a Grant-in-Aid for Young Researcher Scientists, Nihon University School of Dentistry at Matsudo (2015). The authors report no conflicts of interest related to this study.

Author details

Hiroyasu Endo[1]*, Terry D. Rees[2], Hideo Niwa[3], Kayo Kuyama[4], Maya Oshima[5], Tae Serizawa[5], Shigeo Tanaka[5], Morio Iijima[6], Masamichi Komiya[5] and Takanori Ito[1]

*Address all correspondence to: endo.hiroyasu@nihon-u.ac.jp

1 Department of Oral Diagnosis, School of Dentistry at Matsudo, Nihon University, Japan

2 Department of Periodontics, Texas A&M College of Dentistry, Dallas, TX, USA

3 Department of Head and Neck Surgery, School of Dentistry at Matsudo, Nihon University, Japan

4 Department of Oral Pathology, School of Dentistry at Matsudo, Nihon University, Japan

5 Department of Oral Surgery, School of Dentistry at Matsudo, Nihon University, Japan

6 Department of Removable Prosthodontics, School of Dentistry at Matsudo, Nihon University, Japan

References

[1] Casiglia J, Woo SB, Ahmed AR. Oral involvement in autoimmune blistering diseases. Clinics in Dermatology. 2001;**19**:737-741

[2] Chan LS, Ahmed AR, Anhalt GJ, et al. The first international consensus on mucous membrane pemphigoid: Definition, diagnostic criteria, pathogenic factors, medical treatment, and prognostic indicators. Archives of Dermatology. 2002;**138**:370-379

[3] Rashid KA, Gurcan HM, Ahmed AR. Antigen specificity in subsets of mucous membrane pemphigoid. The Journal of Investigative Dermatology. 2006;**126**:2631-2636. DOI: 10.1038/sj.jid.5700465

[4] Calabresi V, Carrozzo M, Cozzani E, et al. Oral pemphigoid autoantibodies preferentially target BP180 ectodomain. Clinical Immunology. 2007;**122**:207-213. DOI: 10.1016/j.clim.2006.10.007

[5] Bernard P, Antonicelli F, Bedane C, et al. Prevalence and clinical significance of anti-laminin 332 autoantibodies detected by a novel enzyme-linked immunosorbent assay in

mucous membrane pemphigoid. JAMA Dermatology. 2013;**149**:533-540. DOI: 10.1001/jamadermatol.2013.1434

[6] Ahmed AR, Hombal SM. Cicatricial pemphigoid. International Journal of Dermatology. 1986;**25**:90-96

[7] Hanson RD, Olsen KD, Rogers RS 3rd. Upper aerodigestive tract manifestations of cicatricial pemphigoid. The Annals of Otology, Rhinology, and Laryngology 1988;**97**:493-499

[8] Lamey PJ, Rees TD, Binnie WH, Rankin KV. Mucous membrane pemphigoid. Treatment experience at two institutions. Oral Surgery, Oral Medicine, Oral Pathology, and Oral Radiology. 1992;**74**:50-53

[9] Endo H, Rees TD, Kuyama K, Kono Y, Yamamoto H. Clinical and diagnostic features of mucous membrane pemphigoid. The Compendium of Continuing Education in Dentistry. 2006;**27**:512-516 quiz 517-518

[10] Endo H, Rees TD, Niwa H, Kuyama K, Yamamoto H, Ito T. Desquamative gingivitis as an oral manifestation of mucous membrane pemphigoid: Diagnosis and treatment. In: Vega JP, editor. Advances in Dermatology Research. New York, USA: Nova Science Publishers; 2015. pp. 73-86. ISBN: 978-1-63482-226-8. Available from: https://www.novapublishers.com/catalog/product_info.php?products_id=54901 Accessed: 2017-09-23

[11] Amagai M, Klaus-Kovtun V, Stanley JR. Autoantibodies against a novel epithelial cadherin in pemphigus vulgaris, a disease of cell adhesion. Cell. 1991;**67**:869-877

[12] Amagai M, Tsunoda K, Zillikens D, Nagai T, Nishikawa T. The clinical phenotype of pemphigus is defined by the anti-desmoglein autoantibody profile. Journal of the American Academy of Dermatology. 1999;**40**:167-170

[13] Endo H, Rees TD, Matsue M, Kuyama K, Nakadai M, Yamamoto H. Early detection and successful management of oral pemphigus vulgaris: A case report. Journal of Periodontology. 2005;**76**:154-160. DOI: 10.1902/jop.2005.76.1.154

[14] Endo H, Rees TD, Hallmon WW, et al. Disease progression from mucosal to mucocutaneous involvement in a patient with desquamative gingivitis associated with pemphigus vulgaris. Journal of Periodontology. 2008;**79**:369-375. DOI: 10.1902/jop.2008.070258

[15] Amagai M. Autoimmunity against desmosomal cadherins in pemphigus. Journal of Dermatological Science. 1999;**20**:92-102

[16] Chams-Davatchi C, Valikhani M, Daneshpazhooh M, et al. Pemphigus: Analysis of 1209 cases. International Journal of Dermatology. 2005;**44**:470-476. DOI: 10.1111/j.1365-4632.2004.02501.x

[17] Lamey PJ, Rees TD, Binnie WH, Wright JM, Rankin KV, Simpson NB. Oral presentation of pemphigus vulgaris and its response to systemic steroid therapy. Oral Surgery, Oral Medicine, and Oral Pathology. 1992;**74**:54-57

[18] Scully C, Paes De Almeida O, Porter SR, Gilkes JJ. Pemphigus vulgaris: The manifestations and long-term management of 55 patients with oral lesions. The British Journal of Dermatology. 1999;**140**:84-89

[19] Sirois DA, Fatahzadeh M, Roth R, Ettlin D. Diagnostic patterns and delays in pemphigus vulgaris: Experience with 99 patients. Archives of Dermatology. 2000;**136**:1569-1570

[20] Suresh L, Neiders ME. Definitive and differential diagnosis of desquamative gingivitis through direct immunofluorescence studies. Journal of Periodontology. 2012;**83**:1270-1278. DOI: 10.1902/jop.2012.110627

[21] Endo H, Rees TD, Niwa H, et al. Desquamative gingivitis as the initial presentation of autoimmune bullous diseases. In: Karpinski TM, editor. Health and Diseases of Oral Cavity. Poznan, Poland: JBBooks; 2017. pp. 2-21. DOI: 10.5281/zenodo.918266. Available from: http://books.tmkarpinski.com/10-Karpinski-2017.pdf [Accessed: 2017-09-23]

[22] Rees TD. Vesiculo-ulcerative diseases and periodontal practice. Journal of Periodontology. 1995;**66**:747-748

[23] Endo H, Rees TD. Diagnosis and management of desquamative gingivitis. In: Panagakos FS, Davies RM, editors. Gingival Diseases—Their Aetiology, Prevention and Treatment. Rijeka, Croatia: InTech; 2011. pp. 171-188. DOI: 10.5772/22864 Available from: http://www.intechopen.com/articles/show/title/diagnosis-and-management-of-desquamative-gingivitis [Accessed: 2017-02-09]

[24] Endo H, Rees TD, Niwa H, et al. Desquamative gingivitis. In: Manakil JF, editor. Insights into Various Aspects of Oral Health. Rijeka, Croatia: InTech; 2017. pp. 3-27. DOI: 10.5772/intechopen.69268. Available from: Bhttps://www.intechopen.com/books/insights-into-various-aspects-of-oral-health/desquamative-gingivitis [Accessed: 2017-09-23]

[25] Rees TD, Burkhart N. Desquamative Gingivitis [Internet]. 2016. Available from: https://www.dentalcare.com/en-us/professional-education/ce-courses/ce481 [Accessed: 2017-02-09]

[26] Lo Russo L, Fedele S, Guiglia R, et al. Diagnostic pathways and clinical significance of desquamative gingivitis. Journal of Periodontology. 2008;**79**:4-24. DOI: 10.1902/jop.2008.070231

[27] Mignogna MD, Fortuna G, Leuci S, Ruoppo E, Marasca F, Matarasso S. Nikolsky's sign on the gingival mucosa: A clinical tool for oral health practitioners. Journal of Periodontology. 2008;**79**:2241-2246. DOI: 10.1902/jop.2008.080217

[28] Higgins GT, Allan RB, Hall R, Field EA, Kaye SB. Development of ocular disease in patients with mucous membrane pemphigoid involving the oral mucosa. The British Journal of Ophthalmology. 2006;**90**:964-967. DOI: 10.1136/bjo.2006.092528

[29] Thorne JE, Anhalt GJ, Jabs DA. Mucous membrane pemphigoid and pseudopemphigoid. Ophthalmology. 2004;**111**:45-52. DOI: 10.1016/j.ophtha.2003.03.001

[30] Alexandre M, Brette MD, Pascal F, et al. A prospective study of upper aerodigestive tract manifestations of mucous membrane pemphigoid. Medicine (Baltimore). 2006;**85**: 239-252. DOI: 10.1097/01.md.0000231954.08350.52

[31] Higgins TS, Cohen JC, Sinacori JT. Laryngeal mucous membrane pemphigoid: A systematic review and pooled-data analysis. The Laryngoscope. 2010;**120**:529-536. DOI: 10.1002/lary.20763

[32] Nair PS, Moorthy PK, Yogiragan K. A study of mortality in dermatology. Indian Journal of Dermatology, Venereology and Leprology. 2005;**71**:23-25

[33] Rees TD. Desquamative gingivitis/mucocutaneous diseases commonly affecting the gingiva. In: Harpenau LA, Kao RT, Lundergan WP, Sanz M, editors. Hall's Critical Decisions in Periodontology and Dental Implantology. 5th ed. Shelton, Connecticut: People's Medical Publishing House; 2013. pp. 68-73

[34] Endo H, Rees TD, Allen EP, et al. A stab-and-roll biopsy technique to maintain gingival epithelium for desquamative gingivitis. Journal of Periodontology. 2014;**85**:802-809. DOI: 10.1902/jop.2014.130428

[35] Mignogna MD, Lo Muzio L, Bucci E. Clinical features of gingival pemphigus vulgaris. Journal of Clinical Periodontology. 2001;**28**:489-493

[36] Mobini N, Nagarwalla N, Ahmed AR. Oral pemphigoid. Subset of cicatricial pemphigoid? Oral Surgery, Oral Medicine, Oral Pathology, Oral Radiology, and Endodontology. 1998;**85**:37-43

[37] Sano SM, Quarracino MC, Aguas SC, et al. Sensitivity of direct immunofluorescence in oral diseases. Study of 125 cases. Medicina Oral, Patología Oral y Cirugía Bucal. 2008; **13**:E287-E291

[38] Rinaggio J, Crossland DM, Zeid MY. A determination of the range of oral conditions submitted for microscopic and direct immunofluorescence analysis. Journal of Periodontology. 2007;**78**:1904-1910. DOI: 10.1902/jop.2007.070095

[39] Hoang-Xuan T, Robin H, Demers PE, et al. Pure ocular cicatricial pemphigoid. A distinct immunopathologic subset of cicatricial pemphigoid. Ophthalmology. 1999;**106**:355-361

[40] Chan LS, Yancey KB, Hammerberg C, et al. Immune-mediated subepithelial blistering diseases of mucous membranes. Pure ocular cicatricial pemphigoid is a unique clinical and immunopathological entity distinct from bullous pemphigoid and other subsets identified by antigenic specificity of autoantibodies. Archives of Dermatology. 1993; **129**:448-455

[41] Malik M, Gurcan HM, Christen W, Ahmed AR. Relationship between cancer and oral pemphigoid patients with antibodies to alpha6-integrin. Journal of Oral Pathology & Medicine. 2007;**36**:1-5. DOI: 10.1111/j.1600-0714.2006.00483.x

[42] Di Zenzo G, Carrozzo M, Chan LS. Urban legend series: Mucous membrane pemphigoid. Oral Diseases. 2014;**20**:35-54. DOI: 10.1111/odi.12193

[43] Amagai M, Tanikawa A, Shimizu T, et al. Japanese guidelines for the management of pemphigus. Committee for guidelines for the management of pemphigus disease. The Journal of Dermatology. 2014;**41**:471-486. DOI: 10.1111/1346-8138.12486

[44] McMillan R, Taylor J, Shephard M, et al. World workshop on oral medicine VI: A systematic review of the treatment of mucocutaneous pemphigus vulgaris. Oral Surgery, Oral Medicine, Oral Pathology, Oral Radiology. 2015;**120**:132-142.e61. DOI: 10.1016/j.oooo.2015.01.022

[45] Harman KE, Albert S, Black MM. Guidelines for the management of pemphigus vulgaris. The British Journal of Dermatology. 2003;**149**:926-937

[46] Mimouni D, Nousari CH, Cummins DL, Kouba DJ, David M, Anhalt GJ. Differences and similarities among expert opinions on the diagnosis and treatment of pemphigus vulgaris. Journal of the American Academy of Dermatology. 2003;**49**:1059-1062. DOI: 10.1016/S0190

8

Optical Diagnostics to Improve Periodontal Diagnosis and Treatment

Fardad Shakibaie and Laurence Walsh

Abstract

The performance of clinicians undertaking periodontal assessment or periodontal therapy can be improved by using optical methods as adjuncts to visual inspection and periodontal probing. Subtle changes that occur over time in periodontal tissues that are below the detection limit of visual examination or periodontal probing can be found and tracked accurately over time using 3D imaging, fluorescence spectroscopy, and optical coherence tomography. During debridement of teeth and dental implants, the effective removal of subgingival microbial biofilms and dental calculus deposits can be enhanced using magnifying loupes and operating microscopes and by novel methods based on the interactions of light with bacterial deposits, such as differential reflectometry and light-induced fluorescence. While such techniques can also be used using initial case assessment, their primary purpose is for checking debridement procedures, since the point when bacterial deposits are no longer present represents an endpoint for treatment. The concept of real-time feedback has been developed, using fluorescence readings to control the removal of deposits. Overall, optical methods can support traditional periodontal diagnosis and improve treatment planning and clinical periodontal care.

Keywords: periodontal diagnosis, fluorescence imaging, laser-induced fluorescence, porphyrins, fluorescence spectroscopy, differential reflectometry, optical coherence tomography

1. Introduction

The standard approaches that are used in periodontal diagnosis are less than perfect in terms of their clinical performance. Tactile assessment of periodontal soft tissues and root surfaces using periodontal probes of various types provides useful information, but the results are influenced by the design of the probe, the probing force applied, and the extent of inflammation in the tissue

Technology	Clinical applications
3D Optical scanning	Monitor graft sites
	Track recession over time
	Track gingival enlargement over time
Optical spectroscopy	Distinguish periodontitis sites from gingivitis
	Distinguish peri-implantitis from peri-implant mucositis
OCT	All of the above applications, plus the following:
	Measure the thickness of the gingival tissues
	Assess biological width
	Detect deposits of subgingival calculus
	Early detection of bone loss and bone formation

Table 1. Applications of optical diagnostic systems for periodontal patient assessment.

[1–3]. It is not possible to relate periodontal probing measurements to precise histological measurements of actual sulcus or pocket depths. During clinical probing, the periodontal tissues are compressed and displaced, and the junctional epithelium may or may not be perforated [4, 5].

There are also issues with being able to reliably detect subgingival calculus on root surfaces using tactile feedback from a periodontal probe [6, 7]. While supragingival calculus is easily seen, deposits of subgingival calculus are hidden from view and are difficult to detect [8, 9].

Given these limitations, there has been long standing interest in additional methods that could be used to augment traditional periodontal clinical examination (**Table 1**). Using optical methods has the major advantage of patient safety, since light with low photon energy is nonionizing (unlike dental X-rays). This chapter summarizes the use of optical diagnostic devices in periodontics, for the assessment of periodontal soft or hard tissues (including the subgingival surfaces of tooth roots and dental implants), and discusses the use of such devices to better inform the clinician during subgingival debridement. By better monitoring the progress of debridement during a treatment session, the frequency of iatrogenic problems such as instrument-induced damage to the treated surfaces and excessive removal of root structure should be reduced.

2. Assessment of periodontal tissues at baseline and recall periodontal examinations

2.1. Three dimensional optical scanning

Intra-oral 3D scanners that are used to scan tooth preparation for CAD-CAM restorations also record exquisite details of the form and color of the periodontal soft tissues. Periodontal parameters of interest that can be measured from such scans include the height and width of areas of recession, the changes in contours of sites that have undergone grafting or augmentation procedures, and the progressive development of areas of gingival enlargement. By comparing measurements from 3D scans over time, the clinician can track subtle changes in soft tissue architecture between dental appointments [10, 11].

Studies comparing clinical measurements with digital measurements taken from intra-oral 3D scans, or from 3D scans of study models, have shown that digital measurements taken from 3D scans are more reliable than those taken in the clinical measurements [12]. A series of 3D scans will document changes in tissue volume and color over time, making it an ideal way to track outcomes of grafting procedures. One can predict that data from 3D intra-oral scans will become the new gold standard in periodontal practice for monitoring patients being treated surgically for muco-gingival problems or who have undergone surgery for gingival overgrowth. It has been suggested that high definition color 3D intra-oral scans could even eventually replace both intraoral photographs and study models. This trend has already been seen in orthodontics [13].

2.2. Optical spectroscopy using near-infrared light

This optical method is a simple, yet powerful addition to the diagnostic armamentarium of periodontal practice. It has been used for many years in medicine and agriculture for the noninvasive assessment of the composition of biological tissues. In periodontics, a portable spectrometer can be used to measure blood flow and inflammation in the periodontal tissues. Optical spectroscopy using near-infrared light provides information on tissue oxygenation, the various forms of hemoglobin present, and tissue edema. There are higher concentrations of deoxyhemoglobin (and thus less tissue oxygenation) at sites of periodontitis, compared to sites with gingivitis or healthy sites [14]. Thus, in any one patient, this method can be used to discriminate between sites with periodontitis, as opposed to sites with gingivitis [15–17]. The same approach can be used to monitor peri-implant disease, because tissue oxygenation at peri-implantitis sites is lower than at healthy sites [18, 19], even when the patient is a smoker.

2.3. Optical coherence tomography

For detailed examination of periodontal hard and soft tissues, optical coherence tomography (OCT) is superior to other approaches because it can provide the three dimensional tissue contour information of an intra-oral 3D scan, as well as cross-sectional images at high resolution that are comparable to histology.

The use of OCT systems for imaging of hard and soft tissues in the oral cavity has been investigated for more than 20 years. Dental OCT systems work on the same principles as their medical OCT counterparts, such as the systems used in ophthalmology, but they require specially designed delivery systems for use in the confined environment of the mouth. The light source in a typical OCT system is a near infrared diode laser that emits light with a wavelength between 850 and 1310 nm. This light penetrates well through teeth, bone, and soft tissues [20]. OCT images have very high resolution (1–15 μm), with a level of detail that surpasses other clinical imaging systems, including ultrasound and radiography [20, 21].

The first dental OCT system suitable for intra-oral use was built in 1998, and was used to obtain high resolution images of periodontal tissues in the laboratory setting. The OCT images revealed details of the cemento-enamel junction and the interface between the teeth and the gingival tissues [21, 22]. When used in the clinical setting, this OCT system provided visual recordings of periodontal tissue contour, sulcular depth, and connective tissue attachment [23, 24], and provided a cross-sectional "optical biopsy" of tissue, up to a depth of 3 mm from the surface [25, 26]. In later OCT systems, the penetration was increased to 4 mm by using longer wavelengths of light (up to 1325 nm) [27].

Using OCT, the thickness of the gingival tissues and the constituent epithelial and connective tissues can be measured, as well as the biological width and the position of alveolar bone crest [28], and the location of any deposits of subgingival calculus, to a high resolution that surpasses traditional methods [29, 30].

The high resolution of OCT allows cellular level details to be seen, including subtle changes in the width of the periodontal ligament, or in the depth of the gingival sulcus [31–34]. Early detection of bone loss is possible. OCT can also be used for checking debridement, and for monitoring the response to periodontal treatment [35].

As the technology for deploying OCT systems into intra-oral handpieces improves, it will become more accessible for use in clinical dental practice as a noninvasive method for imaging the microstructural detail of periodontal tissues *in situ*. Over time, it could replace some current applications of radiology or other diagnostic approaches, as has occurred in some fields of medicine [36].

3. Optical devices for assessing subgingival deposits and monitoring their removal during periodontal debridement

3.1. Conventional optical magnification devices

During closed periodontal debridement or open debridement, improved visibility for ensuring that all deposits are removed properly can be gained using optical magnifying devices, such as operating microscopes and telescopic loupes. Operating microscopes are particularly useful during surgical periodontal therapy, because the lighting is coaxial, giving a well-illuminated site [37–39]. In contemporary specialist periodontal practice, telescopic loupes are more popular than operating microscopes [40].

Fiber optic periodontal endoscopes ("perio-scopes") are an important further part of the armamentarium. These devices are a modification of medical endoscope technology, and use a small rigid optical element or a fixed, fused fiber optic bundle. In both cases, the tip is less than 1 mm in diameter, so that it can be fitted inside a periodontal pocket with only minimal reflection of the adjacent soft tissues. The images from a perio-scope are displayed on a video monitor. In some perio-scopes, a dual lumen allows irrigation of the periodontal environment to improve the clarity of the field that is being viewed [41].

Because effective debridement is difficult in deep pockets and furcation areas [42], perio-scopes are particularly useful for monitoring the removal of subgingival deposits in such locations [41, 43, 44]. Perio-scope images will also show scratches and gouges of the root surface created by instruments. These types of surface irregularities make tactile assessment of root surfaces challenging, as the roughness could be misinterpreted as indicating that calculus deposits are still present [41]. The benefits of using a perio-scope have been shown in clinical studies using teeth destined for removal during a complete dental clearance. In these studies, the quality of subgingival debridement of interproximal root surfaces was improved when perio-scopes were used, with a significantly reduced area of residual deposits compared to conventional debridement [43, 44].

To use a perio-scope effectively, the clinician has to learn how to position and manipulate the imaging tip while viewing the image [43, 44]. Interpreting the image requires training, as the typically dark color of subgingival calculus may be less apparent due to variations in lighting as the perio-scope tip approaches the surface of the calculus. The clinician must use considerable care when moving the perio-scope tip, to prevent damage to the optical components. In some cases, using gas shielding or irrigation during viewing is necessary to gain a clear image and overcome problems of fogging and fouling of the optics during use [45].

3.2. Differential reflectometry

In this optical approach, the root surface is illuminated through a narrow optical tip that is similar in size to a periodontal probe. Two light sources are used, typically visible red light (623 nm) and near infrared light (880 nm). The spectral distribution of the reflected light is analyzed to detect the presence of calculus. The readout indicates when calculus is present, via an audible alert tone. Differential reflectometry is more accurate than tactile assessment for assessing deposits of subgingival calculus on the root surfaces of teeth than a periodontal probe [46].

3.3. Laser fluorescence using visible red light and the DIAGNOdent™

As a means to detect subgingival deposits of calculus remaining after debridement, laser-induced fluorescence (LF) seems ideal, since it can provide a numerical assessment of the volume of the remaining deposits in real time, using an optical probe that is similar in shape to a periodontal probe. LF readings are highly reproducible over time. When using LF at intervals during debridement, LF scores will reduce as calculus is removed. When the LF score reaches the threshold for a healthy root surface, the clinician has reached the endpoint of complete removal of calculus.

When LF is undertaken using 655 nm visible red laser light as the excitation source, the remaining deposits of subgingival calculus emit strong near infrared fluorescence at 720 nm, but these do not occur with sound root surfaces [47]. Using visible red excitation means that the light penetrates through blood and is not masked by any bleeding from the site [48].

In the DIAGNOdent™ Classic and the DIAGNOdent™ Pen (KaVo, Biberach, Germany), the 655 nm light is generated by an In:Ga:As:P diode laser. This light then elicits the near infrared fluorescence from the bacterial porphyrins contained within the subgingival calculus deposits [49]. The optical pathway is designed so that reflected light and any ambient light (from daylight and operatory lighting) is removed using a high-pass (680 nm cutoff) filter. The longer near infrared wavelengths of light pass through the filter to reach a time-gated detector. Finally, the intensity of the fluorescent radiation is presented to the user as a digital value (on a 0–99 scale). Once the LF reading has reduced to the baseline value for cementum or healthy dentine (e.g. an LF score of 7), no further calculus deposits remain, and the endpoint for instrumentation has been reached [50, 51]. Key clinical aspects of using LF devices are summarized in **Table 2** below.

In terms of overall performance, LF is superior to both differential reflectometry and conventional periodontal probing for detecting subgingival calculus [52, 53]. The usefulness of LF has led to the concept of fluorescence-controlled ablation of subgingival bacterial deposits. The debridement component is undertaken using a pulsed Er:YAG laser which generates middle infrared light that is strongly absorbed in water [54]. The Er:YAG laser gives effective calculus removal when low energy pulses are applied onto the root surface at a shallow angle [55–57]. In addition to physically removing calculus and biofilms, the Er:YAG laser pulses have little or no effect on the surfaces of teeth or dental implants. The laser pulses inactivate or vaporize bacteria, and reduce the biological activity of bacterial endotoxins [58–60].

In the KEY3™ laser system (KaVo, Biberach, Germany), the firing of Er:YAG laser pulses is controlled using the LF readings, which provide the feedback for the "autopilot". When used with LF control, the laser debridement process causes no adverse thermal effects on root surfaces [59, 60]. The treated root surfaces are biocompatible, and new cementum formation and the formation of new connective tissue attachment can occur following treatment [61]. Clinical studies of root surface instrumentation have shown that superior removal of subgingival calculus occurs, but without any undesirable surface alterations caused by instrumentation [62, 63]. This means that fluorescence-controlled Er:YAG laser debridement of root surfaces is a direct but superior replacement for conventional closed periodontal debridement undertaken with hand or ultrasonic instruments [64–66].

The same concepts of LF guidance can be applied to subgingival implant surfaces. Er:YAG laser treatment guided by LF removes microbial contamination. The lased surface is biocompatible, and supports adhesion and growth of osteoblasts [67, 68].

When using LF, it is essential that the clinician interprets correctly the readings that guide their decision around when to stop treatment. The LF readings from the DIAGNOdent Classic, Pen, and KEY3 laser correlate to the surface area and volume of subgingival calculus deposits [69].

- Keep the optical components (tips) free of visible contamination
- Calibrate the fluorescence system daily as per the manufacturer's instructions
- Hold the working tip with a light touch and do not apply strong force against the surface being assessed
- When working around restorations, be aware of endogenous fluorescence of restorative materials
- Teeth with discoloration from first and second generation tetracycline antibiotics will have elevated background fluorescence
- Lesions of root surface caries will give strong fluorescence readings
- Ensure that the correct threshold value is being used for the instrument readings

Table 2. Major aspects of clinical technique when using laser fluorescence for detection of subgingival calculus and dental plaque biofilms.

Thus, if readings remain high at a particular site, deposits remain and further debridement is needed. Depending on which LF device is being used, the clinician may need to adjust their decision point. The reason for this is that there are subtle performance differences between the three systems. The KEY3 gives superior accuracy and reproducibility over the DIAGNOdent Pen and the DIAGNOdent Classic [52, 69, 70]. The threshold LF reading for the boundary between a healthy root surface (or implant surface) and bacterial deposits is 5 for the DIAGNOdent Classic, but 7 for the DIAGNOdent Pen and KEY3 laser.

3.4. Fluorescence detection of dental calculus using other wavelengths of light

The fluorescence concepts that underpin LF can be applied using nonlaser light sources, using wavelengths of light other than those in the visible red portion of the spectrum to excite the target tissue. Ultraviolet light (315–400 nm), violet light (405 nm) and visible blue light (400–420 nm) will all generate fluorescence emissions in the visible red region [71–75] (**Figure 1**). The major fluorophores are the porphyrins, particularly protoporphyrin IX, which emits at 633 nm [73]. This approach has been used for detecting mature deposits of supragingival plaque and calculus.

In an intra-oral camera, a long pass orange filter placed over the imaging sensor will remove reflected light [72]. This direct imaging approach cannot however be used for viewing subgingival surfaces during patient examination or during debridement.

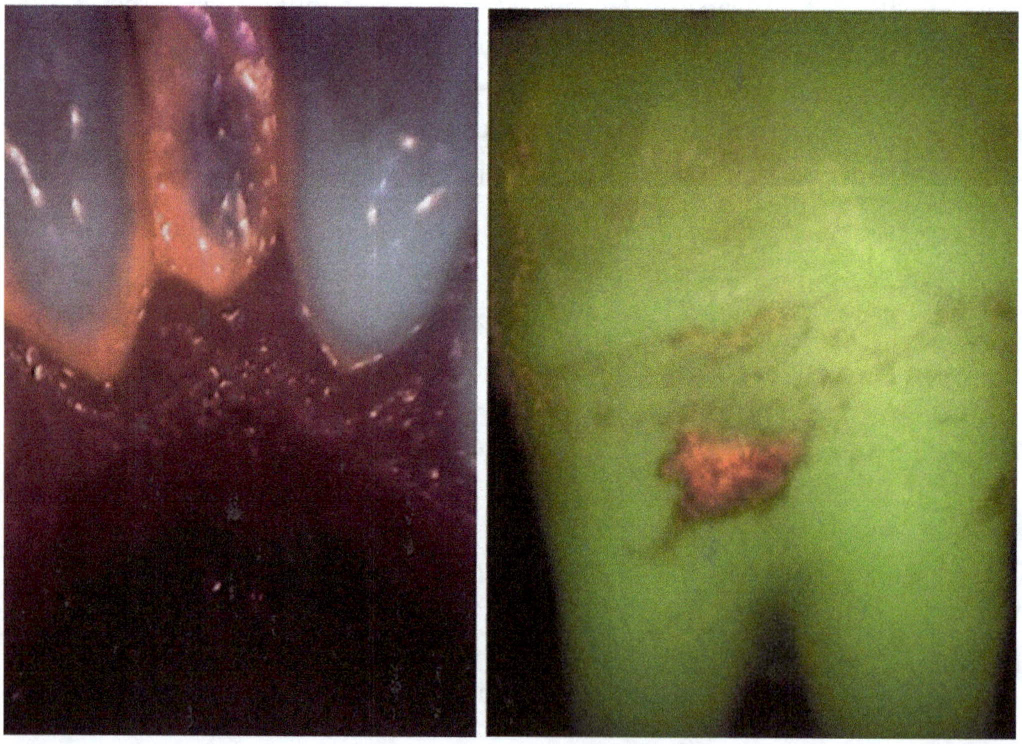

Figure 1. Visible red fluorescence emissions produced by calculus when excited with 405 nm violet light. Left side, supragingival calculus deposits on lingual aspects of mandibular incisor teeth, prior to a debridement visit. Right side, subgingival calculus deposits in the buccal furcation area of an extracted mandibular molar tooth. This location would not be visible using an intra-oral camera unless the patient was having periodontal flap surgery.

4. Conclusions

Optical methods are promising diagnostic technologies that can be used to augment traditional periodontal examination. A key factor that supports the use of optical devices as diagnostic adjuncts is that they are safe, and employ nonionizing radiation, thus making them suitable for frequent use in clinical practice on the same patient. 3D scanning, fluorescence spectroscopy and OCT can all provide valuable information on periodontal soft tissues and their relationship to teeth and dental implants. Light-induced fluorescence can provide improved detection of subgingival calculus during debridement.

Acknowledgements

This work was supported by grants from the Australian Society of Periodontology Research Foundation (APRF) and the Australian Dental Research Foundation (ADRF). Both authors report no conflicts of interest relating to the work described in this chapter.

Author details

Fardad Shakibaie and Laurence Walsh*

*Address all correspondence to: l.walsh@uq.edu.au

School of Dentistry, The University of Queensland, Brisbane, Australia

References

[1] van der Velden U. Influence of periodontal health on probing depth and bleeding tendency. Journal of Clinical Periodontology. 1980;**7**:129-139. DOI: 10.1111/j.1600-051X.1980.tb01956.x

[2] Mombelli A, Graf H. Depth-force-patterns in periodontal probing. Journal of Clinical Periodontology. 1986;**13**:126-130. DOI: 10.1111/j.1600-051X.1986.tb01444.x

[3] Garnick JJ, Silverstein L. Periodontal probing: Probe tip diameter. Journal of Periodontology. 2000;**71**:96-103. DOI: 10.1902/jop.2000.71.1.96

[4] Listgarten MA. Periodontal probing: What does it mean? Journal of Clinical Periodontology. 1980;**7**:165-176. DOI: 10.1111/j.1600-051X.1980.tb01960.x

[5] Jansen J, Pilot T, Corba N. Histologic evaluation of probe penetration during clinical assessment of periodontal attachment levels. An investigation of experimentally induced

periodontal lesions in beagle dogs. Journal of Clinical Periodontology. 1981;**8**:98-106. DOI: 10.1111/j.1600-051X.1981.tb02349.x

[6] Clerehugh V, Abdeia R, Hull PS. The effect of subgingival calculus on the validity of clinical probing measurements. Journal of Dentistry. 1996;**24**:329-333. DOI: 10.1016/0300-5712(95)00095-X

[7] Hefti AF. Periodontal probing. Critical Reviews in Oral Biology and Medicine. 1997;**8**:336-356

[8] Anerud A, Löe H, Boysen H. The natural history and clinical course of calculus formation in man. Journal of Clinical Periodontology. 1991;**18**:160-170. DOI: 10.1111/j.1600-051X.1991.tb01128.x

[9] Pippin DJ, Feil P. Interrater agreement on subgingival calculus detection following scaling. Journal of Dental Education. 1992;**56**:322-326

[10] Lehmann KM, Kasaj A, Ross A, Willershausen I, Schmidtmann I, Staedt H, Scheller H. A novel method for evaluating periodontal recession: A feasibility study. International Journal of Computerized Dentistry. 2011;**14**:297-307

[11] Lehmann KM, Kasaj A, Ross A, Kämmerer PW, Wagner W, Scheller H. A new method for volumetric evaluation of gingival recessions: A feasibility study. Journal of Periodontology. 2012;**83**:50-54. DOI: 10.1902/jop.2011.110143

[12] Schneider D, Ender A, Truninger T, Leutert C, Sahrmann P, Roos M, Schmidlin P. Comparison between clinical and digital soft tissue measurements. Journal of Esthetic and Restorative Dentistry. 2014;**26**:191-199. DOI: 10.1111/jerd.12084

[13] Rossini G, Parrini S, Castroflorio T, Deregibus A, Debernardi CL. Diagnostic accuracy and measurement sensitivity of digital models for orthodontic purposes: A systematic review. American Journal of Orthodontics and Dentofacial Orthopedics. 2016;**149**:161-170. DOI: 10.1016/j.ajodo.2015.06.029

[14] Liu KZ, Xiang XM, Man A, Sowa MG, Cholakis A, Ghiabi E, Singer DL, Scott DA. In vivo determination of multiple indices of periodontal inflammation by optical spectroscopy. Journal of Periodontal Research. 2009;**44**:117-124. DOI: 10.1111/j.1600-0765.2008.01112.x

[15] Xiang X, Sowa MG, Iacopino AM, Maev RG, Hewko MD, Man A, Liu KZ. An update on novel non-invasive approaches for periodontal diagnosis. Journal of Periodontology. 2010;**81**:186-198. DOI: 10.1902/jop.2009.090419

[16] Ge Z, Liu KZ, Xiang X, Yang Q, Hui J, Kohlenberg E, Sowa MG. Assessment of local hemodynamics in periodontal inflammation using optical spectroscopy. Journal of Periodontology. 2011;**82**:1161-1168. DOI: 10.1902/jop.2011.100632

[17] Zhang C, Xiang X, Xu M, Fan C, Sowa MG, Liu KZ. Assessment of tissue oxygenation of periodontal inflammation in patients with coronary artery diseases using optical spectroscopy. BMC Oral Health. 2014;**14**:25. DOI: 10.1186/1472-6831-14-25

[18] Nogueira-Filho G, Xiang XM, Shibli JA, Duarte PM, Sowa MG, Ferrari DS, Onuma T, de Cardoso LA, Liu KZ. On site noninvasive assessment of peri-implant inflammation by optical spectroscopy. Journal of Periodontology. 2011;**46**:382-388. DOI: 10.1111/j.1600-0765.2011.01361.x

[19] Liu KZ, Duarte PM, Santos VR, Xiang X, Xu M, Miranda TS, Fermiano D, Gonçalves TE, Sowa MG. Assessment of tissue oxygenation of periodontal inflammation in smokers using optical spectroscopy. Journal of Clinical Periodontology. 2014;**41**:340-347. DOI: 10.1111/jcpe.12225

[20] Colston BW Jr, Everett MJ, Sathyam US, DaSilva LB, Otis LL. Imaging of the oral cavity using optical coherence tomography. Monographs in Oral Science. 2000;**17**:32-55

[21] Colston BW Jr, Everett MJ, Da Silva LB, Otis LL, Stroeve P, Nathel H. Imaging of hard- and soft-tissue structure in the oral cavity by optical coherence tomography. Applied Optics. 1998;**37**:3582-3585

[22] Colston B, Sathyam U, Dasilva L, Everett M, Stroeve P, Otis L. Dental OCT. Optics Express. 1998;**3**:230-238. DOI: 10.1364/OE.3.000230

[23] Otis LL, Everett MJ, Sathyam US, Colston BW Jr. Optical coherence tomography: A new imaging technology for dentistryJournal of the American Dental Association 2000;**131**: 511–514. DOI: 10.14219/jada.archive.2000.0210

[24] Otis LL, Colston BW Jr, Everett MJ, Nathel H. Dental optical coherence tomography: A comparison of two in vitro systems. Dento Maxillo Facial Radiology. 2000;**29**:85-89. DOI: 10.1038/sj/dmfr/4600507

[25] Feldchtein F, Gelikonov V, Iksanov R, Gelikonov G, Kuranov R, Sergeev A, Gladkova N, Ourutina M, Reitze D, Warren J. In vivo OCT imaging of hard and soft tissue of the oral cavity. Optics Express. 1998;**3**:239-250. DOI: 10.1364/OE.3.000239

[26] Gimbel C. Optical coherence tomography diagnostic imaging. General Dentistry. 2008;**56**: 750-757

[27] Mota CC, Fernandes LO, Cimões R, Gomes AS. Non-invasive periodontal probing through Fourier-domain optical coherence tomography. Journal of Periodontology. 2015; **86**:1087-1094. DOI: 10.1902/jop.2015.150047

[28] Park JY, Chung JH, Lee JS, Kim HJ, Choi SH, Jung UW. Comparisons of the diagnostic accuracies of optical coherence tomography, micro-computed tomography, and histology in periodontal disease: An ex vivo study. Journal of Periodontal and Implant Science. 2017; **47**:30-40. DOI: 10.5051/jpis.2017.47.1.30

[29] Tung OH, Lee SY, Lai YL, Chen HF. Detection of subgingival calculus through oral gum in vitro using two-photon fluorescence microscopy. Conference Proceedings IEEE Engineering in Medicine and Biology Society 2008;**2008**:4051-4054. DOI: 10.1109/IEMBS.2008.4650099

[30] Archana V. Calculus detection technologies: Where do we stand now? Journal of Medicine and Life. 2014;**7**(2):18-23

[31] Hsieh YS, Ho YC, Lee SY, Lu CW, Jiang CP, Chuang CC, Wang CY, Sun CW. Subgingival calculus imaging based on swept-source optical coherence tomography. Journal of Biomedical Optics. 2011;**16**:071409. DOI: 10.1117/1.3602851

[32] Kao MC, Lin CL, Kung CY, Huang YF, Kuo WC. Miniature endoscopic optical coherence tomography for calculus detection. Applied Optics. 2015;**54**:7419-7423. DOI: 10.1364/AO.54.007419

[33] Baek JH, Na J, Lee BH, Choi E, Son WS. Optical approach to the periodontal ligament under orthodontic tooth movement: A preliminary study with optical coherence tomography. American Journal of Orthodontics and Dentofacial Orthopedics. 2009;**135**:252-259. DOI: 10.1016/j.ajodo.2007.10.037

[34] Fernandes LO, Mota CCBO, de Melo LSA, da Costa Soares MUS, da Silva Feitosa D, Gomes ASL. In vivo assessment of periodontal structures and measurement of gingival sulcus with optical coherence tomography: A pilot study. Journal of Biophotonics. 2017;**10**:862-869. DOI: 10.1002/jbio.201600082

[35] Hsieh YS, Ho YC, Lee SY, Chuang CC, Tsai JC, Lin KF, Sun CW. Dental optical coherence tomography. Sensors (Basel). 2013;**13**:8928-8949. DOI: 10.3390/s130708928

[36] Kakizaki S, Aoki A, Tsubokawa M, Lin T, Mizutani K, Koshy G, Sadr A, Oda S, Sumi Y, Izumi Y. Observation and determination of periodontal tissue profile using optical coherence tomography. Journal of Periodontal Research. 2018;**53**:188-199. DOI: 10.1111/jre.12506

[37] Tibbetts LS, Shanelec D. Periodontal microsurgery. Dental Clinics of North America. 1998;**42**:339-359

[38] Belcher JM. A perspective on periodontal microsurgery. International Journal of Periodontics and Restorative Dentistry. 2001;**21**:191-196

[39] Hegde R, Sumanth S, Padhye A. Microscope-enhanced periodontal therapy: A review and report of four cases. The Journal of Contemporary Dental Practice. 2009;**10**:E088-E096

[40] Sitbon Y, Attathom T. Minimal intervention dentistry II: Part 6. Microscope and microsurgical techniques in periodontics. British Dental Journal. 2014;**216**:503-509. DOI: 10.1038/sj.bdj.2014.356

[41] Stambaugh RV, Myers G, Ebling W, Beckman B, Stambaugh K. Endoscopic visualization of the submarginal gingiva dental sulcus and tooth root surfaces. Journal of Periodontology. 2002;**73**:374-382. DOI: 10.1902/jop.2002.73.4.374

[42] Breininger DR, O'Leary TJ, Blumenshine RV. Comparative effectiveness of ultrasonic and hand scaling for the removal of subgingival plaque and calculus. Journal of Periodontology. 1987;**58**:9-18. DOI: 10.1902/jop.1987.58.1.9

[43] Reinhardt RA, Johnson GK, Tussing GJ. Root planing with interdental papilla reflection and fiber optic illumination. Journal of Periodontology. 1985;**56**(12):721-726

[44] Johnson GK, Reinhardt RA, Tussing GJ, Krejci RF. Fiber optic probe augmented sonic scaling versus conventional sonic scaling. Journal of Periodontology. 1989;**60**:131-136. DOI: 10.1902/jop.1989.60.3.131

[45] Harrel SK, Wilson TG Jr, Rivera-Hidalgo F. A videoscope for use in minimally invasive periodontal surgery. Journal of Clinical Periodontology. 2013;**40**:868-874. DOI: 10.1111/jcpe.12125

[46] Shakibaie F, Walsh LJ. Differential reflectometry versus tactile sense detection of subgingival calculus in dentistry. Journal of Biomedical Optics. 2012;**17**:106017. DOI: 10.1117/1.JBO.17.10.106017

[47] Kurihara E, Koseki T, Gohara K, Nishihara T, Ansai T, Takehara T. Detection of subgingival calculus and dentine caries by laser fluorescence. Journal of Periodontology. 2004;**39**:59-65. DOI: 10.1111/j.1600-0765.2004.00712.x

[48] Folwaczny M, Heym R, Mehl A, Hickel R. Subgingival calculus detection with fluorescence induced by 655 nm InGaAsP diode laser radiation. Journal of Periodontology. 2002;**73**:597-601. DOI: 10.1902/jop.2002.73.6.597

[49] Shakibaie F, George R, Walsh LJ. Applications of laser induced fluorescence in dentistry. International Journal of Dental Clinics. 2011;**3**:26-29

[50] Krause F, Braun A, Frentzen M. The possibility of detecting subgingival calculus by laser-fluorescence in vitro. Lasers in Medical Science. 2003;**18**:32-35. DOI: 10.1007/s10103-002-0241-7

[51] Krause F, Braun A, Jepsen S, Frentzen M. Detection of subgingival calculus with a novel LED-based optical probe. Journal of Periodontology. 2005;**76**:1202-1206. DOI: 10.1902/jop.2005.76.7.1202

[52] Shakibaie F, Walsh LJ. Laser fluorescence detection of subgingival calculus using the DIAGNOdent classic versus periodontal probing. Lasers in Medical Science. 2016;**31**:1621-1626. DOI: 10.1007/s10103-016-2027-3

[53] Shakibaie F, Walsh LJ. DIAGNOdent pen versus tactile sense for detection of subgingival calculus: An in vitro study. Clinical and Experimental Dental Research. 2015;**1**:26-31. DOI: 10.1002/cre2.5

[54] Bornstein ES. Why wavelength and delivery systems are the most important factors in using a dental hard-tissue laser: A literature review. The Compendium of Continuing Education in Dentistry. 2003;**24**:837-838

[55] Folwaczny M, Mehl A, Haffner C, Benz C, Hickel R. Root substance removal with Er:YAG laser radiation at different parameters using a new delivery system. Journal of Periodontology. 2000;**71**:147-155. DOI: 10.1902/jop.2000.71.2.147

[56] Folwaczny M, Thiele L, Mehl A, Hickel R. The effect of working tip angulation on root substance removal using Er:YAG laser radiation: An in vitro study. Journal of Clinical Periodontology. 2001;**28**:220-226. DOI: 10.1034/j.1600-051x.2001.028003220.x

[57] Folwaczny M, George G, Thiele L, Mehl A, Hickel R. Root surface roughness following Er:YAG laser irradiation at different radiation energies and working tip angulations. Journal of Clinical Periodontology. 2002;**29**:598-603. DOI: 10.1034/j.1600-051X.2002.290703.x

[58] Eberhard J, Ehlers H, Falk W, Açil Y, Albers HK, Jepsen S. Efficacy of subgingival calculus removal with Er:YAG laser compared to mechanical debridement: An in situ study. Journal of Clinical Periodontology. 2003;**30**:511-518. DOI: 10.1034/j.1600-051X.2003.00052.x

[59] Ishikawa I, Aoki A, Takasaki AA. Potential applications of erbium:YAG laser in periodontics. Journal of Periodontology. 2004;**39**:275-285. DOI: 10.1111/j.1600-0765.2004.00738.x

[60] Ishikawa I, Aoki A, Takasaki AA. Clinical application of erbium:YAG laser in periodontology. Journal of the International Academy of Periodontology. 2008;**10**:22-30

[61] Schwarz F, Jepsen S, Herten M, Aoki A, Sculean A, Becker J. Immunohistochemical characterization of periodontal wound healing following nonsurgical treatment with fluorescence controlled Er:YAG laser radiation in dogs. Lasers in Surgery and Medicine. 2007;**39**:428-440. DOI: 10.1002/lsm.20509

[62] Schwarz F, Sculean A, Berakdar M, Szathmari L, Georg T, Becker J. In vivo and in vitro effects of an Er:YAG laser, a GaAlAs diode laser, and scaling and root planing on periodontally diseased root surfaces: A comparative histologic study. Lasers in Surgery and Medicine. 2003;**32**:359-366. DOI: 10.1002/lsm.10179

[63] Herrero A, García-Kass AI, Gómez C, Sanz M, García-Nuñez JA. Effect of two kinds of Er: YAG laser systems on root surface in comparison to ultrasonic scaling: An in vitro study. Photomedicine and Laser Surgery. 2010;**28**:497-504. DOI: 10.1089/pho.2009.2527

[64] Sculean A, Schwarz F, Berakdar M, Romanos GE, Arweiler NB, Becker J. Periodontal treatment with an Er:YAG laser compared to ultrasonic instrumentation: A pilot study. Journal of Periodontology. 2004;**75**:966-973. DOI: 10.1902/jop.2004.75.7.966

[65] Schwarz F, Bieling K, Venghaus S, Sculean A, Jepsen S, Becker J. Influence of fluorescence-controlled Er:YAG laser radiation, the vector system and hand instruments on periodontally diseased root surfaces in vivo. Journal of Clinical Periodontology. 2006;**33**:200-208. DOI: 10.1111/j.1600-051X.2005.00889.x

[66] Badran Z, Demoersman J, Struillou X, Boutigny H, Weiss P, Soueidan A. Laser-induced fluorescence for subgingival calculus detection: Scientific rational and clinical application in periodontology. Photomedicine and Laser Surgery. 2011;**29**:593-596. DOI: 10.1089/pho.2010.2951

[67] Kreisler M, Kohnen W, Christoffers AB, Götz H, Jansen B, Duschner H, d'Hoedt B. In vitro evaluation of the biocompatibility of contaminated implant surfaces treated with an Er: YAG laser and an air powder system. Clinical Oral Implants Research. 2005;**16**:36-43. DOI: 10.1111/j.1600-0501.2004.01056.x

[68] Friedmann A, Antic L, Bernimoulin JP, Purucker P. In vitro attachment of osteoblasts on contaminated rough titanium surfaces treated by Er:YAG laser. Journal of Biomedical Materials Research Part A. 2006;**79**:53-60. DOI: 10.1002/jbm.a.30699

[69] Shakibaie F, Walsh LJ. Surface area and volume determination of subgingival calculus using laser fluorescence. Lasers in Medical Science. 2014;**29**:519-524. DOI: 10.1007/s10103-012-1242-9

[70] Shakibaie F, Walsh LJ. Performance differences in the detection of subgingival calculus by laser fluorescence devices. Lasers in Medical Science. 2015;**30**:2281-2286. DOI: 10.1007/s10103-015-1808-4

[71] Buchalla W, Lennon ÁM, Attin T. Fluorescence spectroscopy of dental calculus. Journal of Periodontal Research. 2004;**39**:327-332. DOI: 10.1111/j.1600-0765.2004.00747.x

[72] Shakibaie F, Walsh LJ. Violet and blue light-induced green fluorescence emissions from dental calculus: A new approach to dental diagnosis. International Dental. 2016;**11**:6-13

[73] Hibst R, Paulus R. Molecular basis of red excited caries fluorescence. Caries Research. 2000;**34**:323. DOI: 10.1159/000016607

[74] Shakibaie F, Lamard L, Rubinsztein-Dunlop H, Walsh LJ. Application of fluorescence spectroscopy for microbial detection to enhance clinical investigations. In: Nikiforov N, editors. Photon counting - fundamentals and applications. Intech; 2018. pp. 225-242. DOI: 10.5772/intechopen.73616

[75] Shakibaie F, Walsh LJ. Dental calculus detection using the VistaCam. Clinical and Experimental Dental Research. 2016;**2**:226-229. DOI: 10.1002/cre2.42

9

Chemically Modified Tetracyclines

Anshul Sawhney

Abstract

The use of chemotherapeutic agents or drugs specifically designed to treat periodontal diseases is emerging to aid in this risk assessment and reduction strategy. They include locally applied and systemically delivered antimicrobials and host modulatory thera pies. Tetracyclines are a group of antibiotics produced naturally from certain species of *Streptomyces* or derived semisynthetically. Their advantages were broad-spectrum activ ity, better tolerated, and less toxic to some individuals. Further modifications of these natural products by means of synthetic reactions and reagents led to the production of the clinically used antibiotic tetracycline compounds—minocycline, doxycycline, and methacycline. Tetracyclines are now recognized to have non-antimicrobial properties that may also be therapeutically advantageous. They have anti-inflammatory properties, particularly in the treatment of certain skin diseases. One important aspect is their abil ity to inhibit host collagenolytic enzymes, an effect that inhibits the connective tissue degradation and thus preventing bone resorption. To identify the site of the anticollage nase property, Golub and co-workers in 1991 synthesized 10 different analogs of tetra-cyclines known as chemically modified tetracyclines (CMTs 1-10). All 10 analogs lacked antimicrobial efficacy and inhibited collagenase activity, but only 1 did not. Though not approved for human use by the FDA, preliminary studies using CMT-3 are being inves tigated on humans with cancer.

Keywords: anti-collagenase, anti-inflammatory, collagenolytic enzymes, nonantimicrobial

1. Introduction and background

Host modulation with chemotherapeutic therapy or drugs is a new adjunctive therapeutic option for the management of periodontal diseases. The concept of host modulation was introduced by Williams and Golub et al. and then expanded on by many scholars. Various studies have indicated that host responses believed to be involved in pathogenesis of periodontal diseases may be efficacious in slowing progression of periodontitis. For the management of periodontal diseases, conventional approaches were initially mechanical in nature, as reviewed in the historical section, that is, surgery as well as scaling and root planning. New adjunctive approaches involve modulation of the host response. It has been recognized that genetic, environmental (e.g., tobacco use), and acquired risk factors (e.g., systemic disease) can increase a patient's susceptibility to developing periodontitis. Some of these risk factors can be modified to reduce a patient's susceptibility.

Risk assessment and therapy may include smoking cessation, improved control of diabetes, nutritional supplementation, improved oral hygiene, changes in medication, stress management, and more frequent dental visits.

The use of chemotherapeutic agents or drugs specifically designed to treat periodontal diseases is emerging to aid in this risk assessment and reduction strategy. They include locally applied and systemically delivered antimicrobials and host modulatory therapies which can be used to reduce excessive levels of enzymes, cytokines, and prostanoids as well as to modulate osteoclast and osteoblast function. Golub and colleagues discussed "host modulation with tetracyclines and their chemically modified analogs." When considering the imbalance in destructive or pro-inflammatory mediators versus protective or anti-inflammatory mediators in the diseased state, physicians should contemplate the use of pharmacological agents or host modulatory therapy.

Tetracyclines are a group of antibiotics produced naturally from certain species of *Streptomyces* or derived semisynthetically. Chlortetracycline (**Figure 1**) is the first tetracycline to be fully

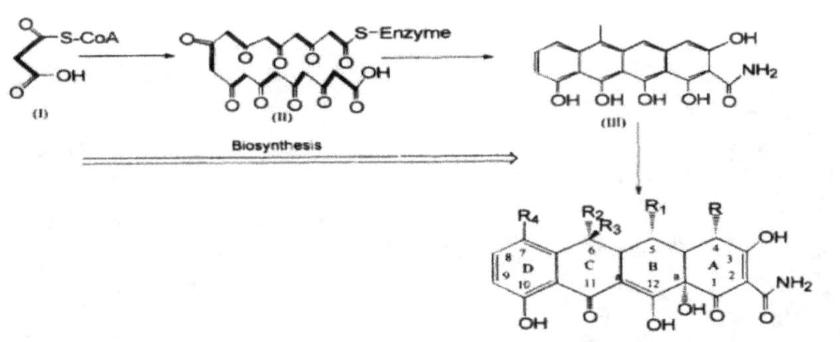

Tetracycline Natural Products	R	R_1	R_2	R_3	R_4
A. Chlortetracycline	$N(CH_3)_2$	H	CH_3	H	Cl
B. Oxytetracycline	$N(CH_3)_2$	OH	CH_3	OH	H
C. Tetracycline	$N(CH_3)_2$	H	CH_3	H	H
Tetracycline Semi-synthetic Compounds					
D. Minocycline	$N(CH_3)_2$	H	H	H	$N(CH_3)_2$
E. Doxycycline	$N(CH_3)_2$	OH	CH_3	H	H
F. Methacycline	$N(CH_3)_2$	OH	$= CH_2$	-	H

Fig. 1—Polyketide synthesis pathway, tetracycline natural products, and tetracycline semi-synthetic compounds: (I) acetate subunits, (II) polyketide intermediates, and (III) pretetramid.

Figure 1. Polyketide synthesis pathway, tetracycline natural products, and semi-synthetic compounds.

characterized both chemically and clinically. Their advantages were broad-spectrum activity, better tolerated, and less toxic to some individuals. Further modifications of these natural products by means of synthetic reactions and reagents led to the production of the clinically used antibiotic tetracycline compounds—minocycline, doxycycline, and methacycline.

2. Advantages of tetracyclines in periodontitis

Chemically modified tetracycline plays an important role in suppressing the concentration of Gram-negative microorganisms in the subgingival plaque. Concentration in the (GCF) was 5-10 times greater than in serum. Tetracyclines are now recognized to have nonantimicrobial properties that may also be therapeutically advantageous. An ability to promote fibroblast and connective tissue attachment to tooth & other surfaces (**Figure 2**), which is relevant to periodontal regeneration. They have anti-inflammatory properties, particularly in the treatment of certain skin diseases like rosacea, dermatitis herpetiformis and epidermolysis bullosa, disorders that are not thought to have a bacterial etiology and their ability to inhibit host collagenolytic enzymes, an effect that inhibits the connective tissue degradation, including bone resorption [1].

2.1. Matrix metalloproteinases (MMPs)

These are a family of enzymes capable of degrading connective tissue matrix. These enzymes are secreted in latent form by fibroblasts, keratinocytes, macrophages and polymorphoneutrophils.

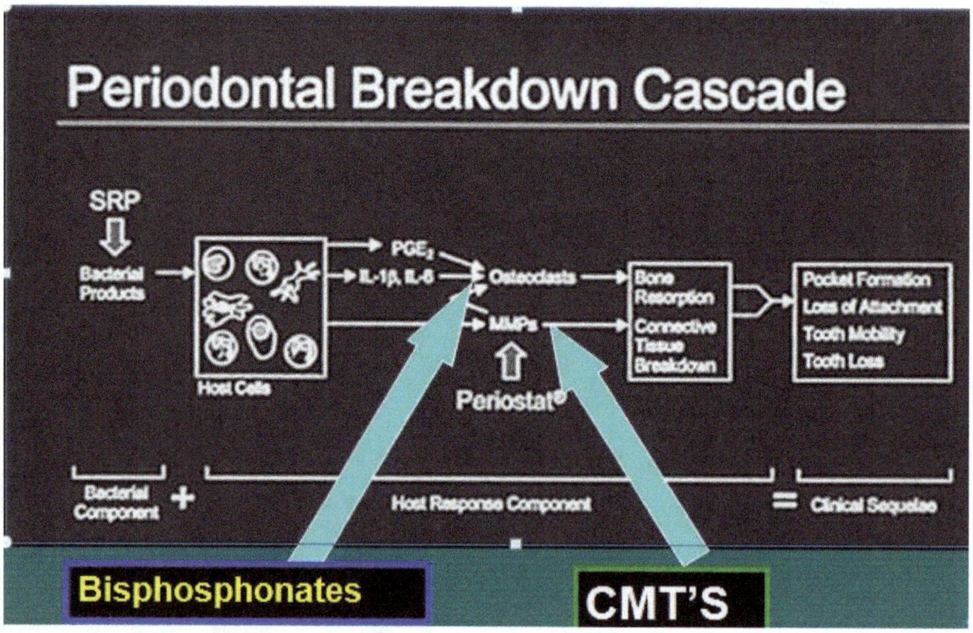

Figure 2. Role of chemically modified tetracycline in periodontitis.

There are about 28 MMPs. There are about 28 MMPs. All MMPs have similar multi-domain structure (**Figure 3**) Ryan et al. [2]:

1. "Pre" region to target for secretion
2. "Pro" region to maintain latency
3. Catalytic region that contains the active zinc-binding site
4. Proline-rich hinge region, which acts as a zinc-binding site

The majority of MMPs have additional domains, such as hemopexin region or fibronectin-like region, which play a role in recognition and in inhibitor binding.

MMPs can be grouped into six:

(a) Collagenase
(b) Gelatinase
(c) Stromelysins
(d) Membrane-type MMPs
(e) Matrilysins
(f) Other MMPs

Activation and regulation of MMPs (**Figure 4**)

Metal ions

Thiol reagents

Detergents

Organomercurials

Oxidants

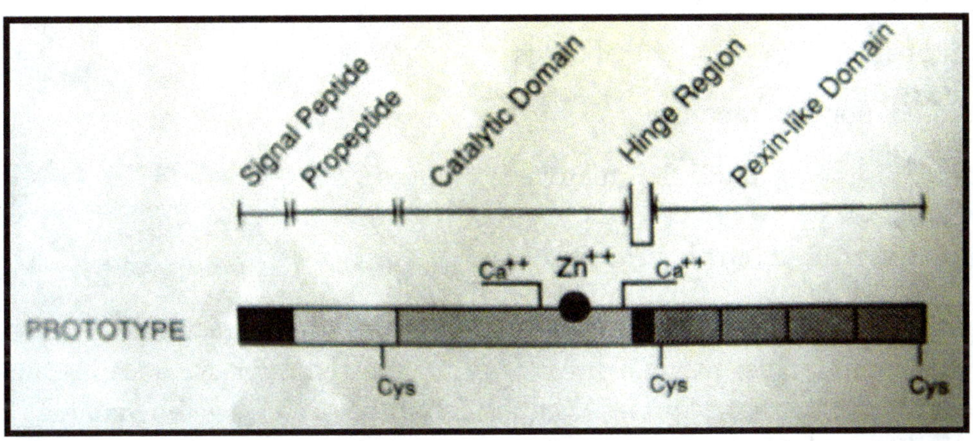

Figure 3. Structure of matrix metalloproteinases (MMPs).

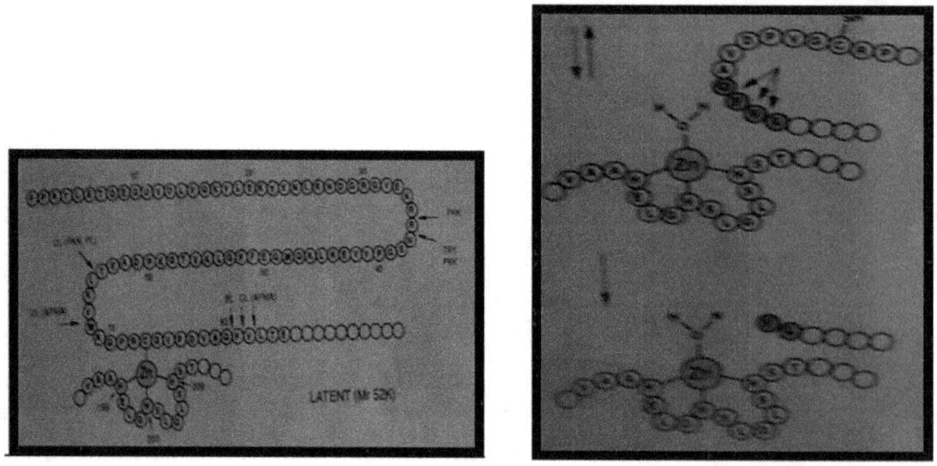

Inactive MMPs **Active MMPs**

Figure 4. Inactive and active MMPs.

Inhibitors of MMPs can be broadly classified as being

- **a.** Nonsynthetic, e.g., endogenous TIMPs
- **b.** Synthetic, e.g., collagen peptidomimetics, non-peptidomimetics, bisphosphonates, tetracycline derivatives like chemically modified tetracyclines (CMTs), and subantimicrobial dose doxycycline (SDD)

2.1.1. Host modulatory therapy

It is a treatment concept that aims to reduce tissue destruction and stabilize or even regenerate the periodontium by modifying or downregulating destructive aspects of host response and upregulating protective or regenerative responses [3, 4].

Various host modulatory agents proposed to block pathways responsible for periodontal tissue destruction are:

1. Inhibition of MMPs through CMTs
2. Inhibition of arachidonic acid metabolites
3. Modulation of bone metabolism
4. Regulation of immune and inflammatory responses

2.2. Chemically modified tetracyclines (CMTs)

The unexpected ability of tetracyclines to inhibit the breakdown of the connective tissue and bone by a nonantimicrobial mechanism was first reported over six decades. Based on the thoroughly explored chemistry of tetracyclines, a number of tetracycline analogs can be synthesized with side-chain deletions or, in some cases, moieties added to the parent tetracycline molecule.

Golub and co-workers (1983, 1987) [5] made the observation that collagenase activity was inhibited by tetracycline.

Their study showed that: in severe hypoglycemic rats, there was a shift to Gram-negative microflora in subgingival plaque with more of endotoxin penetration into subepithelial connective tissue leading to stimulation of host cells.

2.2.1. The diabetic rat model

Golub [5] and co-workers modified their experimental diabetes protocol using tetracycline therapy and germ-free rats to determine whether the Gram-negative microflora increased collagenase levels (**Figure 5**).

As a result of these initial studies, Golub et al. proposed:

1. Collagenase action was inhibited by tetracycline.
2. This property of tetracycline can be useful not only for periodontal disease but also for rheumatoid and osteoarthritis (as well as several cutaneous and other diseases) that involve collagen destruction.

Tetracyclines are known to inhibit collagenase and some other, but not all, matrix metalloproteinases or MMPs from a variety of cells:

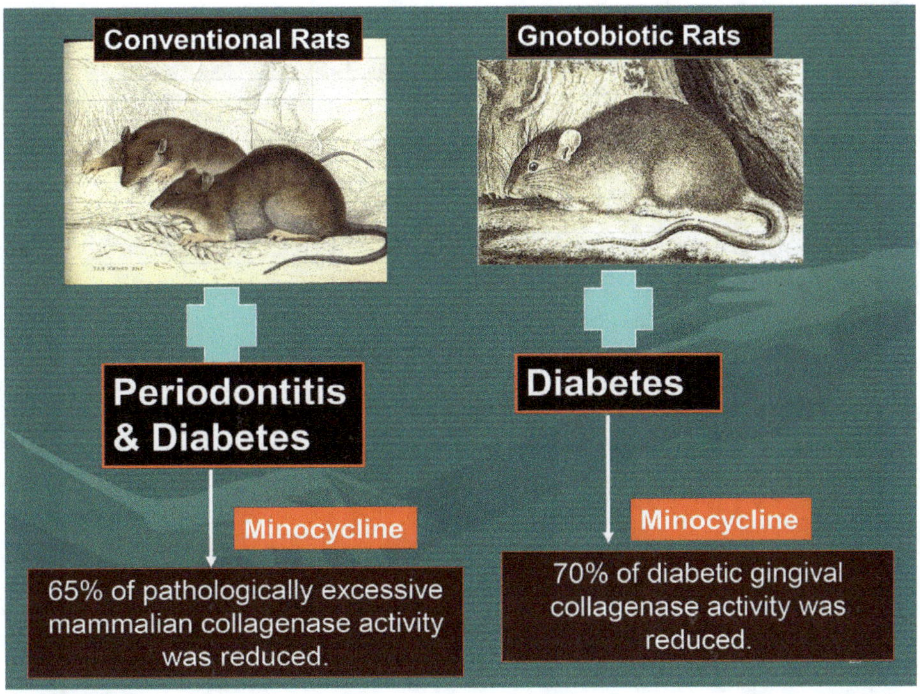

Figure 5. The diabetic rat model.

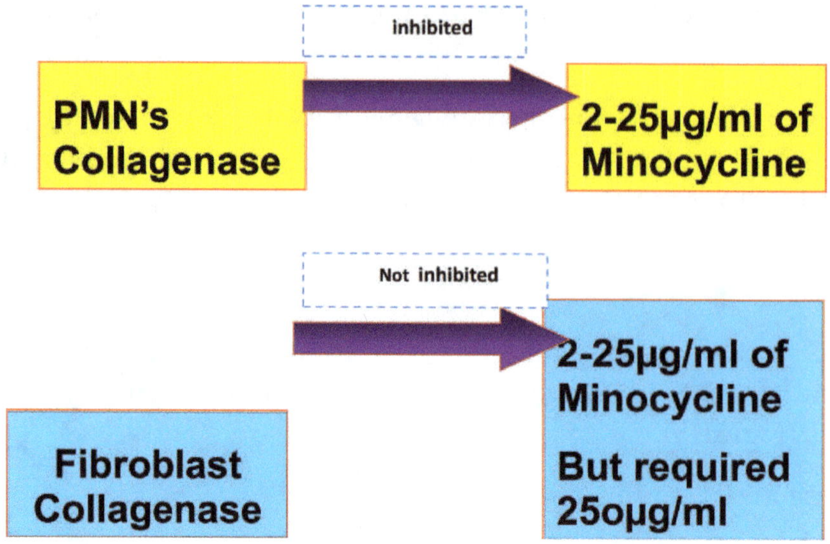

Figure 6. Inhibition mechanism of polymorphoneutrophils (PMNs) and fibroblast collagenase.

- Neutrophils
- Macrophages
- Osteoblasts
- Chondrocytes
- A wide range of tissues: skin, gingiva, cornea, cartilage, and rheumatoid synovium

Tetracyclines inhibit PMN but not fibroblast collagenase [6, 7] (**Figure 6**):

- PMNs are the major sources of collagenase that mediates tissue breakdown instead of fibroblasts.
- During inflammation, collagenolytic activity will be reduced by the use of these drugs but not the collagen turnover.

To identify the site of the anti-collagenase property, Golub and co-workers (1991) [5] synthesized 10 different analogs of tetracyclines known as chemically modified tetracyclines (CMTs 1–10). All 10 analogs lacked antimicrobial efficacy and inhibited collagenase activity, but only 1 did not.

3. Structure of CMT

This modification did not reduce the ability of drug to block the activity of collagenases from a number of tissue sources (PMNs, gingiva, osteoblasts, synovial tissue, lung cancer cells) or its ability to inhibit bone resorption [8] (**Figure 7**). Thus, it was concluded that the C-4 moiety had no role in anti-collagenase action of the drug.

When changes were made at C-11 and C-12 position by converting tetracycline to the pyrazole derivative or CMT-5, the collagenase inhibitory activity was lost.

These carbon groups are thought to be the sites for cation binding at physiologic pH 48, and all collagenases are known to require the cations, calcium and zinc, for their hydrolytic activity.

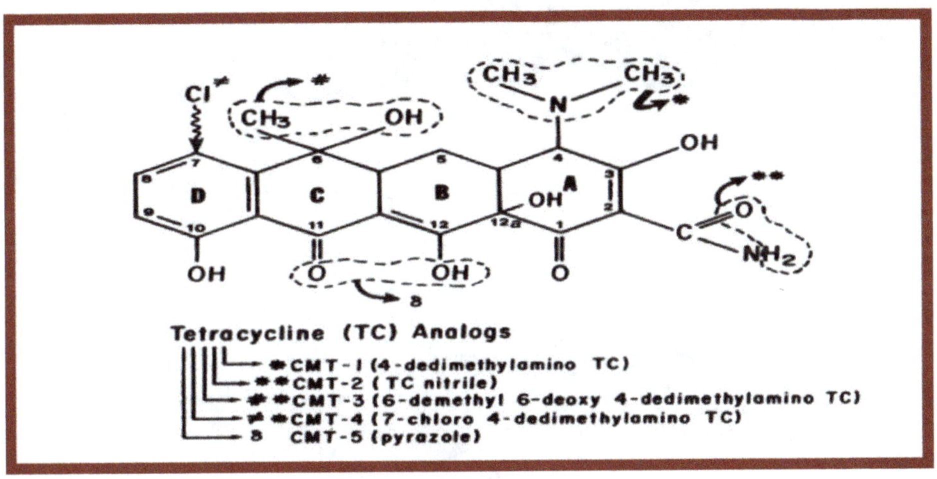

Figure 7. Structure of chemically modified tetracyclines (CMTs).

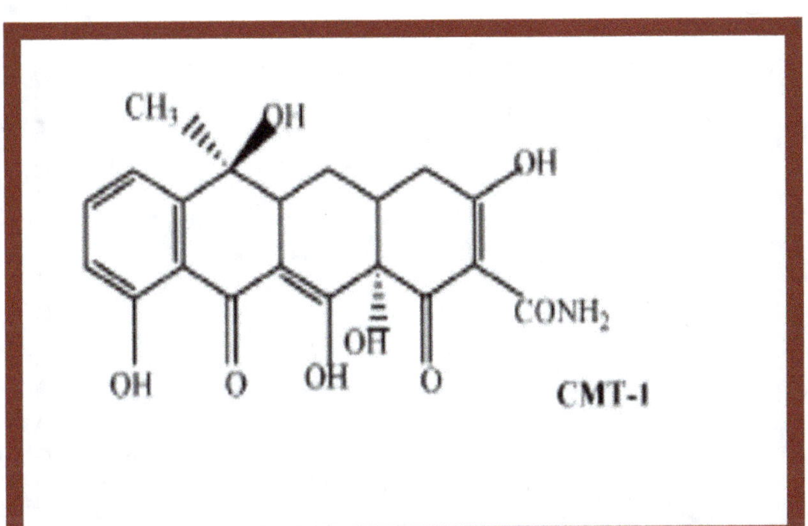

CMT-2 or tetracyclinonitrile was produced by dehydration of the carboxamide residue at carbon 2.

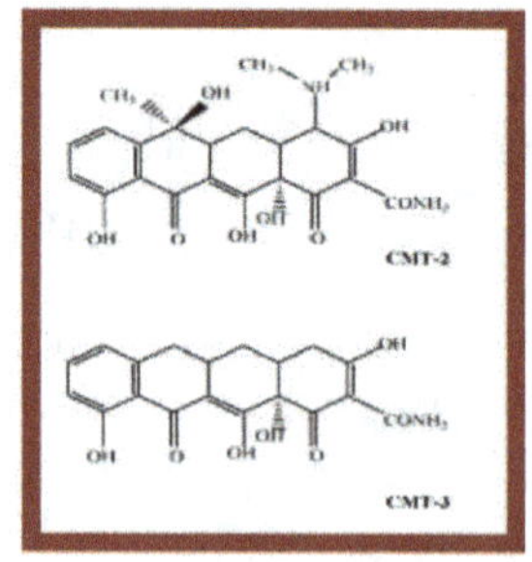

CMT-3 - produced by removing the hydroxyl & methyl groups on carbon 6 & 4.

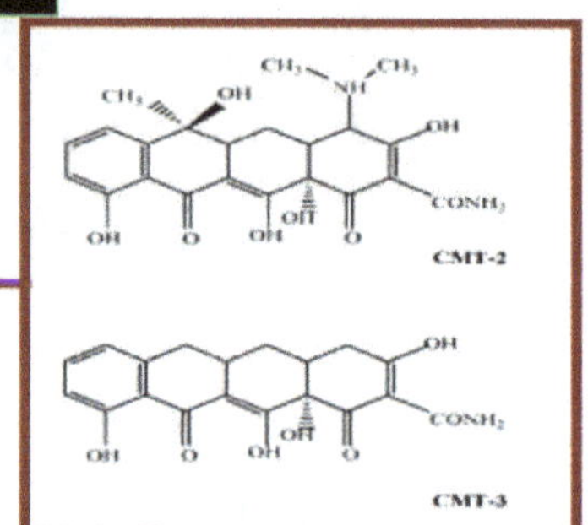

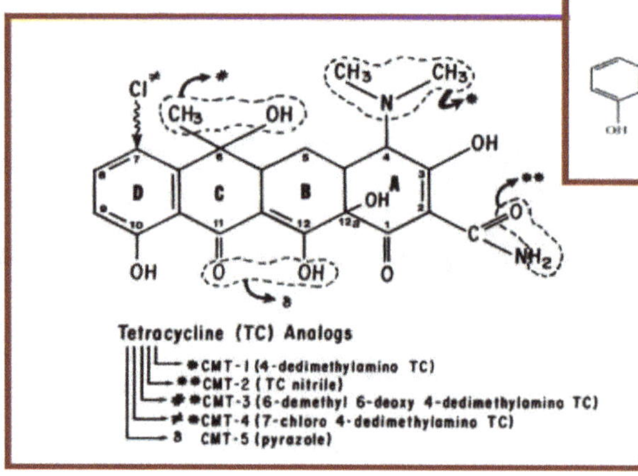

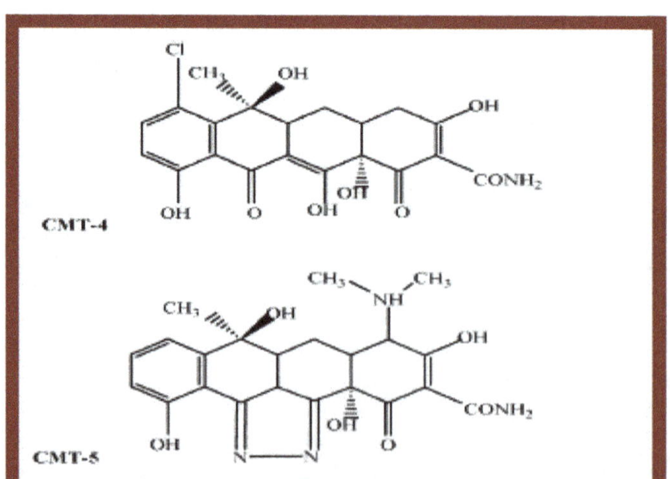

3.1. Mechanism of action of CMTs

a. CMTs bind metal ions, particularly Ca2+ and Zn2+, which are required by enzymes for their normal activity [9] (**Figure 8**).

b. Inhibition of pro-MMPs.

c. CMTs have also been shown to downregulate expression of MMP-2 and MMP-9 [Golub et al. (1991, 1998)].

d. Also, CMTs may inhibit the activation of collagenases (MMP-1, MMP-8, and MMP-13)

e. Inhibit stromelysins (MMP-3, MMP-10, and MMP-11).

f. Inhibit MT-MMPs.

Other mechanisms that have been proposed include:

- Retards cytokine production.
- Reduced serine proteinase and trypsinogen-2 (Pruzanski et al., 1998; Kirkwood et al., 1999).
- Inhibition of protein glycation.
- Inhibition of non-collagenolytic proteases.
- Inhibit secretion of other collagenolytic enzymes like lysosomal cathepsin.
- Scavenges reactive oxygen species.
- Modulates the osteoclast function and inhibits already active MMPs.

Tetracyclines affect several parameters of osteoclast function (**Figure 9**).

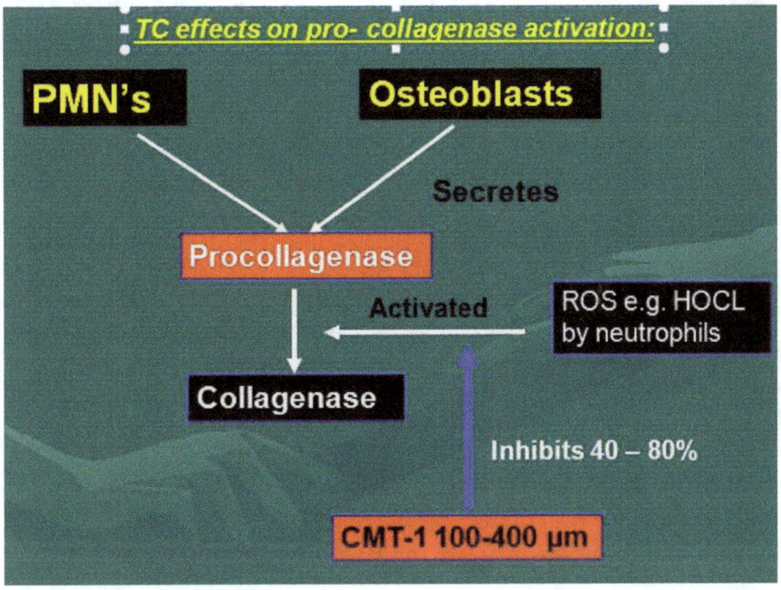

Figure 8. Mechanism of action of chemically modified tetracyclines (CMTs).

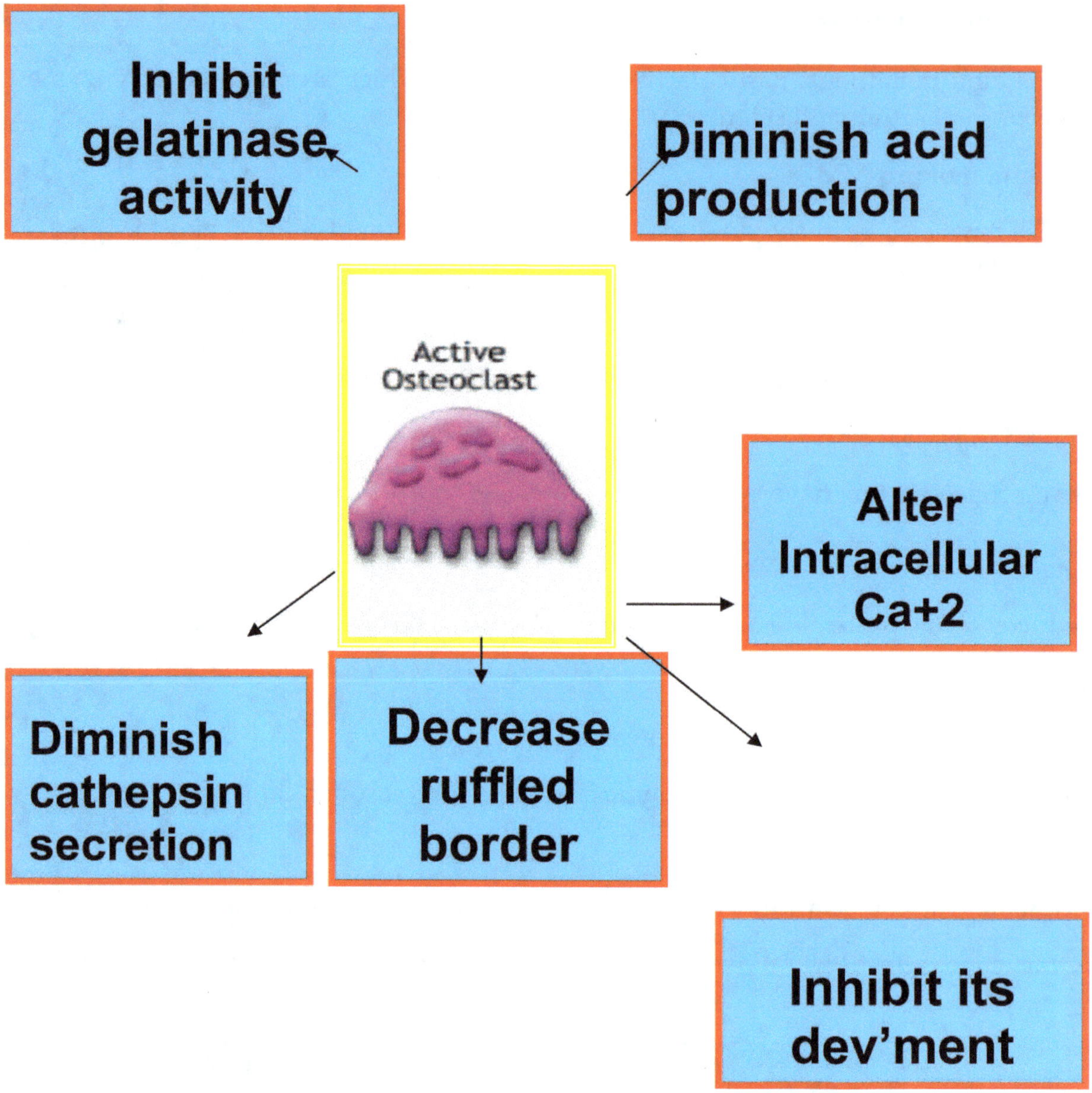

Figure 9. Effect of tetracyclines on osteoclast function.

3.2. Action on *P. gingivalis* and *T. denticola*

- Inhibits Arg- and Lys-gingipain activities and collagenolytic activity of *P. gingivalis*.
- Inhibited trypsin like activity of *T. denticola*.
- CMT-I inhibited serum albumin degradation by *P. gingivalis* and *T. denticola*.
- CMT-1 inhibited the inactivation of $\alpha 1$ proteinase inhibitor by *P. gingivalis*.
- CMT's potential advantages over conventional tetracyclines:
- The recent observations in rats showed that CMT-1 is absorbed after oral administration more rapidly and has a longer serum half-life than tetracycline.

- Their long-term systemic administration does not result in gastrointestinal toxicity.
- No resistance.
- Can be used for prolonged periods.

3.3. Current status of CMTs

- Though not approved for human use by the FDA, preliminary studies using CMT-3 are being investigated on humans with cancer.
- Greenwald et al. recently conducted a synergism study using CMT-1 + flurbiprofen, a standard nonsteroidal anti-inflammatory drug selected primarily because of its reported beneficial effect on bone loss in humans with adult periodontitis and the beagle dog model of periodontal disease.

4. Periostat

It is subantimicrobial dose of doxycycline hyclate (SDD) capsule of 20 mg prescribed for patients with chronic periodontitis twice daily for 3 months, up to a maximum of 9 months of continuous dosing [10]. Indications for periostat are patients who have not responded to non-surgical therapy, patients with generalized recurrent sites of 5 mm or greater pocket depth that bleed on probing, and patients with mild to moderate chronic periodontitis and a high susceptibility to rapid periodontal disease progression. It is the only FDA-approved systemically administered HMT indicated in the treatment of periodontitis [11]. Most patients will have small (i.e., less than 1 mm) additive effect on pocket depth reduction when this systemic approach is added to scaling and root planning. Modulation of host response may be valuable in enhancing effects of antimicrobial agents, such as doxycycline, which are locally released and in periodontitis treatment, especially in smokers.

4.1. Mechanism

The rationale for using SDD is based on the concept of host modulation; that is, it downregulates the activity of destructive responses such as MMP activity and upregulates protective responses as it promotes osteoblastic activity leading to new bone formation by upregulating collagen production.

4.2. Indications

a. Indicated in the management of chronic periodontitis

b. Can be used in patients with Ag periodontitis who are treated nonsurgically

c. Can also be used as an adjunct to periodontal surgery

d. May also be beneficial in cases that are refractory to treatment, as well as in patients with risk factors such as smoking or diabetes, in whom the treatment response might be limited

4.3. Contraindications

SDD should not be used in conditions such as gingivitis and periodontal abscess or when an antibiotic is indicated. The other contraindication of its use is in allergy to tetracycline. Patients taking oral contraceptives may have reduced protection from pregnancy with this therapy.

Host modulation therapy is an emerging treatment concept and can be used in susceptible, high-risk patients in whom a prolonged and excessive host response to microorganisms promotes activity of MMPs and osteoclast. Clinical trials have demonstrated a clear treatment benefit when it is used in combination with phase I therapy. The further development of these agents will help clinicians to treat specific aspects of periodontal diseases by reducing inflammation and inhibiting destructive processes in tissues, which will result in enhanced periodontal stability after conventional periodontal treatment such as scaling root planning (SRP) and surgery.

Ramamurthy et al. (2002) tested doxycycline and five different CMTs to prevent MMP-dependent periodontal tissue breakdown in an adult rat model. CMTs were administered orally at conc. 2 mg/day for 7 days, and gingival biopsies were taken to assess cytokines TNF, IL-1, and MMP-2 and MMP-9. All tetracycline inhibited periodontal breakdown in the following order of efficacy: CMT, 8 > 1 > 3 > doxy >4 > 7.

Long-term (i.e., 9–18 months) administration of SDD does not result in emergence of resistant organism or alteration of subgingival microflora. Various long term studies have been conducted.

Doxycycline 20 mg bid was used in 51 patients with active periodontitis based on pocket depth and increased collagenase at multiple exams showed no clinical attachment loss over 36 months.

Twenty subjects ≤ 45 year old patients with severe generalized periodontitis patients and showing >30% of sites with CAL ≥ 5 mm were given subantimicrobial dose of doxycycline for 6 months. The result showed less clinical attachment loss, probing depth. Gingival index and bleeding on probing were not significant when compared to placebo.

Doxy 20-mg bid for month along with scaling and root planning was done in 208 chronic periodontitis subjects. The patients showed improvements in clinical attachments level and probing depth ≥ 4 mm.

Used 20 mg bid SDD for 9 months + scaling and root planning in 190 adult periodontitis patients, there was a significant improvements in CAL (≥ 2 mm) PD and BOP when compared to placebo group receiving only SRP.

Author details

Anshul Sawhney

Address all correspondence to: dranshul1986@yahoo.co.in

Department of Periodontics, Uttar Pradesh University of Medical Sciences, Saifai, India

References

[1] Golub LM, Sorsa T. Host modulation with tetracyclines and their chemically modified analogs. Current Opinion in Dentistry. 1992;**2**:80

[2] Ryan ME, Preshaw PM. Host modulation. In: Newman, Takei, Carranza, editors. Clinical Periodontology. 10th ed. WB Saunders; 2007. pp. 275-282

[3] Genco RJ. Host response in periodontal disease: Current concepts. Journal of Periodontology. 1992;**63**:338

[4] Kornmann KS. Host modulation as a therapeutic strategy in the treatment of periodontal disease. Clinical Infectious Diseases. 1999;**28**:520

[5] Golub LM, Mc Namara TF, Angelo GD, Greenwald RA, Ramamurthy NS. A non-antibacterial chemically-modified tetracycline inhibits mammalian collagenase activity. Journal of Dental Research. 1987;**66**(8):1310-1314

[6] Ryan ME, Kinney J, Kim Amy S, Giannobile WV. The host modulatory approach. Dental Clinics of North America. 2005;**49**:624-635

[7] Salve GE, Lang NP. Host response modulation in the management of periodontal disease. Journal of Clinical Periodontology. 2005;**32**(suppl. 6):108-129

[8] Devulapalli SN, Sahitya S, Srinivas M, Vasavi K. Chemically modified tetracyclines: The novel host modulating agents. Journal of Indian Society of Periodontology. Jul-Aug 2015;**19**(4)

[9] Wang Y, Morlandt AB, Xu X, Carnes DL, Chen Z, Steffenson B. Tetracycline at subcytotoxic levels inhibits matrix metalloproteinase-2 and -9 but does not remove the smear layer. Journal of Periodontology. 2005;**76**:1129-1139

[10] Greenstein G, Lamster I. Efficacy of subantimicrobial dosing with doxycycline. Journal of the American Dental Association (Chicago, IL). 2001;**132**(4):457-466

[11] Choi DH, Moon IS, Paik JW, Kim YS, Choi SH, Kim CK. Effects of sub-antimicrobial dose doxycycline therapy on crevicular fluid MMP-8, and gingival tissue MMP-9, TIMP-1 and IL-6 Levels in Chronic Periodontitis. Journal of Periodontal Research. 2004;**39**:20-26

10

Supportive Periodontal Therapy for Dental Implant Patients

Krishna Kripal and Kavita Chandrasekaran

Abstract

Some of the early indicators of future implant failure are increased plaque accumulation, bleeding upon probing, increased probing pocket depth, abscess formation, bone loss seen under radiographic, retrograde tooth wear and broken restoration. A periodic supportive periodontal treatment visit allows for early detection and intervention to provide an opportunity to salvage an ailing implant. Presence of biofilm/plaque on the implant may progress to peri-implantitis with bone resorption. Microbial challenge in the oral environment may result in pathological reactions in peri-implant tissues and thereby compromising tissue integration. The long-term success of implants depends on adequate supportive periodontal treatment visits. Prevention of disease is a key factor in the aim of preserving the supporting tissues around implants. Thus, sufficient supportive therapy during maintenance is inevitable in order to achieve optimal results in implant dentistry.

Keywords: implant, implant failure, peri implant mucositis, peri implantitis, supportive periodontal therapy

1. Introduction

Adequate supportive periodontal treatment visits are needed for the long- term success of implants [1]. Some percentage of implants ultimately fail and majority that fail, do so soon after placement [2]. Early indicators of future implant failure includes excessive plaque accumulation, Bleeding on probing, Increased probing depth, suppuration, radiographic bone loss, retrograde wear and broken restorations and hence supportive periodontal visits allows for early intervention to enable clinician to save an ailing implants.

Primary causes of implant failure have been suggested to be plaque, bacterial infection and traumatic occlusal forces [3]. Some of the bacterial species found to be associated with failing implants are reported to be *Aggregatibacter actinomycetemcomitans, Prevotella intermedia, Porphyromonas gingivalis.* Other species shown to be associated are Spirochetes and Fusobacterium. It has been observed that poor oral hygiene facilitates the growth of such anaerobic bacteria and in presence of plaque, the implants may clinically present with peri-implantitis with bone resorption [4]. Several studies have shown the development of the peri-implant infection progressed at a similar rate as the development of periodontitis lesion.

Implant is "any object or material, such as an alloplastic material or other tissues, which is partially or completely inserted and grafted on to the body for the diagnostic, prosthetic and experimental purposes" [5]. As defined by Glossary of Prosthodontics terms. In the late 1950s, Per Ingvar Branemark, a Swedish Professor in Anatomy, studying blood circulation in bone and marrow, developed through a serendipitous finding a historical breakthrough in medicine he predictably achieved an intimate bone to implant apposition that offered sufficient strength to cope with load transfer, he called the phenomenon as "osseointegration" [6].

In 1965 the first patient was treated by means of this approach for a law edentulous jaw. One definition of osseointegration was provided by Albrektson et al. (1981) [7] who suggested that this was a direct structural and functional connection between living bone and the surface of load carrying implants. As defined by Zarb and Albrektson "a process whereby clinically asymptomatic rigid fixation of alloplastic materials is achieved and maintained in bone during functional loading" [8].

A series of screw shaped, commercially pure titanium implants were inserted in the symphysis and left covered for a few months. Commercially pure titanium implants were inserted in the symphysis and left uncovered for a few months. The gingival and mucosal tissues were reopened and titanium abutments were placed, on top of which fixed prosthesis could be screwed. All implants appeared firmly anchored. Since that time millions of people have been treated worldwide using this technique. The implants used sometimes had different geometrics and surface characteristics.

The serendipitous finding of Branemark was that when a hole is prepared in the bone without traumatizing the tissues or overheating, an inserted biocompatible implantable would achieve an intimate bone apposition and micro movements at the interface were prevented during early healing period [6].

A successful outcome of implant therapy depends on number of factors. A satisfactory healing following implant placement is determined by biocompatibility of implant material and surgical technique. Presence of microbes and their interaction with host tissues in the oral environment may result in pathological reaction in the peri-implant tissues and thereby compromising tissue integration. Thus prevention of disease is a key factor in the aim of preserving the supporting tissues around implants.

2. Soft and hard tissue integration

The integration of hard and soft tissues with implants is the result of wound healing process. A blood clot is formed within of the surgical procedure. After a few days, there is infiltration of the clot by vascular structures and abundant inflammatory cells to form a granulation tissue. The continuation of the healing process involves the organization of connective tissue by modification of granulation tissue. This is followed by the formation of bone which in turn results in osseointegration at the recipient site.

Formation of barrier epithelium adjacent to implants and apical to the epithelium the connective tissue that integrates with titanium surface prevents the epithelial migration. The barrier epithelium and connective tissue/implant interface establish a specific biological width of peri implant mucosa.

3. Peri implant mucosa and gingiva

The soft tissue that surrounds the transmucosal parts of implant is termed as peri-implant mucosa. The structure and dimension of this mucosa is similar to that of gingiva around the teeth. The concept of biological width controls the thickness of soft tissue adjacent to both teeth and implants. Some fundamental differences also exist between these two tissue types in terms of gingival fibers, periodontal fibers and periodontal ligament space.

In tooth, a layer of cementum covers the surface of root. From the cementum, the collagen fibers run in a perpendicular direction to the long axis of the tooth and insert into the surrounding hard and soft tissues. But, the implant lacks the cemental layer and, hence, collagen fibers are unable to attach to the implant surface in the same way as around the tooth. Thus, the collagen fibers are aligned in different directions and in the tissue which is in immediate lateral surface to the implant surface. The collagen fibers are orientated parallel to the long axis of the implant. Nevertheless, an effective soft tissue seal to the oral environment is provided by the biological attachment formed by the barrier epithelium and the connective tissue in the mucosa surrounding the implant (**Figure 1**).

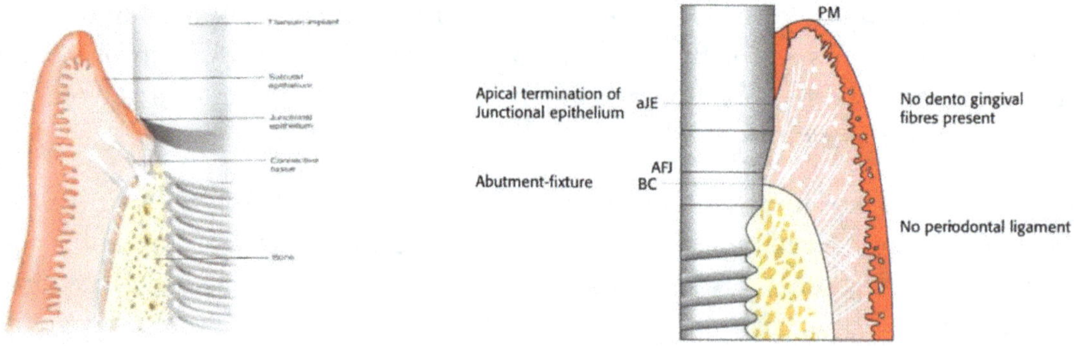

Figure 1. Peri-implant mucosa.

3.1. Examination of peri-implant tissues

Increasing probing depth and loss of clinical attachment are pathognomonic for periodontal disease. Pocket probing is, therefore, a crucial procedure in diagnosis of the periodontium and for the evaluation of periodontal therapy. The major clinical criteria used to determine the success of periodontal treatment are reduction of probing depth and gain of clinical attachment level. The penetration of probe is greatly influenced by various factors such as the roughness of the root surface, the inflammatory state of the periodontal tissues and the firmness of the marginal cuff.

The limitations of probing are – (i) it often fails to identify the histological level of the connective tissue attachment as determined by various studies; (ii) it has a limited reproducibility; variations of 1 mm have to be expected under clinical conditions. The changes that occurred in the past are reflected by measurements of clinical attachment level. Once disease is detectable by clinical attachment level measurement, it is indicative of substantial, and possibly irreversible, tissue changes have already occurred.

Some of the advantages of probing are—the simplicity of the method and the immediate availability of the results. Also, the topographical disease patterns can also be demonstrated. The results from a histological study determining the extent of peri-implant probe penetration in dogs indicate that the density of the peri-implant tissues influences penetration depth. In inflamed tissues around one-stage non submerged implants, periodontal probes penetrated close to the bone level, whereas the probe tips tended to stop at the histological level of connective tissue adhesion if healthy tissues were present [9].

Quirynen et al. [10] found a correlation between the level of bone as seen on radiographs and the extent of peri-implant probe penetration. In the case of screw-type implants, the probe tip appeared to stop 1.4 mm coronally to the bone level. It was observed that the mean discrepancy between probe penetration and the location of the bone margin in radiographs was 1.17 mm in 100 non submerged titanium implants 1 year after implantation. [10] Microbiological studies have shown that there is a marked difference in the composition of the peri-implant microflora between implants with deep and shallow pockets.

Deeper pockets of 5 mm or more can be viewed as protected habitats for putative pathogens and indicate peri-implantitis. The penetration of the probe tip is influenced to some extent by implant shape and surface texture. In some implants, peri-implant probing is impossible due to peculiarities of the shape or design (concavities, shoulders or steps) of the implant. Lack of surface smoothness (such as plasma-coating, sandblasting or the presence of threads) may increase the resistance to probe penetration and may lead to the underestimation of pocket depth. Thus, probing around implant has not gained much acceptance among clinicians as a reliable diagnostic tool.

On the other hand, one may consider it a deficiency of an implant system if its design disables probing. In addition, some authors have expressed concern about the possibility of introducing bacteria into the peri-implant tissues and damaging the implant surface with a metallic periodontal probe while probing. The peri-implant probing should include a fixed reference point on the implant or its suprastructure to measure the relative attachment level.

If peri-implantitis is associated with a marginal recession, then probing depth alone may not accurately reflect peri-implant bone loss, whereas increasing loss of attachment is definitely indicative of peri-implant pathology.

The examination of peri-implant tissues is fundamental in the maintenance and follow-up of implant treated patients. The methods to be applied in the clinical examination of the tissues surrounding implants resemble those used in the examination of the periodontal tissues surrounding teeth. Thus, probing represents one of the critical assessments and includes not only the appraisal of probing pocket depth (PPD) but also the more important detection of bleeding on probing (BOP). Probing peri-implant and periodontal tissues is in most respects similar and is regarded as a predictable and reliable procedure in the effort to distinguish between healthy and diseased tissue, provided that a normal force is applied [9].

When probing healthy tissues around implants and teeth, the probe meets resistance from the peri-implant mucosa/gingiva and the apical extension of the probe into the pocket corresponds to the vertical dimension of the junctional epithelium. Probe penetration of inflamed tissues, however, is different such that the probe reaches a position apical to the epithelial extension, depending on the degree of inflammation (**Figure 2**).

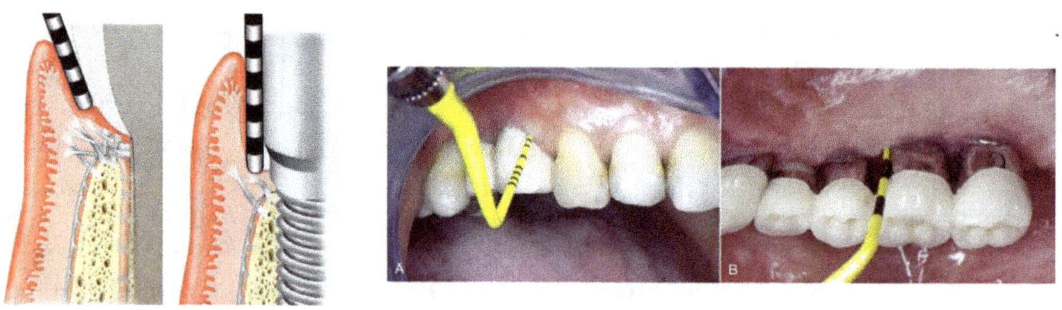

Figure 2. Peri-implant probing.

3.2. Mucosal inflammation

Definition of inflammatory changes of peri-implant tissues should be based on established periodontal index systems such as the Sulcus Bleeding Index or the Gingival Index. Consequently, a modified Bleeding Index has been proposed by Mombelli et al. [11]. Also, a simplified Gingival Index was suggested by Apse et al. for the assessment of soft tissues around implants [12].

In the Gingival Index scores, two important discriminators used are the texture and color of the gingiva. However, in case of implants, these features depend on the normal appearance of the recipient tissues before implantation. They may also be influenced by the properties of the implant surface. Non-keratinized peri-implant mucosa appears redder than keratinized tissues. Therefore, a modification of the original Gingival Index was required for use on implants.

In a longitudinal study conducted by Chaytor [13], only a weak correlation between the Gingival Index scores and changes of marginal bone level was reported. In clinical practice, the reduction of the evaluation of signs and symptoms of inflammation to bleeding on gentle probing on implants may be a reasonable extrapolation from the clinical situation around teeth. In contrast to gingivitis and periodontitis patients, this parameter has not yet been validated for implant situations.

Consequently, for peri-implant lesions, sensitivity, specificity, diagnostic accuracy and predictive values are not available. However, from a biological point of view it may be reasonable to assume that absence of bleeding on probing represents stability of the peri-implant mucosal seal in a similar way as absence of bleeding on gentle probing represents stability and health in periodontal tissue. Further research in required to fill these gaps in knowledge, of the role of this common clinical parameter as an indicator and/or predictor for health and disease (**Tables 1** and **2**).

3.3. Mobility

The establishment and, maintenance of intimate contact between the bone and the implant is a major requirement for implant success. An important criterion for the success of implant therapy is the absence of mobility. Clinically visible mobility of an implant after an appropriate period indicates failure to achieve osseointegration. Presence of mobility at the follow-up visit is a sign of the final stage of peri-implant pathology and indicates complete failure of osseointegration. Implants with less advanced stages of peri-implantitis may still appear immobile due to some remaining osseointegration. Thus, mobility cannot be used to detect early stages of peri-implant pathology. It is advisable to use an electronic device to interpret low degrees of mobility [9].

3.4. Definition and diagnosis of peri-implant disease

Peri-implant mucositis is described as the inflammation limited to soft tissues around a dental implant. It may result from dental plaque colonization and is a reversible inflammatory condition. It does not involve any bone loss, analogous to gingivitis around natural teeth. A diagnosis of peri-implantitis results when the inflammation spreads apically, causing progressive loss of osseointegrated supporting bone, analogous to periodontitis around natural teeth. The

Score 0	No detection of plaque
Score 1	Plaque only recognized by running a probe across the smooth marginal surface of the implant. Implants covered by plasma spray in this area always score 1
Score 2	Plaque can be seen by the naked eye
Score 3	Abundance of soft matter

Table 1. Assessment of plaque accumulation by a modified Plaque Index [11].

Score 0	No bleeding when a periodontal probe is passed along the gingival margin adjacent to the implant
Score 1	Isolated bleeding spots visible
Score 2	Blood forms a confluent red line on margin
Score 3	Heavy or profuse bleeding

Table 2. Assessment of bleeding tendency by a modified Sulcus Bleeding Index [11].

practitioners essentially require to be familiar with these diagnostic terms when assessing the long-term success of implants and peri-implant health.

It is also important to accurately identify the etiology and chronology of bone loss around implants for better diagnosis and treatment plan. Bone loss may result from surgical trauma or technique, such as pressure necrosis from inadequate osteotomy preparation or coronal bony voids from excessive counter sinking. It must be differentiated from bone loss resulting from bacterial plaque mediated by an immune-inflammatory reaction. Implants placed using a subcrestal platform position have been shown to have a deeper baseline probing depths than those placed supracrestally; thus, it is important to know the baseline probing depth after initial healing to allow monitoring for changes over time.

Various studies in literature have reported the incidence and prevalence of peri-implantitis. Berglundh et al. [14] found that the incidence of peri-implantitis was up to 14.4% and appeared to be related to the number of years for which the fixtures were in service. Additionally, Roos-Jansaker et al. [15] reported that of all implant cases which were not enrolled in a regular post treatment periodontal maintenance program, 16% demonstrated peri-implantitis by 7–9 years after implant placement. The incidence of peri-implantitis may be underestimated because only few studies exist with follow-up longer than 10 years.

Dental implants have been shown to be successful in patients with severe periodontitis. Similarity between the bacterial profile around implants and natural teeth has been demonstrated by several researchers. Moreover, dental implants may harbor a complex microbiota with a large proportion of known periodontal pathogens, which have been associated with the onset of peri-implant mucositis and peri-implantitis [16]. Additionally, long term follow-up studies that examined dental implants in patients with a history of periodontitis, have suggested a higher incidence of soft-tissue inflammation (mucositis) and peri-implantitis, as well as a slightly higher failure rate [17]. These findings suggest that the patients with dental implants require regular and careful evaluation at selected periodontal maintenance intervals to detect any clinical signs and symptoms of peri-implant disease at an early stage.

Probing depths should be recorded to detect the inflammation in the peri-implant mucosa. It helps to identify bleeding or suppuration during examination. While the probing pocket depth (PPD) may vary around implants, such assessments are secondary to bleeding on probing (BOP). Sites with PPD ≥ 6 mm, however, may indicate pathology and thus require meticulous examination. For peri-implantitis, bone loss can be assessed through radiographs in addition to the PPD and BOP. The radiograph for this purpose should be obtained after the delivery of the prosthesis [18].

4. Histopathology of peri-implant disease

4.1. Mucositis

The similarity between inflammatory lesions in peri-implant mucositis and gingivitis has been revealed by various animal experiments and analyses of human biopsy material. The development of inflammatory lesions in the connective tissue in the marginal portion of the gingiva or peri-implant mucosa as a response to microbial challenge follows the same pattern and the composition of inflammatory cells in both the lesions. While gingivitis and mucositis are reversible conditions, periodontitis and peri-implantitis are not. The inflammatory lesion in the former conditions can be completely resolved after the institution of appropriate infection control measures [14, 19] (**Figure 3**).

4.2. Peri-implantitis

Peri-implantitis lesions differ from mucositis lesions in that they exhibit characteristics that are markedly different from their periodontal counterparts. The inflammatory lesion in periodontitis is contained within the sub-epithelial connective tissue compartment of the gingiva and is separated from the alveolar bone by a 1 mm-wide zone of dense connective tissue. Furthermore, the area of soft tissue affected with pocket formation is lined by a pocket epithelium. The epithelium in its most apical portion is in contact with the root surface and thereby effectively sheds off the biofilm of bacteria in the pocket.

In peri-implantitis, bacteria survive in the inflammatory lesion within the pocket compartment. But the entire extension of the pocket usually remains uncovered by a pocket epithelium. Thus, the apical third of the inflamed tissue in the pocket comes to lie in direct contact with the biofilm. Another dissimilarity to periodontitis is the extension of the lesion in peri-implantitis. The lesion in peri-implantitis is seen to extend to a position closer to the bone surface, while the lesion in periodontitis is usually separated from the crestal bone by a zone of connective tissue. An understanding of the difference in the lesions observed in periodontitis and peri-implantitis will help clinician to select the appropriate treatment strategy (**Figure 4**).

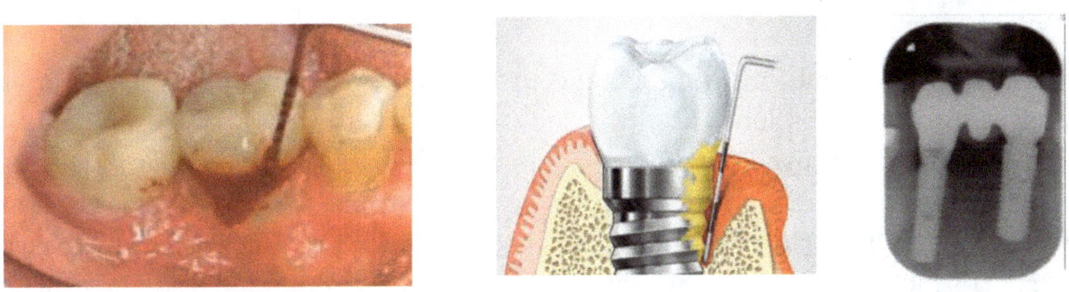

Figure 3. Peri-implant mucositis.

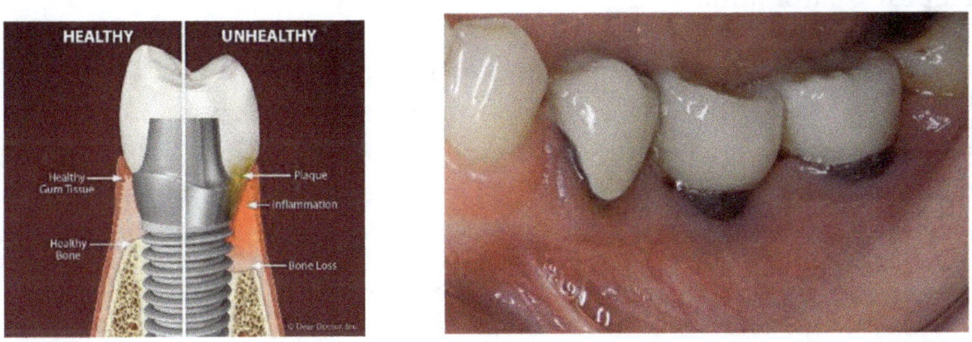

Figure 4. Peri-implantitis.

5. Guidelines for follow-up of implant treated patients

5.1. Supportive therapy: infection control

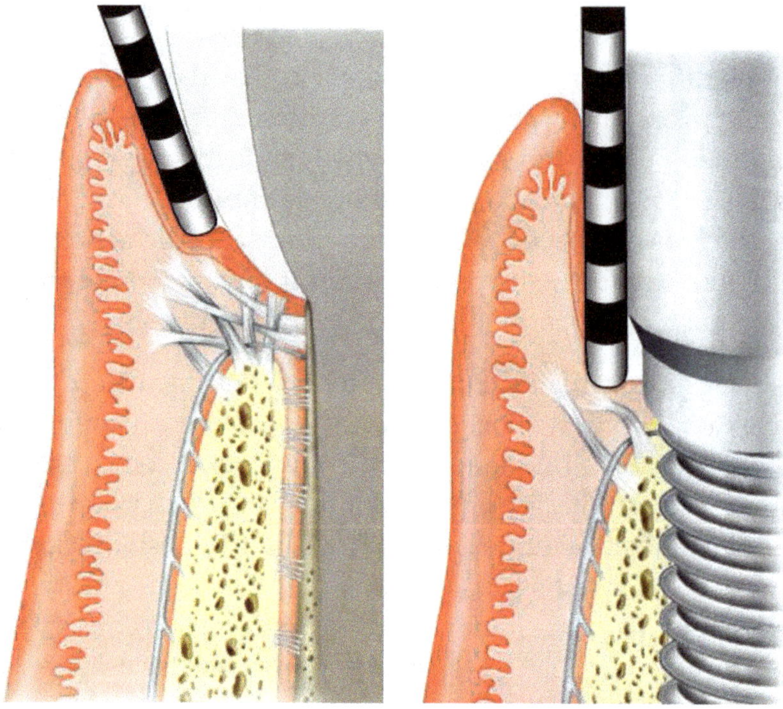

Following the completion of the surgical and prosthetic procedures in implant therapy, it is imperative to inform the patient about the self-performed infection control procedures [20]. Different types of toothbrushes and/or floss are available to suit the varying designs of the prosthetic reconstruction. The patient should be taught to use the mechanical cleaning aids properly and efficiently to clean the implant and adjacent parts of the prosthesis. The cleansing should be performed twice a day. The prosthesis should be designed in a such way as to allow access for self-performed and professional infection control [20].

5.2. Radiographic examination

The implant sites should be evaluated with radiographs carried out at two time points - at the time of the delivery of the prosthesis and at the one-year follow up. Any alteration in the marginal bone level should be recorded during the first year in function of an implant. This change may be associated with the remodeling of bone after implant installation. This information will serve as a baseline value for evaluation of bone level at subsequent visits.

The following radiographic parameters are in currently in use for evaluation of dental implants:

i. Assessment of alterations in height of peri-implant bone

ii. Computer-assisted evaluation of changes in peri-implant bone height

iii. Assessment of quality of peri-implant bone

iv. Photodensitometric evaluation of peri-implant bone quality

v. Bone mineral content (dual-photon absorptiometry)

5.3. Clinical examination

Clinical examinations should be performed at all annual follow- up visits. Besides examining the function of the prosthesis, BOP, PPD and plaque assessment should also be carried out. If the probing indicates peri-implant disease (BOP positive and PPD ≥ 6 mm), a radiographic examination is called for to reveal possible bone loss. In the absence of clinical findings of pathology in peri-implant tissues, radiographic examination should be avoided.

The re-evaluation of implant-treated patients should be designed in accordance with evaluation of risk factors for peri-implant disease. Subjects with a history of severe should be recalled in every 2–6 months after the delivery of the prosthesis. Routine maintenance therapy is imperative for maintenance of the peri-implant health. Implant maintenance therapy includes considering the patient's overall health in addition to the assessment and monitoring of implant(s).

Implants fail from a loss of integration generally due to bacterial infection, occlusal overload, or a poorly designed prosthesis. The role of a dental hygienist and dentist is thus essential in preventing and controlling bacterial infection, including careful instrumentation and polishing of implant(s) once in every 3-4 months.

5.3.1. Step 1: assessment of the patient's medical history

At each appointment, medical history and overall health of the patient should be updated and reviewed. Any changes in the health status of the patient can influence negatively the success of implants or treatment provided. If the diabetic status of the patient is not under good control, this can increase the risk of peri-implantitis and ultimately implant failure. Overall good general health is one of the keys to the success of the implant(s).

Implant dentistry is true interdisciplinary dentistry, requiring close collaboration with the surgical practice, the dental laboratory, and the patient's physician [20].

5.3.2. Step 2: assessment of implants

Implant assessment starts with a visual soft tissue examination of the peri-mucosal seal and should be carried out at every maintenance appointment. Any signs of inflammation or bleeding or suppuration should be recorded. It is important to record any clinical symptoms present, such as pain and mobility of the implant. Obtaining accurate radiographs will enable the clinician to evaluate the crestal bone level appropriately [20].

5.3.2.1. Visual assessment of soft tissue

The soft tissue should be examined for color, texture, form, bleeding, and inflammation. The assessment and any tissue changes should be recorded and photographs should be taken. This photograph or digital image can be used to educate the patient and can be an excellent visual tool to reinforce the importance of good home care.

5.3.2.2. Protocol for assessment of inflammation

Soft tissue assessment includes redness, inflammation, or bleeding, check for the presence of calculus deposits around the implant. Peri-implant infections can progress more rapidly than infection around natural teeth. In presence of an infection, the dental hygienist or dentist will evaluate for pain, mobility. All the data that is gathered is made available to the dentist to develop a treatment plan. The plan may include shortening the interval between implant maintenance visits, possible antibiotics, a radiograph, and/or the dentist may refer the patient for an evaluation by a specialist.

5.3.2.3. Examination upon probing

Some researchers recommend not to probe around the implant, or wait for 3 months, following abutment attachment, to avoid disrupting the formed peri-mucosal seal. The peri-mucosal seal is fragile and probe penetration induces pathogens and jeopardize the success of the implant, a number of considerations and guidelines should be followed when probing the tissue surrounding an implant. A flexible plastic probe is recommended to avoid any scratching of the implant's surface and reduces the potential for trauma to the peri-mucosal seal. Secondly, the probe should be used as a measuring device for recording inflammation or to measure exposed implant threads for monitoring.

A baseline measurement should be established by identifying a monitor marker on the restoration and should be gently probed to check the clinical parameters. This information should be recorded in the patient's notes along with any signs of inflammation present at the first implant maintenance appointment (3 months following prosthesis placement).

5.3.2.4. Signs of failing implant

Presence of infection, pain, mobility, or unacceptable bone loss are the signs of failing implants. Pain or discomfort may be the important signs, before it is evident on a radiograph. In presence of pain, the dentist needs to evaluate the cause i.e. whether it is due to occlusal trauma or infection. An occlusal adjustment may be required to be performed since an implant is held in place by bone not by the periodontal ligament and does not respond like a natural tooth to occlusal trauma.

Mobility following osseointegration can occur because of a loose fixed restoration, infection, fractured abutment thread, an implant fracture or trauma. In case the mobility is due to a loose crown, it may be possible to re-cement it or rescrew it (depending on the type of abutment). If mobility of the implant itself or a broken screw, this is a greater cause for concern. A radiographic assessment is needed.

5.3.2.5. Monitoring the implant

This final step in monitoring the dental implant(s) is the radiographic assessment using a measurable device is recommend to accurately monitor the crestal bone level around the implant(s) and to verify that the restoration is seated properly. The abutment can be visually confirmed through indentations in implant shown in the radiographs, or the screw that is clearly in focus, which should appear as a clear line. This is indicative of a properly seated abutment.

Further radiographs can be taken to determine any crestal bone loss around the implant and to measure the same if present. A measurement of 0.5–1 mm. horizontal bone loss is acceptable in the first year, with an anticipated 0.1 mm of bone loss each subsequent year. If more than 1 mm of horizontal or vertical bone loss is detected in the first year, an evaluation by the implant surgeon is recommended.

5.3.3. Step 3: instrumentation and polishing of dental implants

Following careful assessment of implant, the dental hygienist or dentist should ascertain the presence of calculus on the implant or abutments. Minimal, or indeed no, instrumentation is required for an implant with a healthy gingival attachment. Calculus or microbial deposits are primarily supragingival and are safe for instrumentation. Care must be taken to avoid scratching or roughening the implant surface, as this may result in bacterial accumulation and subsequent inflammation [20].

5.3.3.1. Protocol for safe instrumentation

There is a difference in instrumentation around an implant and natural tooth. Natural teeth are anchored in the bone by the periodontal ligament and sulcular epithelium, whereas the implants are osseointegrated to bone. For instrumentation of a natural tooth, the instrument blade is adapted to the tooth surface and gently inserted between the sulcular epithelium and the side of the tooth or root. To remove calculus deposits, vertical, horizontal, and oblique stokes are used.

5.3.3.2. Dental implant instrumentation

A thorough instrumentation of implants requires the removal of microbial deposits without creating any alteration of the surface of implant or adversely affecting its biocompatibility. Scratches and gouges may be created on the surface that will affect the titanium-oxide layer, reducing the corrosion-resistant nature of a titanium implant. The implant surface may also get contaminated with trace elements from the remaining scaler material, which compromises the long-term osseointegration of the implant.

The suggested materials for use on implant surface are plastic, graphite and titanium scalers. Some studies had revealed that these instruments do not scratch or gouge implant surface. Titanium is the metal of choice because it produces instruments which are thinner than plastic or graphite instruments and provides more strength to dislodge calculus. They are also more biocompatible with other metals. This avoids leaving trace elements from a scaler on the implant surface.

According to Dmytryk, Fox and Moriarty [21], *"Although the use of a plastic curette did not significantly roughen the implant surface there was concern that some of the plastic material may have been smeared or deposited on the implant surface, perhaps altering the biocompatibility of the titanium surface."*

The results of these research studies throw light on the fact that more studies are needed to evaluate the effects of debris left behind on the implant surface, and the biocompatibility of this debris with the titanium implant surface. Stainless steel instruments and metallic power scaler tips have been shown to gouge or scratch the implant surface and are therefore contraindicated. However power scalers and air powder abrasive systems can be used with specific tips, sleeves and powder formulated for implants. Care should be taken when using a plastic sleeve with the tip of a power scaler to prevent aspiration of the plastic tip, in case it gets dislodged [19].

5.3.3.3. Plastic, graphite and titanium coated implant scalers

Implant Prophy™ from TESS are designed from materials like polycarbonate plastic and include Gracey and Columbia designs. Implacare™, Hu-Friedy instruments are featured with a sturdy handle and plastic disposable tips in various designs. Premier Dental Facial implant scalers are made of non-metallic, autoclavable graphite. Titanium-coated Suvan-O'Hehir implant scoop curettes are available from G. Hartzell and Son [20].

5.3.3.4. Titanium implant scalers

An instrument called Implant Pro™ from Brasseler is available in the Langer series with titanium tips that can be replaced from time to time. Nordent makes ImplaMate™, also in the Langer series, Barnhart and universal scalers. The newest in the market are the Wingrove Series, made by Paradise Dental Technologies (PDT), which are designed with a uniquely processed titanium that will refrain from any scratches or leaving any debris behind on implants. These are available in a series of three professionally designed scalers which can be adapted to specifically meet all the challenges of maintaining an implant.

Few of the challenges include removing calculus from a variety of implants and restorative choices. Some are narrow base implants (narrow platform is used for lower incisors, congenially missing laterals, and area with limited available bone) while others have a wide base or wide platform. There is difficulty to gain access to high water bridges as well as full-arch cement or screw retained implants. Also an instrument with small diameter is required to fit under a Hader clip bar or around O-ring ball or locator abutment that can be used for debridement of over dentures.

It is very critical to select an appropriate instrument to remove calculus deposits that will not harm the implant surface during debridement. For narrow base posterior implants or implants that replace two adjacent teeth, an instrument with a longer blade will be advantageous. It can be used under the more bulbous shaped crowns and even under the framework of a high water bridge or full arch implant retained prosthesis. The scaling stroked should be short and horizontal. The calculus present on these implants, crowns or frameworks can be dislodged effectively.

For wide base posterior implants, a universal posterior implant scaler is recommended with short vertical strokes to remove the calculus. For instrumenting any exposed implant threads; anterior or posterior, a shorter radius blade tip of an instrument is suggested which can be used carefully in a side-to-side motion, covering one thread at a time.

For patients with over denture implant abutment, the denture has to be removed to assess the O-rings or clips inside the denture for loss or wear. These O-rings or plastic retention clips should be replaced if worn out, or replaced at least once a year.

For instrumenting the abutments under an over denture, a thinner radius blade tip is adapted under a Hader clip bar in a side to side stroke. An instrument tip with a shorter radius is recommended, used with short vertical strokes around a ball or locator abutment to dislodge any calculus. It is important to understand the unique and different designs of implant and to have a proper armamentarium for the safe implant maintenance. This will allow the clinician to provide patients with ideal implant care with a predictable long-term success of their implants [20].

5.3.3.5. Polishing of restorations on dental implant

Soft rubber tip, with appropriate nonabrasive paste to polish the implants. Aluminum oxide, tin oxide, APF-free prophy paste, and low-abrasive dentifrice are all considered acceptable polishing abrasives for implants. Coarse abrasive polishing pastes and acidulated phosphate fluoride (APF) products are contraindicated, as they may etch surface of implants.

6. CIST protocol for management of recurrent disease during maintenance of dental implants

Conventional periodontal therapy should be done when inflammation develops around an implant. The therapy should include the efforts to improve patient's oral hygiene, with methods similar to those used for natural teeth. Lang et al. [22] suggested a novel, systematic stepwise approach for the prevention and treatment of peri-implant diseases. This approach is referred to as the cumulative interceptive supportive therapy (CIST) protocol.

It is based on periodic monitoring with implementation of treatment as thresholds for a particular condition are met. The first step is protocol (A), then (B) and, if conditions continue to worsen, the patient may require more advanced treatment, i.e. execution of protocol (C), and finally (D) by a specialist who has implant training for it. To control inflammation in peri-implant mucositis, that is, implants with minimal increase in pocket depth, slight (+) bleeding on probing, marginal erythema, plaque, and/or calculus, Protocol (A) is implemented.

The endpoint of the therapy is resolution of inflammation with careful mechanical debridement (using plastic curettes and rubber cup prophylaxis), swabbing with 0.12% chlorhexidine twice daily, and a review of home care and patient motivation. Protocol (B) is carried out for conditions that exhibit features similar to mucositis but with deeper pocket depths (4–5 mm) but without loss of supporting bone.

The treatment should include the therapies of protocol (A), plus locally delivered antibiotic (minocycline microspheres, doxycycline gel) at the infected implant site(s). Studies in the recent past have shown the use of minocycline microspheres may be beneficial in treatment of peri-implant mucositis and peri-implantitis. For management of early peri-implantitis,

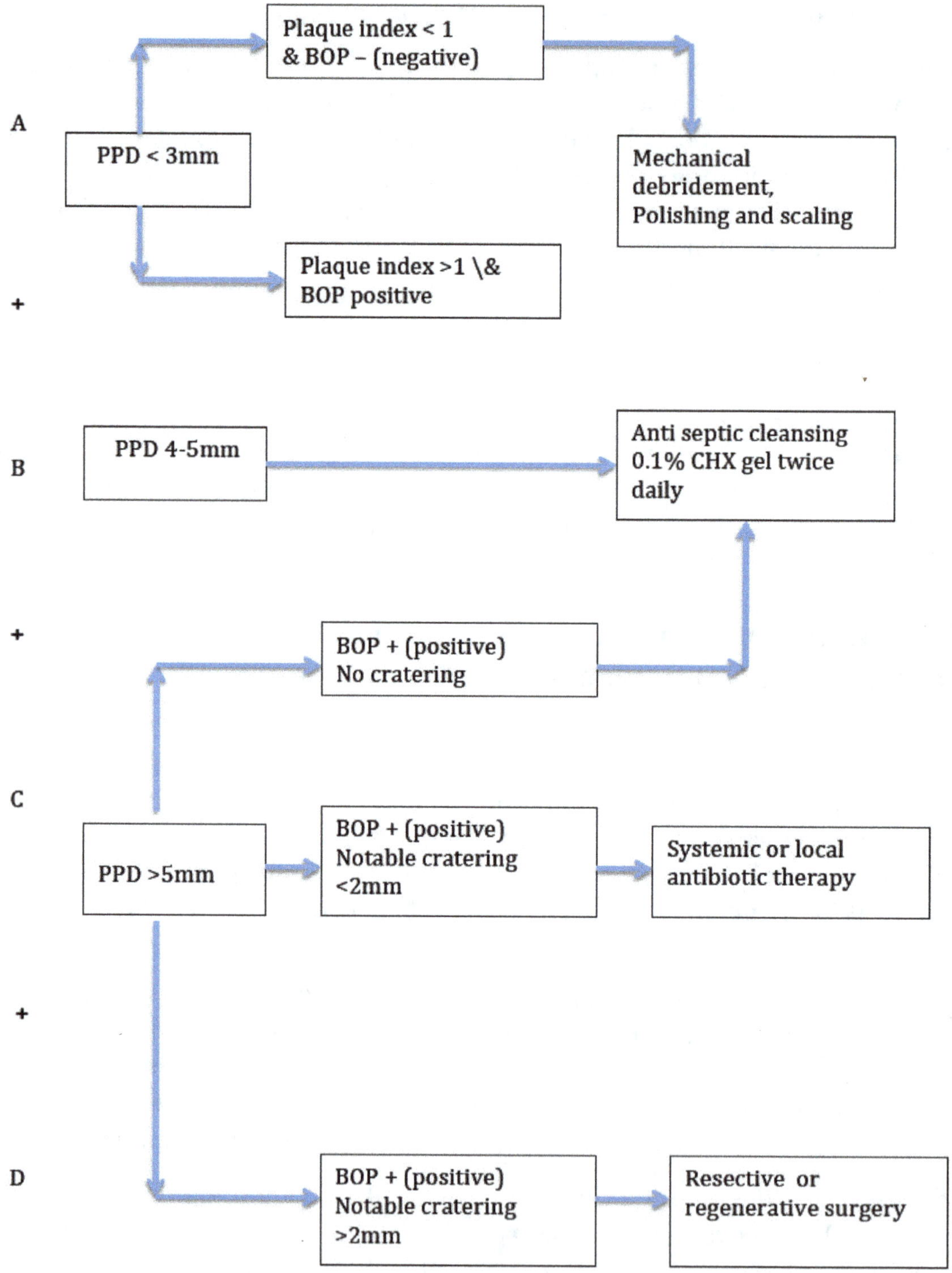

Figure 5. CIST protocol.

Protocol (C) is used, which consists of a more intensive approach and is used in conditions where there is radiographic evidence of osseointegrated bone loss of <2 mm and probing pocket depths >5 mm. The strategy should comprise a combination of the modalities for protocols (A) and (B) with the addition of systemic antibiotic therapy (metronidazole 250 mg *t.i.d.* for 7 days or amoxicillin 500 mg *t.i.d.* for 10 days).

Furthermore, periodontal surgical access for surface de- contamination (citric acid 1–2 min or tetracycline 250 mg, 5 mL for 5 min) should be considered. In cases of frank peri-implantitis that reveal probing depths (>5 mm), (+) bleeding on probing, plaque/calculus, and peri-implant bone loss of >2 mm, Protocol (D) is initiated along with other three protocols.

This treatment modality comprises periodontal surgical intervention for chemical disinfection, osseous resection, and/or guided bone regeneration (GBR). GBR is a procedure to attempt for salvaging the implant through bone regeneration techniques with the use of resorbable or nonresorbable semipermeable membranes and a bone substitute or replacement graft (such as freeze-dried bone allograft or anorganic bovine bone). In clinical practice, the protocol of CIST is targeted for early detection and methodical sequential treatment, which may help rescue and even reverse the fate of the ailing or failing endosseous dental implant [23] (**Figure 5**).

The four steps are:

1. Antiseptic therapy, CIST protocol A & B
2. Antibiotic therapy, CIST protocol A + B
3. Antibiotic therapy, CIST protocol A + B + C
4. Regenerative or resective therapy, CIST protocol A + B + C + D.

Author details

Krishna Kripal[1] and Kavita Chandrasekaran[2]*

*Address all correspondence to: dr.ckavita@gmail.com

1 Rajarajeswari Dental College and Hospital, Bangalore, India

2 Department of Periodontology, Rajarajeswari Dental College and Hospital, Bangalore, India

References

[1] Albrektsson T, Dahl E, Enbom L, Engevall S, Engquist B, Erikksson AR, Feldmann G, Freiberg N, Glantz PO, Kjellman 0 CL, Kvint S, Kondell PA, Palmquist J, Werndah1 L, htrand P. Osseointegrated oral implants—A Swedish multicenter study of 8139 consecutively inserted Nobelpharma implants. Journal of Periodontology. 1988;**59**:287-296

[2] Branemark P-I, Breine U, Adell R, Hansson BO, Lindstrom J, Olsson A. Osseointegrated implants in the treatment of the edentulous jaw. Experience from a 10-year period. Scandinavian Journal of Plastic and Reconstructive Surgery and Hand Surgery. 1977;**2**(16): 1-132

[3] Buser D, Hf W, Bragger U, Balsiger C. Tissue integration of one-stage IT1 implants: 3-Year results of a longitudinal study with hollow-cylinder and hollow-screw implants. Journal of Oral & Maxillofacial Implants. 1991;**6**:405-412

[4] Rosenberg E, Torosian J. Slots 1. Microbial differences in 2 clinically distinct types of failures of osseointegrated implants. Clinical Oral Implants Research. 1991;**2**:135-144

[5] Glossary of Prosthodontic Terms

[6] Brånemark PI, Adell R, Breine U, Hansson BO, Lindström J, Ohlsson A. Intra-osseous anchorage of dental prostheses. I. Experimental studies. Scandinavian Journal of Plastic and Reconstructive Surgery. 1969;**3**(2):81-100

[7] Albrektsson T, Brånemark PI, Hansson HA, Lindström J. Osseointegrated titanium implants. Requirements for ensuring a long-lasting, direct bone-to implant anchorage in man. Acta Orthopaedica Scandinavica. 1981;**52**(2):155-170

[8] Zarb GA, Albrektsson T. Osseointegration–A requirement for the periodontal ligament? Editorial. International Journal of Periodontics and Restorative Dentistry. 1991;**11**:88-91

[9] Berglundh T, Lindhe J. Dimension of the periimplant mucosa. Biological width revisited. Journal of Clinical Periodontology. 1996;**23**(10):971-973

[10] Quirynen M, Van Steenb Berghe D, Jacobs R, Schotte A, Darius P. The reliability of pocket probing-around screw-type implants. Clinical Oral Implants Research. 1991;**2**:186-192

[11] Mombelli A, Mac VO, Schurch E, Lang NP. The microbiota associated with successful or failing osseointegrated titanium implants. Oral Microbiology and Immunology. 1987;**2**:145-151

[12] Apse F, Zarb GA, Schmitt A, Lewis DW. The longitudinal effectiveness of osseointegrated dental implants. The Toronto study: Peri-implant mucosal response. The International Journal of Periodontics & Restorative Dentistry. 1991;**11**:95-111

[13] Chaytor DV. The longitudinal effectiveness of osseointegrated dental implants. The Toronto study: Bone level changes. The International Journal of Periodontics & Restorative Dentistry. 1991;**11**:113-125

[14] Berglundh T, Lindhe J, Marinello C, et al. Soft tissue reaction to de novo plaque formation on implants and teeth. An experimental study in the dog. Clinical Oral Implants Research. 1992;**3**:1-8

[15] Roos-Jansaker AM. Long-time follow up of implant therapy and treatment of Peri-Implantitis. Swedish Dental Journal. Supplement. 2007;**188**:7-66

[16] Pontoriero R, Tonelli MP, Carnevale G, et al. Experimentally induced peri-implant mucositis. A clinical study in humans. Clinical Oral Implants Research. 1994;**5**(4):254-259

[17] Roos-Jansåker AM, Renvert H, Lindahl C, et al. Nine- to fourteen-year follow-up of implant treatment. Part iii: Factors associated with peri-implant lesions. Journal of Clinical Periodontology. 2006;**33**(4):296-301

[18] Lindhe J, Meyle J. Peri-implant diseases: Consensus report of the sixth European workshop on periodontology. Journal of Clinical Periodontology. 2008;**35**(Suppl. 8):282-285

[19] Ericsson I, Berglundh T, Marinello C, Liljenberg B, Lindhe J. Long-standing plaque and gingivitis at implants and teeth in the dog. Clinical Oral Implants Research. 1992;**3**(3):99-103

[20] Ochsenbein C. Retreatment. Periodontology. 1996;**2000**(12):129-132

[21] Dmytryk JJ, Fox SC, Moriarty JD. The effects of scaling titanium implant surfaces with metal and plastic instruments on cell attachment. Journal of the Pancreas: JOP. 1990;**61**:491-496

[22] Lang B, Worthington P, Lavelle W. Osseointegration in Dentistry: An Introduction. Chicago, IL: Quintessence; 1994. p. 121

[23] Schumaker ND, Metcall BJ, Toscano NT, Holtzclaw DJ. Periodontal and periimplant maintenance: A critical factor in longterm treatment success. Compendium. 2009;**30**:2-13

11

Involvement of Heat-Shock Proteins During Periodontal Ligament Remodeling

Rina Muraoka, Keisuke Nakano,
Hidetsugu Tsujigiwa, Hitoshi Nagatsuka,
Hirokazu Matsuda, Mihoko Tomida,
Norimasa Okafuji, Kazuhiro Yamada and
Toshiyuki Kawakami

Abstract

Mechanical stress induces various molecules such as heat-shock protein (HSP), which causes structural changes in the proteins in periodontal ligament (PDL). We carried out an experiment to induce traumatic occlusion in mouse PDL and analyzed the expression of HSPs. HSPs investigated acts differently depending on the time of expression. HSPs are constitutively expressed in the PDL and defend cells from stress and maintain homeostasis under normal conditions. During bone addition to the PDL on the tension side, HSP27 and HSP47, HSP70 also acts as molecular chaperone, which assists the maturation of bone morphogenetic proteins and aids osteoblast activation. In HSP 70 and HSP 47, mechanical stress is applied to the PDL on the tension side for a short period of time for alveolar bone repairing, and when abnormality occurs in the collagen structure fibroblasts of PDL, it functions at the injured site, whereby extracellular that promotes abnormal collagen secretion and stores the modified protein in the endoplasmic reticulum, there by controlling the decalcification of PDL. In other words, HSP47 and HSP70 are expressed in PDL fibroblasts on the pressure side damaged by application of mechanical stress and contribute to the repair of collagen tissue by activating PDL fibroblasts, supporting recovery from cell damage.

Keywords: periodontal ligament, mechanical stress, homeostasis, heat-shock proteins, HSP, fibroblasts, collagen tissue, immunohistochemistry, occlusal trauma

1. Introduction

The periodontal tissue responds to different types of stimulus such as mechanical stress and inflammation, to maintain homeostasis, and expresses various proteins to bring about active remodeling of the periodontal tissue [1–12]. Periodontal connective tissue remodeling occurred due to traumatic occlusal overload [13, 14]. Heat-shock proteins (HSPs) reply to mechanical stress, and it is learned about as the main protein manifested by various systems and organiza tions. HSP is also led by an inflammation, a physical stress, a chemical stress and a pathological change in heat shock [15]. But, the function of each HSP is still unclear. HSP participates in defense and restoration of an injury cell, and it is thought that it contributes to the control of cellular function [16–18]. The main ingredient of a cell outside matrix of PDL is the collagen, and this acts on it so that mechanical stress of bite force and the mechanical correction power may be eased. When a collagen fiber of PDL suffers damage by mechanical stress, and mechanical stress is freed once, a collagen fiber returns to the original shape. However, many points are unclear about the cell protein which contributes to recovery mechanism. In the remodeling course, the fibroblasts play an important role, such as collagen synthesis. HSP47 is a collagen-binding stress protein that acts as a collagen-specific molecular chaperone during the biosynthesis and secre tion of procollagen. Type I collagen is a major component of periodontal ligaments [19–21].

We focused on collagen synthesis and HSP47, which are essential to the development of mouse and humans. We developed an experimental model by exposing the periodontal tissue to occlusal overload, and the expression of HSP47 was determined using immunohis tochemistry (IHC). Then, we carried out an immunohistochemical investigation of HSP47 expression state in mouse PDL tissue after applying a mechanical stress and during the recovery of the PDL.

2. Materials and methods

Before the experiments: Anesthesia was induced in the mouse by inhalation of a gaseous mixture of isoflurane and air (preanesthetic concentration 4.0%). The experiment animal were using gas anesthesia system for insensitivity to pain by the administration of lower concentra tion gases before experiment. Gas anesthesia system was control with the fixed current veloc ity, it was became stable, and the experiment was conducted under the maintained opiate. The upper part of body of a mouse was lifted and fixed on the experimental platform after anesthesia. General anesthesia was maintained during an experiment using an induction pipe through a nose of a mouse (maintenance anesthetic density 1.0%). The upper and lower jaw of the mouse was fixed on the laboratory table to do while opening the mouth of a mouse during an experiment. We prepared the specimen after completing loading occlusal trauma and mechanical stress on the maxillary molar part of the mouse.

Experimental animals: Seventy 8-week-old male ddY mouse (body weight 35 ± 5 g) was used in this study. The mouse was kept in an environment controlled by an air-conditioning unit, in metal cages with bedding on the floor.

This study was planned according to the Matsumoto Dental University (MDU) Experimental Animal Guidelines. This protocol followed the MDU Experimental Animal Study Guidelines and was approved by Animal Study Experimental Committee of MDU (Approval No. 179-10, 233-13).

2.1. Load mechanical stress from the vertical direction

Experiments 1 and 2: We made a hole in an occlusal surface of the upper jaw first molar using one-quarter sizes of round bur. After that, stainless micro screw of head diameter 1.7 mm, head thickness 0.5 mm, official diameter 1.0 mm and the full length 3.5 mm was planted. This makes the mandibular first molar opposite cause a prematurity, and an occlusal trauma has been caused. The experimental period continued for 30 days. A change in the periodontal ligament was observed on 1, 4, 7 and 14 days. The untreated maxillary first molar of the mouse served as the control group (Experiment 1). Then after, the micro plus screw was removed at 4 days after implantation and the subsequent tissue changes were observed (Experiment 2).

2.2. Load mechanical stress from lateral direction

Experiments 3 and 4: A separator was inserted by the method of Waldo [22] in order to apply persistent mechanical stress to the upper molar PDL region of the mouse (**Figure 1**). The one from which a rubber weir seat was severed in a square of 2.0 × 2.0 mm of folding into two was employed as a separator. The upper part molar range of the mouse is sequence of three teeth, and the first molar and the second molar from the near heart side are the third molar. Therefore, a separator was inserted between the first molar of upper right and the second molar. HSP manifestation was estimated using two experimental systems by this study. Mechanical stress has been loaded with the passage of time using a separator. Mechanical stress was released at most 24 h later, and lumping was removed by the upper part molar of a periodontal tissue of a mouse of the range of the problem. We decided to observe total of

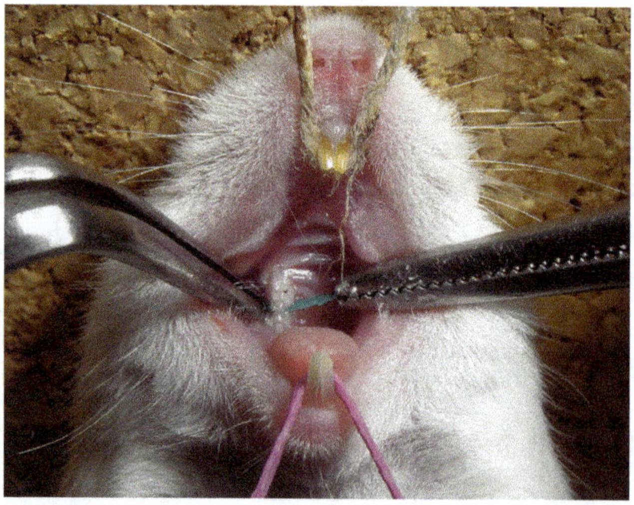

Figure 1. The situation of the insertion. The upper jaw was immobilized by fixing a kite string, and the position of the lower jaw was immobilized by fixing a rubber band. Quotation alteration of literatures #1.

six experimental duration, a group for 10 min (10 min), a group for 20 min (20 min), a group for 1 h (1 h), a group for 3 h (3 h) and a group for 9 h (9 h) and 24 h (24 h) and used five experimental animals per one group. It should be noted that only water was given to a mouse to prevent a separator being dropped during impressing of mechanical stress (Experiment 3).

After loading a mechanical stress by a separator during the 3 hours, and then the stress was released. In the shortest experimental time, an organization that around the maxillary molar and incisers of the mouse have been extracted after 20 minutes later from remove separator. In the longest experimental time was 1 week immediately after removal of a separator. The group in which the tissue was removed immediately after removing the separator (3 h + 0 min, 3 h + 0 min), a 20 min after removing the separator group (3 h + 20 min), a 1 h after removing the separator group (3 h + 1 h), a 3 h after removing the separator group (3 h + 3 h), a 9 h after removing the separator group (3 h + 9 h), a 24 h after removing the separator group (3 h + 24 h), a 3 day after removing the separator group (3 h + 3 d), and a 1 week after removing the separator group (3 h + 1 w), with five mice per group.

A mechanical stress was loaded for 3 hours, and it was released, then we were permitting that the mouse could consuming water and solid feed freely till the end of an experimental period (Experiment 4).

The periodontal tissue of the upper left molar from the same individual mouse (the opposite, untreated side) was used as a control group. For both the experimental and control groups, the distal buccal root of the upper first molar was the observation site by this experiments.

2.3. Tissue preparation

In the four experiments described earlier, the mouse upper molar periodontal tissue was excised together with the jawbone, promptly fixed and immersed for 24 h in a fixing solution. Then after, specimens were decalcified in 10% EDTA solution for 3 weeks. Next, it was embedded in paraffin.

Experiments 1 and 2: This was followed by embedding in paraffin, deparaffinization in xylene and vertical sectioning of the root portion with a thickness of 4 μm.

Experiments 3 and 4: A series of horizontal 5-μm thick sections was produced for the PDL region of the roots in question and immune histochemically examined.

3. Histopathology

Specimens were stained with hematoxylin and eosin and were examined under the light microscope.

3.1. Histopathological examination: vertical sectioning of the root portion

Experiment 1: Dense amount of PDL fibroblasts and spindle cells were seen in the control group. Capillaries were congested with red blood cells. PDL fibers were irregularly arranged (**Figure 2A**). At alveolar bone, osteoclasts were noticeable. The furcation is lined by acellular cementum. First a histopathology view of an experimental group is described. At day 1, capillaries shevel hyperemia were filled with red blood cells dilated. At day 4, hyperemia was observed stronger than day 1. The amount of deeply stained cells with round shape nuclei increased (**Figure 2B**). A lot of osteoclasts were observed on the glassy surface of the alveolar bone. At day 7, the cytological density reduced compared to day 4. Further, osteoclasts appeared in between fibroblasts (**Figure 2C**). Howship's lacunae formed in borders of resorbed alveolus bone and cementum (**Figure 2D**). Resorption of cementum was part of the acellular cementum. At day 14, bone resorption and osteoclasts in lacunae have become more evident as compared to day 7, and resorbed cementum also increased. The PDL at the furcation area in the control group runs in an orderly fashion from the tooth to the alveolar bone. But, the fibroblasts were sort of irregular. It can be speculated that the occlusal force to the furcation was in an equilibrium state.

It was inferred that congestion and vasodilation occurred from day 1. Since there was an increase in hyperemia at day 4, excessive occlusal load caused tissue reaction by a rise in blood supply. But, the blood vessels did not show any change at day 7, and this is considered to be affected by the HSP47. On the other hand, the osteoclasts in Howship's lacunae as well as bone resorption continued to rise. The osteoclasts expressed by occlusal trauma have been derived from bone marrow [13]. According to this result, the osteoclasts observed at day 7 were probably bone marrow derived cells. The enlargement of Howship's lacunae at day 14 compared to day 7 suggested that the activity of the osteoclasts was elicited excessive load.

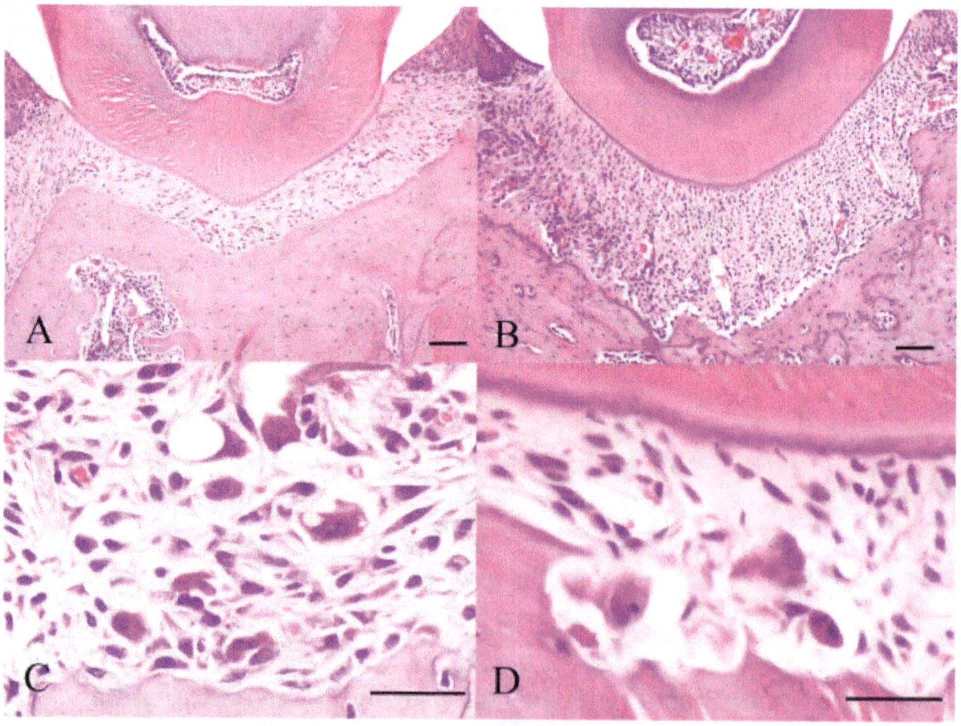

Figure 2. Histopathology of Experiment 1. Control specimen (A), Experimental day 4 specimen (B), Experimental day 7 specimen (C) and Experimental day 14 specimen (D). The inset scale bar indicates 50 μm. Quotation alteration of literatures #14.

Experiment 2: In the control group, strong hyperemia was seen at day 4 (Experimental group 1). At day 3 of the experimental group, significant vasodilation were observed compared to control group. Osteoclasts were scattered in the alveolar bone and some formed clusters in Howship's lacunae (**Figure 3A**). At day 6, capillaries were decreased in hyperemia, and fewer osteoclasts were noted. Fibroblasts were deeply stained with hematoxylin stain and have round shape nucleus. At day 10 of the experimental group, Howship's lacunae were more observed compared to day 6. Fibroblasts and dilating capillaries were no longer conspicuous at day 30. These histological findings at day 30 of the experimental group are similar to the control group in experiment 1 (**Figure 3B**).

To summarize this finding, at the experimental group of day 3, hyperemia was not so prominent compared to control group, and when occlusal overload was released, hyperemia declined as well. At day 6 and 10, osteoclasts were reduced. The osteoclasts were induced by the implantation of micro screw at day 4, and these activities continued even if the micro screw was removed.

Howship's lacunae were enlarged at day 10 compared to day 6. The constant activity of osteoclasts was brought about by the influence of occlusal overload which allowed the cells to proceed to the activity which already began. This result means that osteoclasts was increased due to occlusal overload and continued to increase even when the occlusal overload was removed. The congestion or vasodilation was no longer observed at day 30 of the experiment. It can be inferred that the periodontal ligament was restored to its equilibrium state at day 30 of the experimental group.

3.2. Histopathological examination: horizontal sectioning of the root portion

Experiment 3: The distal buccal root of the upper jaw first molar was horizontally examined. At the control group, the mesial side of root had a slight deviation where the PDL width is about 50 μm. The distal side of PDL in between the alveolar bone and the distal buccal root of the left maxillary first molar were relatively arranged in order (**Figure 4**, C-H, C-T). In contrast, the mesial side PDL of the distal buccal root and the PDL fibroblasts were observed in a diagonal orientation (**Figure 4**, C-P).

At the experimental group, the PDL located near by the separator were called the tension side (PDL of the distal side at the distal buccal root of right maxillary first molar); the PDL located

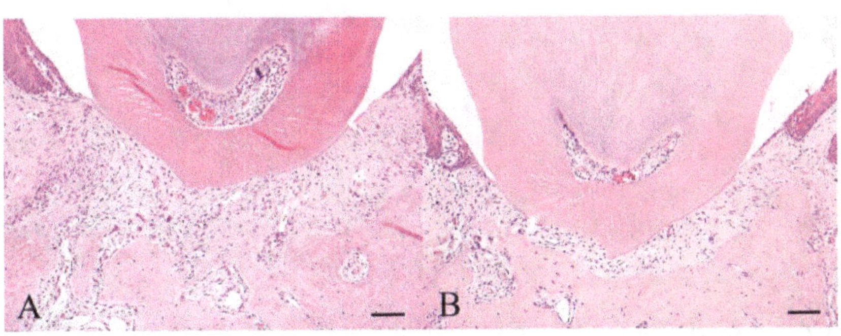

Figure 3. Histopathology of Experiment 2. Experimental day 3 specimen (A) and Experimental day 30 specimen (B). The inset scale bar indicates 50 μm. Quotation alteration of literatures #14.

at opposite side were called the pressure side (PDL of the mesial side PDL at the distal buccal root of the maxillary first molar). The 20 min group of the tension side, difference between the tension and pressure side became apparent (**Figure 4**, 20m-H, 20m-T, 20m-P). 1 h group

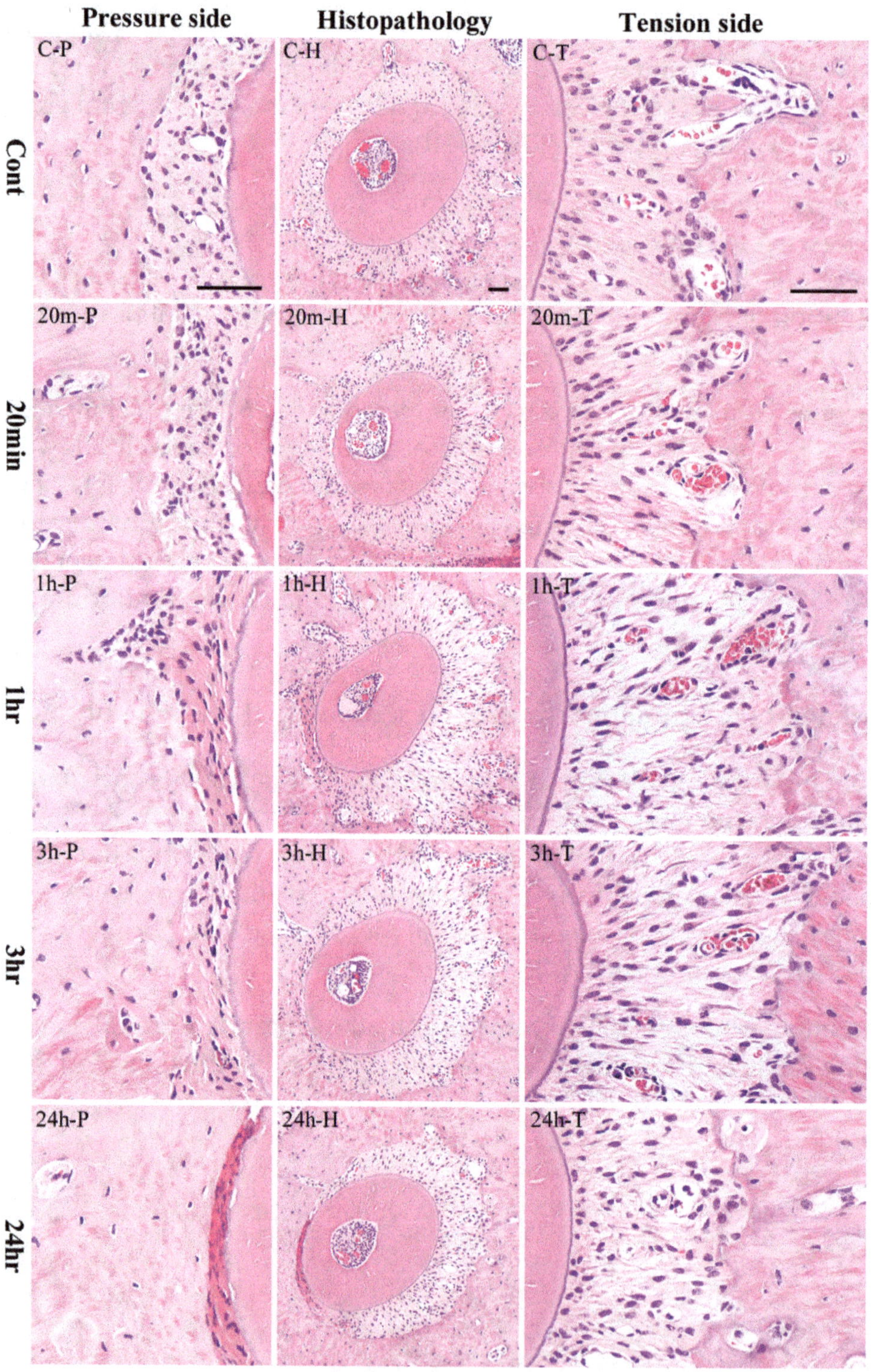

Figure 4. Histopathology of Experiment 3. Center histopathological image shows the alveolar bone socket morphology. Left and right histopathological image shows high power view of pressure side and tension side. The most upper row is the control group (cont), and the following is the experimental groups of 20 min (20 min), 1 h (1 h), 3 h (3 h) and 24 h (24 h). The inset scale bar indicates 50 μm. Quotation alteration of literatures #2.

of the tension side, the root moved further to the mesial direction (**Figure 4**, 1h-H). The PDL width created a greater traction and the fibers had been stretched considerably (**Figure 4**, 1h-T). The 1 h group of the pressure side, the PDL cells showed various degenerative changes. Furthermore, osteoblasts lining the bone surface were reduced in number; the cytoplasm and nucleus became flattened by pressure and distinction among surrounding fibroblasts became difficult (**Figure 4**, 1h-P). The 3 h group of the tension side, the root continued to move mesially and the width of the PDL space increased (**Figure 4**, 3h-H). The number of fibroblasts decreased compared to the 1 h group. Oval-shaped osteoblasts are observed lining the surface of the alveolar bone (**Figure 4**, 3h-T). The 3 h group of the pressure side, the PDL space further became narrower; degenerative changes were more severe that distinction of PDL cells was difficult. PDL fibroblasts increased its eosinophilic staining; they had fewer nuclei per unit area. Osteoblasts lining bone surfaces were also fewer (**Figure 4**, 3h-P). The 9 h group of the tension side, the root stopped moving in the mesial direction and the width of the PDL did not further increase. The gap in between collagen bundles was reduced. The 9 h group of the pressure side, eosinophilic staining of the PDL further increased; the number of PDL fibroblasts decreased. Moreover, some obscure spaces partly in the fiber bundles showed hematoxylin staining caused by karyolysis. The 24 h group of the tension side, osteoblasts lining the alveolar bone surface are oval or short cuboidal in shape. Dilated vessels and scattered hemorrhages can be observed (**Figure 4**, 24h-H, 24h-T). The 24 h group of the pressure side, the PDL became strongly eosinophilic. Strong nuclear chromatin condensation or pyknosis has been observed in PDL fibroblasts, karyorrhexis is very evident (**Figure 4**, 24h-P).

4. Immunohistochemistry

Experiments 1 and 2: This was followed by embedding in paraffin, deparaffinization in xylene and vertical sectioning of the root portion with a thickness of 4 μm. After deparaffinization, the slides were treated in incubator at 60°C for 30 min. Specimens were subjected to proteolytic enzyme, immersed in 0.03% hydrogen peroxide methanol solution for 3 min, followed by endogenous peroxidase activation for 10 min. Anti-HSP47 was the primary antibody (1/2000 dilution). Polyclonal anti-rabbit was the secondary antibody [14]. Then after, slides were washed with PBS and then subjected to DAB color development for 3 min. Finally, counterstaining was done by immersing the specimen in hematoxylin for 1 s.

Experiments 3 and 4: A series of horizontal 5-μm thick sections was produced for the PDL region of the roots in question and immune histochemically examined. The immunohistological study was carried out using Dako Envision+Kit. Anti-rabbit HSP47 polyclonal antibody was the primary antibody (1/1000 dilution) [1]. The specimens were counterstained with hematoxylin. The negative controls were treated by using the same experimental protocol, but without the primary antibody.

4.1. Immunohistochemical examination: vertical sectioning of the root portion

Experiment 1: HSP47 was slightly detected in the cytoplasm of fibroblasts in the control group (**Figure 5A**). Other cells that were scattered in the periodontal ligament were also positive to

HSP47 (**Figure 5B**). At day 1, HSP47 expression was detected more in fibroblasts in epithelial attachment, the intensity was similar to those in the control group. At day 4, HSP47 was detected in the entire periodontal ligament. Strong expression was detected in the fibroblast with which covered an alveolar bone in particular (**Figure 5C**). More expression of HSP47 was increased on day 7 more than day 4. HSP47 was also detected by a vascular endothelial cell. The strongest expression of HSP47 was detected by a cell of fibroblasts on day 14 (**Figure 5D**).

In the control group, periodontal ligaments expressed HSP47 even though they were at equilibrium. Only few cells in junctional epithelium and subepithelial connective tissue showed positive reaction. This result means that HSP47 was co-expressed at cells of nonstress condition in which the protein was regulated at the transcription level. Moreover, we mentioned that the weak expression of HSP47 [5, 6] in normal tissues was considered to be involved in the maintenance of homeostasis in the periodontal tissue. From day 1, fibroblasts near the epithelial attachment expressed HSP47. The findings were similar to our study of horizontal sectioning of the root portion where HSP70 was initially detected on tension side of PDL after loading orthodontic force. This result suggests that HSP47 is initially involved in remodeling of collagen fibers on tension side upon mechanical stress application. HSP47 was increased at a cell on the alveolar bone in particular on day 4. Compression of a PDL was clear because a collagen fiber received restoration. HSP47 has begun to show conspicuously in an endothelial cell on day 7. This suggests that becoming a capillary depends on surplus occlusal load. Although there was no increase in congestion at day 4, but HSP47 was still considered to be involved in the process. HSP47 had peaked on day 14 and kept being increased by a continuous load. You can guess the collagen fibers to keep restoring under the existence of a

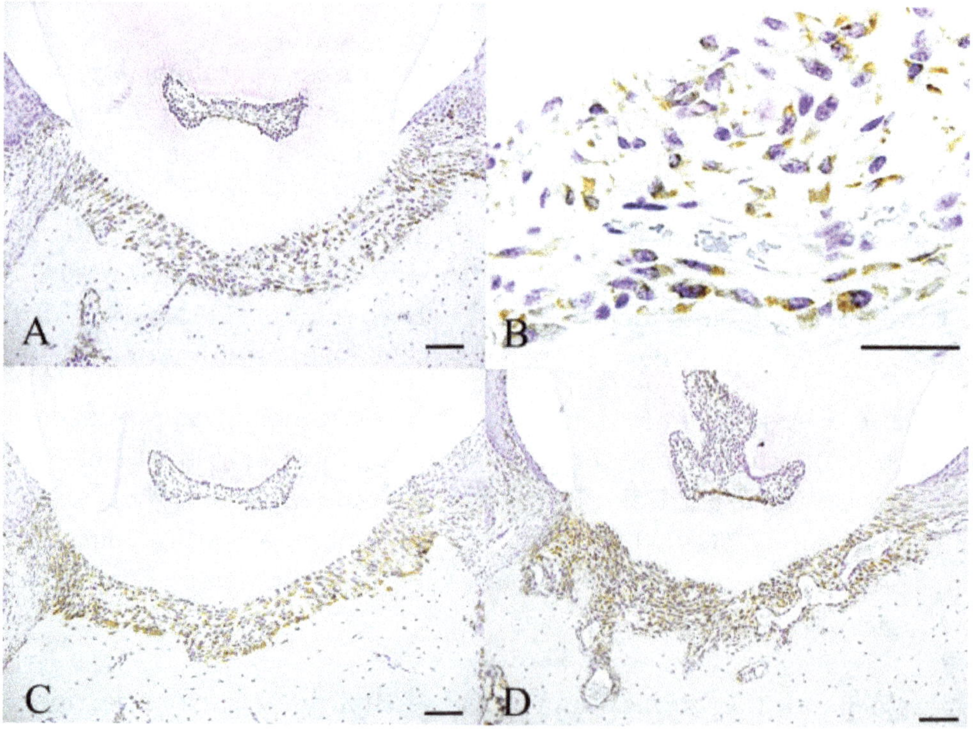

Figure 5. Immunohistochemical features of Experiment 1. Control specimen (A, B), Experimental day 4 specimen (C) and Experimental day 14 specimen (D). The inset scale bar indicates 50 μm. Quotation alteration of literatures #14.

traumatic occlusion. Fibrosis follows a continuous stress by successive accumulation of a collagen fiber. These suggest that manifestation of HSP47 always participated in a physiological remodeling of a periodontal ligament by the excessive occlusal load.

Experiment 2: At day 3, the number of fibroblasts that expressed HSP47 was similar to the control group (**Figure 6A**). Some cells scattered in the periodontal ligament also expressed HSP47. The manifested strength on day 6 was increased more than day 3 (**Figure 6B**). Most of a positive cell possesses round nuclei. At day 10, the number of the cell which indicates positive reaction decreased more than the sixth day (**Figure 6C**). A small number of scattered cells were positive and this was equal to opposition on day 30 (**Figure 6D**). On day 3, HSP47 was slightly stronger than the control group suggesting the progressive repair of damaged collagen.

Though excessive occlusal load was removed, the cell with which I cover an alveolar bone kept manifesting expressions of HSP47 on day 4. HSP47 kept being increased on day 6 and decreased on day 10. Thus, HSP47 tends to be increased with the over time. But on day 30, the expression of HSP47 was like the contrasting group and that a cell had returned to equilibrium state. The previous studies had shown the increase in HSP expression caused by mechanical stress and decrease upon mechanical load release. Our data suggested that HSP47 expressed by damaged epidermis during wound healing, and damaged cells caused by mechanical trauma also express HSP47 [23]. Continuous expression of HSP47 prevented a disturbance of epidermal cells, abnormal cell division, rupture of a blood vessel and other

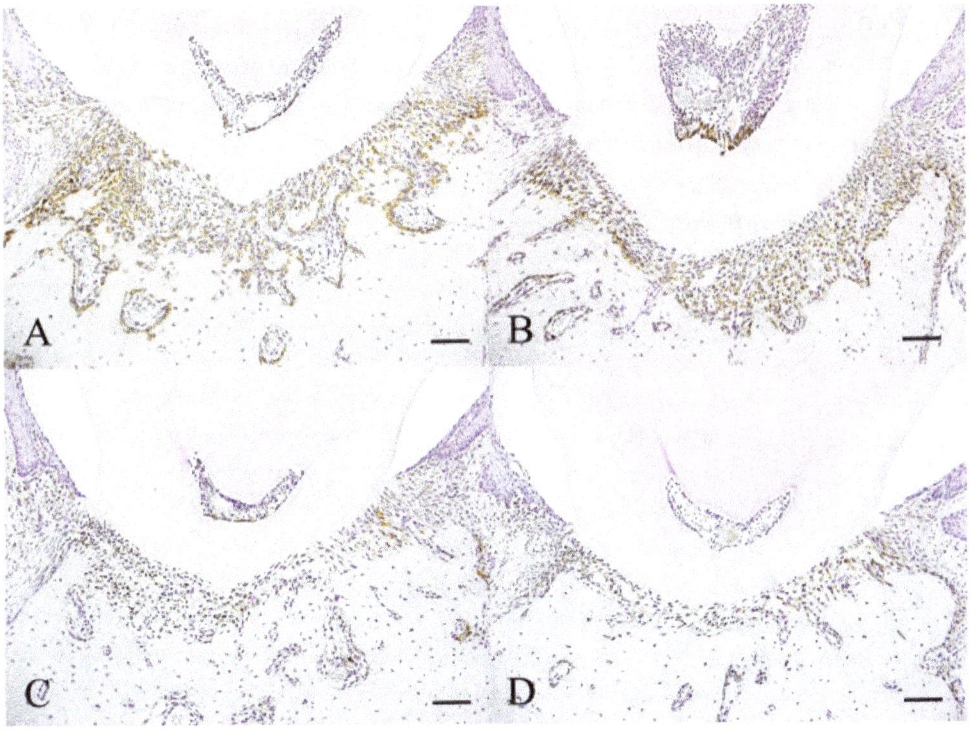

Figure 6. Immunohistochemical features of Experiment 2. Experimental day 3 specimen (A), Experimental day 6 specimen (B), Experimental day 10 specimen (C) and Experimental day 30 specimen. The inset scale bar indicates 50 μm. Quotation alteration of literatures #14.

occurrence of apoptosis. The continuous HSP expression from day 1 to the day 14 was a defending reply. The abnormal function of HSP47 was observed by the collagen bundles of the periodontitis damaged.

4.2. Immunohistochemical examination: horizontal sectioning of the root portion

Experiment 3: In the PDL tissue from mouse in the control group, HSP47 expression was detected in the cell cytoplasm of the PDL collagen bundles uniformly over the entire PDL (**Figure 7**).

In the PDL tissue from mouse in the experimental group, the distal side of the PDL on the side in which the separator was inserted was the tension side and the proximal PDL on the opposite side was the pressure side. After loading mechanical stress over time up to 24 h by inserting a separator, histological analysis of the mouse periodontal tissue was performed (**Figure 8**).

In the 10 and 20 min group, there was hardly any clear difference in the intensity of HSP47 expression when compared with the control group. There was a clear difference in the width of the PDL on the tension side and PDL on the pressure side by a 1 h group. HSP47 manifestation in expansion PDL on the tension side was stronger than HSP47 manifestation in opposition. PDL space on the pressure side shrunk and was small by a 3 h group, and the width of the PDL space on the side pulled it and expanded more, and PDL fiber in this territory was extended conspicuously. PDL fiber was sparsely by the part of PDL, and there was a place where PDL fiber breaks and causes space. But the manifestation of HSP47 on the tension side was stronger than that of the control group. The expansion width of tension side PDL observed by a 3 h group was maintained by a 9 h group. However, the intensity of HSP47 expression showed localized changes in the 9 h group. Stronger HSP47 manifestation was observed on the pressure side more than the tension side. A stronger HSP47 reply was observed in PDL on the tension side by a 24 h group. However, on the pressure side, HSP47 expression disappeared because the PDL fibroblasts were strongly compressed, but HSP47 expression was detected in the PDL fibroblasts adjoining the compressed PDL.

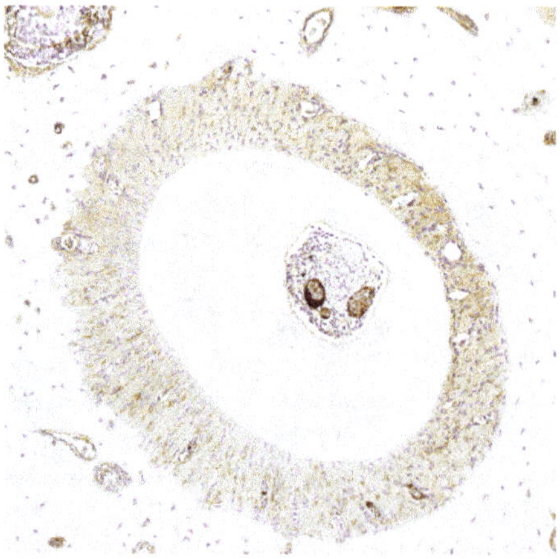

Figure 7. Immunohistochemical results of the control group. IHC staining profile of HSP47 in control specimens. The inset scale bar indicates 50 μm. Quotation alteration of literatures #1.

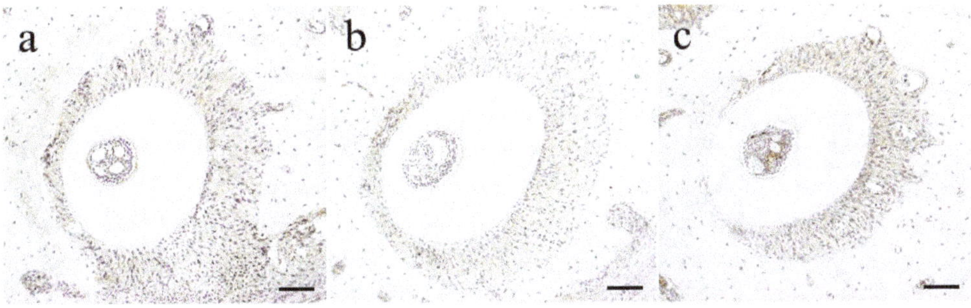

Figure 8. Immunohistochemical results of Experiment 3 at horizontal sectioning of the root portion. (a) 3 h group, (b) 9 h group and (c) 24 h group. The inset scale bar indicates 50 μm. Quotation alteration of literatures #1.

Summarize the results of immunohistochemical experiment 3. So early time, a positive HSP47 response appeared in the PDL on the tension side, and the same level expression of HSP47 was keeped for 9 hours. The 24 hours group indicated the manifested strength of HSP47 the most highest in the all experimental group. A positive immunohistochemistry-like HSP47 response in the tension side indicated strong step-by-step increase with the passage of time. The low manifested position was maintained about immunohistochemistry-like HSP47 positive reaction on the pressure side, and there were no manifested conspicuous changes after stress loaded. But strong positive reaction was detected by a group for 9 hours. A PDL fibroblast was compressed hard by a group for 24 hours, but HSP47 manifestation disappeared on the pressure side because strong HSP47 manifestation was detected in a PDL fibroblast which neighbors compressed PDL. In the 24 hours group, HSP47 expression disappeared in the pressure side because of the PDL fibroblasts were strongly compressed. But intense HSP47 expression was detected in the PDL fibroblasts adjoining the compressed PDL.

Experiment 4: After 3 h of mechanical stress loading, separator was removed. Mouse periodontal tissue of upper jaw was removed for the passage of time until after 1 week. An immunohistochemistry analysis of HSP47 manifestation with the passage of time in the mouse PDL organization of the territory concerned was performed. Just after having removed separator for 3 h + 0 min after impressing mechanical stress for 3 h, a manifested local change in HSP47 was observed at the tension side and the pressure side of mouse PDL. The manifestation of HSP47 in PDL on the tension side was higher than the control group. Manifestation of HSP47 on the pressure side did not change and was while being weak. In the 3 h + 20 min group the intensity of HSP47 expression in the whole around the root of the tooth was also similar to 3 h + 0 min group. The strength of HSP47 manifestation in PDL on the tension side was maintained more than a group in 3 h + 0 min and 3 h + 20 min by a group for 3 + 1 h. Manifestation of HSP47 was increased in PDL on the pressure side, and there was not a clear difference between the pressure side and the tension side in the strength of HSP47 manifestation. HSP47 manifestation was similar on both sides. The location of the root of the alveolar socket returned to an initial position substantially by a group for 3 + 3 h, and the width of PDL was convalescent. HSP47 manifestation in the pressure side and the tension side was increased more than that of a group for 3 + 1 h. HSP47 manifestation in PDL on the pressure side was stronger than something which can be put in PDL on the tension side. There were no changes in HSP47 manifestation by a group for 3 + 9 h. However, 24 h after removing separator (3 + 24 h), HSP47 expression was again noticeably increased over the entire PDL. A positive HSP47 response was also noted in the osteoblasts and the bone cells of

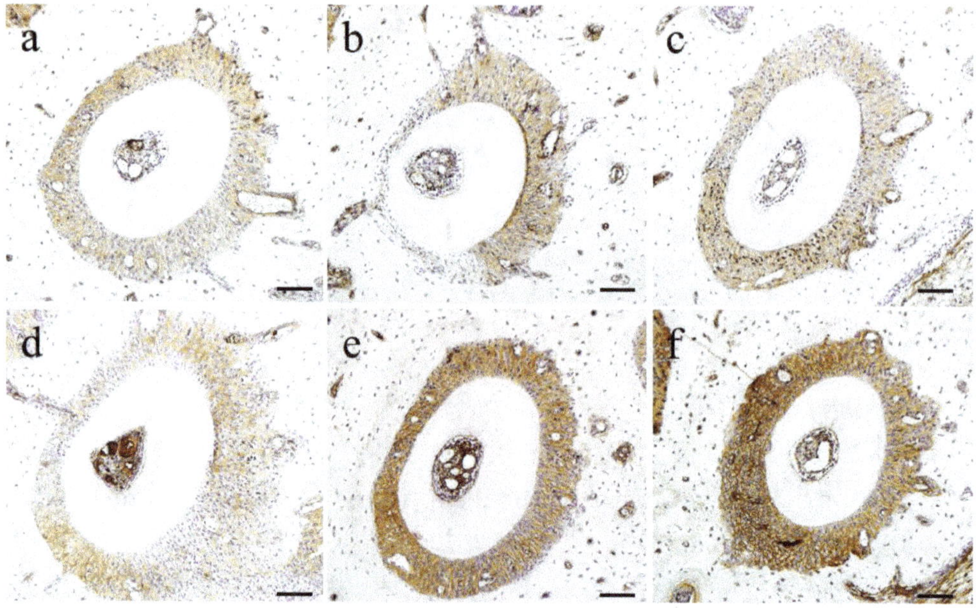

Figure 9. Immunohistochemical results of Experiment 4. (a) Control group, (b) 3 h + 0 min group, (c) 3 + 3 h group, (d) 3 + 9 h group, (e) 3 + 24 h group and (f) 3 h + 1 w group. The inset scale bar indicates 50 μm. Quotation alteration of literature #1.

the alveolar bone. The same response was also observed 3 days after remove separator (3 h + 3 d). HSP47 expression remained strong over the entire PDL 1 week after remove separator (3 h + 1 w). However, expression of HSP47 was weaker than 24 h after release separator.

Summarize the immunohistochemical experiment 4. So early, a positive HSP47 response appeared in the PDL on the tension side, and the same level expression of HSP47 was kept for 9 h. The 24 h group indicated the manifested strength of HSP47 the most highest in all experimental groups. A positive immunohistochemistry-like HSP47 response on the tension side indicated strong step-by-step increase with the passage of time. The low-manifested position was maintained about immunohistochemistry-like HSP47 positive reaction on the pressure side, and there were no manifested conspicuous changes after stress loaded. But a strong positive reaction was detected by a group for 9 h. A PDL fibroblast was compressed hard by a group for 24 h, but HSP47 manifestation disappeared on the pressure side because strong HSP47 manifestation was detected in a PDL fibroblast which neighbors compressed PDL (**Figure 9**).

5. Discussion

Long-term excessive occlusal force and occlusal trauma has an influence on the PDL. An occlusal trauma has a destructive influence on a periodontal tissue [24–27]. It has been studied variously about a relation between a traumatic occlusion and bone resorption. Glickman et al. [28] reported that an inflammatory change is caused by pathogenicity bacteria in a serious periodontitis syndrome with a progressive bone resorption, but influence by both of the excessive occlusal force and occlusal trauma. They were experimented with the rat to which the excessive occlusal load has been added by Kaku et al. [29]. It was transplanted to the upper jaw first molar for micro plus screw with average head diameters to generate high occlusal contact uniformly in that experiment. It was possible to reduce the torque by tightening micro plus screw cross recessed up during the experimental period. The too early contact which makes a molar cause the excessive occlusal load was also easy to produce because the gliding movement of the jaw of a mouse was easy relatively. A result suggested that increase of a fibroblast as the part of the remodeling of a periodontal tissue depends on adaptation to the excessive occlusal load. We considered that a histology-like change in a fibroblast is increased significantly on day 4 and prepared a different experimental system about this regard. When paraphrasing, the implantation of the micro plus screw to cause a traumatic occlusion was possible by the day 4. So we were examined about that histological and expression of HSP47 after traumatic occlusion. Osteoclast was induced by transplantation of a micro plus screw on day 4, and even if a micro plus screw was removed, the way continued. On the other hand, a fixed way of an osteoclast was brought by influence of occlusal overload, and it was possible to advance toward the activity that a cell has already been begun by that. This was indicated by expansion of a glandular cavity of Howship's on day 10 more than day 6. Increase of an osteoclast depends on occlusal overload, and even if a load is removed, this means that it kept being increased. Becoming or a hemangiectasis with the histology-like features like the contrasting group was no longer observed on day 30. It is possible to guess a root of the periodontal ligament to have been convalescent in equilibrium state on day 30.

In summary of experiment about the vertical sectioning of the root portion, there is a possibility that a collagen fiber in a periodontal ligament is destroyed for a continuous occlusal overload. This was clear by increase of HSP47 expression by arrangement of a micro plus screw. HSP47 is maintained by a fibroblast for restoration of the damaged collagen fibers. Simultaneously, though a load to stress was released, an osteoclast keeps being increased. The osteoclast which appeared on the alveolar bone surface is probably caused by sustained activity and it is activated. We presumed increase of an osteoclast to happen after load application on day 4. It kept being increased until day 6 of experimental 2, but HSP47 decreased on day 10. Therefore, HSP47 shows after a period of certain activities that a damaged collagen fiber is restored. The activity of HSP47 returned to equilibrium state on day 30, and expression of HSP47 decreased significantly.

We focused on the collagen fiber which is a main component of a PDL and check manifested movement of HSP47 which is peculiar molecular chaperone in the collagen. HSP localized in the endoplasmic reticulum in the fibroblasts of the PDL.

Heat-shock protein is one kind of proteins by which manifestation is reinforced with a stress [16]. HSP is the stress protein caused by an inflammation, a physical stress, a chemical stress and a pathological change in a heat shock. A stress response functions as the universal and basic defense mechanism which participates in a biological defense response. HSP was the protein from which even the state that has no stress ranges to a cell of equilibrium state widely, and it was indicated clearly by in vitro and in vivo experiment that HSP is the indispensable protein to various cellular function of a cell differentiation, multiplication, survival and maintenance of function [17, 30, 31]. HSP are polypeptides which are classified by molecular weight, and each has different functions. Many HSPs suppress protein modifications as well as repair of modified proteins. They are molecular chaperones [30] having a so-called anti-apoptosis function to escape cell death [17, 18]. Periodontal ligament is the fibrous connective tissue which is surrounding the dental root. A tooth is fixed on an alveolar bone and mechanical stress of the occlusal pressure is received periodically. The biological metabolic half-life of PDL is very short in 1 day. PDL is composed of much cell type like a fibroblast, an osteoblast, an epithelium stationary stem cell of an osteoclast, a cementoblast, cementoclasts and Malassez, a mastocyte and a macrophage. A blood vessel, a nerve and a matrix protein outside the collagen fibers and the cell of an oxytalan fiber and a sugar protein exist. The type I collagen is the main ingredient (90%) about an ingredient of a periodontal film, there is less type III collagen (10%), and type V collagen is present in very small quantities. The collagen is one of general fibrous proteins most at the interior of the body of an animal. The collagen is formed to construct more than one numerator out of in vivo. A polypeptide of the amino acid 1000 combined is included in the collagen molecule of which the unit of the collagen is composed. Three α chains form a spiral and form the collagen fibers.

HSP47 defends a cell against a stress and supports maturity of the collagen in the cell and secretion. When normal synthesis is failed for a stress of the different type, and abnormality has occurred to the collagen structure; HSP47 obstructs a cell external secretion of the abnormal collagen and stores a modified protein in an endoplasmic reticulum. It was reported that indispensable molecular chaperone is HSP47 to form the collagen with the right three chains reported by Nagata et al. [32, 33] in 1986. Abnormality occurs to formation of a collagen fiber including the type I collagen by a collagen-specific molecular chaperone HSP47 lost knockout mouse. Abnormality is admitted by basic film formation with abnormality of the type IV collagen, and a mouse is embryonal fatality [34, 35]. Therefore, HSP47 is the molecular chaperone indispensable to normal occurrence in a mammal and a histogenesis. Accordingly, it was thought that HSP47 would be similarly expressed in the periodontal ligament in vivo when mechanical stress such as excessive occlusal force or orthodontic force is loaded.

Some researchers did experiments on animals to establish an immunohistological basis for a orthodontic treatment at the past. They were a basic research about a tooth movement of orthodontic treatment and the mechanism in the root in order to clarify aspects of bone absorption and addition and the underlying mechanism which has a clear have long history. After loading the mechanical stress which imitated the orthodontic treatment, we studied the various proteins manifested in a periodontal tissue of a mouse using the experiment that horizontal sectioning of the root portion [1–12]. However, almost no cellular responses related to harmful influential restoration of mechanical stress to a PDL fibroblast during an orthodontic treatment is studied. Therefore, we focused on manifested HSP to oppose various types of cell damage. Expression of HSP peptides occurs within an extremely short time in PDL cells subjected to mechanical stress over time [2, 4–6, 8, 11, 12]. Therefore, we infrared HSP47 which contributes to a cell differentiation was manifested by a short time relatively and that a manifested strong change in HSP47 might be observed within 24 h. The experimental periods of these experiments were set to enable comparison with the data obtained by Watanabe et al. [11, 12] Matsuda et al.[4, 8], and prior reports [2, 5, 6, 9], from 10 min to a maximum time of 24 h after inserting a separator. Moreover, in order to investigate the recovery of the PDL from damage caused by the mechanical stress, after loading a mechanical stress to the mouse PDL tissue for only 3 h, HSP47 expression was observed over time up to a maximum time of 1 week after releasing the stress. This results show that, in the PDL at the control group (distal buccal root of untreated mouse upper left first molar), HSP47 expression was noted in the cell cytoplasm of the PDL collagen bundles uniformly over the entire periodontal membrane and remained low level. At the normal circumstances, teeth are subjected to mechanical stress caused by mastication several thousand times per day. Under these circumstances, the supporting PDL tissue maintains its physiological functions. These findings in the control group PDL agree with reports that other HSP such as HSP27 and HSP70 are present even in the absence of stress [17, 36, 37] and act to maintain physiological functions in the PDL tissue [2, 5, 6]. It appears that, like these proteins, HSP47 is also expressed in the absence of stress and serves as an element of the mechanism underlying the physiological functions of the PDL tissue and maintains the homeostasis of the PDL.

Next, in the experimental groups subjected to mechanical stress over time for up to 24 h, HSP47 expression was detected in the PDL on the tension side from a very early time and gradually increased over time with the greatest increase in the 24 h group. No marked change was detected in HSP47 expression on the pressure side, after loading stress, expression of HSP47 was maintained low level. However, a strong positive HSP47 response was observed in the 9 h group. However, on the pressure side in the 24 h group, HSP47 expression was absent because the PDL fibroblasts were strongly compressed, but intense HSP47 expression was detected in PDL fibroblasts adjoining the compressed PDL. When examining the time course of HSP47 expression after loading a mechanical stress, HSP47 expression occurred with the same timing as the expression of proteins such as Runx2, Msx2, ALP, BMP, Smad and P-Smad reported by Watanabe et al. and Matsuda et al., which contribute to controlling bone formation by activating osteoblasts [4, 8, 11, 12]. These data suggest that during addition of a bone to PDL on the tension side. HSP47 also has a molecular chaperone function, assisting the maturation of bone morphogenetic proteins and supporting osteoblast activation.

Further, we observed expression of HSP47 at different time points after loading a mechanical stress to the mouse PDL tissue for only 3 h and releasing the stress up to at most 1 week. HSP47 was manifested highly in PDL on the tense side at the very early stage of the later when mechanical stress was freed, but manifestation in a periodontal film on the pressure side was while being still weak. However as time passed, the width of the compressed PDL was gone back in the previous early stage width before applying stress, and HSP47 expression in the PDL on the pressure side increased, and 3 h after release, when the position of the root in the alveolar bone had almost returned to the initial state, HSP47 expression was stronger in the periodontal membrane on the pressure side than that in the periodontal membrane on the tension side. After 24 h releasing the stress, expression of HSP47 notably increased over the entire PDL, and expression of HSP47 remained at a high level over the entire PDL until 1 week after release the stress. These reactions are thought to have been caused by the mechanical stress on the PDL. We previously reported that HSP70, expressed on a pressure side, which has been subjected to intense cell damage, may contribute to osteoclast differentiation on the pressure side, suppresses modification of nascent protein therein and fulfills the function of carrying out management and repair of modified proteins, which cannot be regenerated [6]. It is conjectured that HSP47 which, like HSP70, has a function in tissue repair, is expressed in PDL fibroblasts on the pressure side damaged by applying a mechanical stress, contributes to repairing collagen tissue by activating PDL fibroblasts and contributes to the recovery from cell damage. Moreover, as previously mentioned, HSP47 manifested by the fibroblasts on the tension side probably has a molecular chaperone function, which assists the maturation of bone morphogenetic proteins and aids osteoblast activation. However, when mechanical stress is loaded to the PDL on the tension side during time which is not enough for bone addition, cell damage forms, and there is a possibility that abnormality occurs to the collagen structure of the PDL fibroblast. By functioning at the damage site, HSP47 obstructs a cell external secretion of the abnormal collagen, stores a modification protein in an endoplasmic reticulum and controls decalcification which is the feature of PDL by that by functioning by a damage part.

6. Conclusions

The results suggest that HSP47 is actively involved in homeostasis of periodontal tissue subjected to mechanical stress and occlusal overload. In other words, HSP47 is constitutively expressed in the PDL and defends cells from different types of stress and maintains homeostasis under normal conditions.

There is a possibility that a collagen fiber in the PDL is destroyed for mechanical stress and a continuous occlusal overload. HSP47 is manifested in the PDL fibroblast damaged by application of mechanical stress. HSP47 contributes to restoration of the collagen organization by activating a PDL fibroblast and supports a recovery from cell damage.

HSP47 was suggested that in the course of the alveolar bone addition to the PDL at the tension side, that also acts as molecular chaperone and that support the maturation of bone morphogenetic proteins and aids osteoblast activation.

Further, HSP47 inhibits extracellular secretion of abnormal collagen, stores the modified protein in the endoplasmic reticulum, thereby controlling decalcification of the PDL.

HSP47 acts differently depending on the time of expression in PDL.

Acknowledgements

This research was partially supported in part by JSPS KAKENHI Grant Numbers 23792456, 26861804, 26463104 and 25463204 from the Japan Society for the Promotion of Science (JSPS).

Author details

Rina Muraoka[1]*, Keisuke Nakano[2], Hidetsugu Tsujigiwa[3], Hitoshi Nagatsuka[2], Hirokazu Matsuda[1], Mihoko Tomida[1,4], Norimasa Okafuji[1,4], Kazuhiro Yamada[1,4] and Toshiyuki Kawakami[4]

*Address all correspondence to: rina.muraoka@mdu.ac.jp

1 Matsumoto Dental University School of Dentistry and Hospital, Shiojiri, Japan

2 Okayama University Graduate School of Medicine, Dentistry and Pharmaceutical Sciences, Okayama, Japan

3 Faculty of Science, Okayama University of Science, Okayama, Japan

4 Matsumoto Dental University Graduate School of Oral Medicine, Shiojiri, Japan

References

[1] Muraoka R, Nakano K, Yamada K, Kawakami T. HSP47 as a possible molecular chaperone for the collagen synthesis in the mouse periodontal ligament cells due to orthodontic force. International Journal of Dentistry and Oral Science. 2017;**4**(1):387-394. DOI: 10.19070/2377-8075-1700078

[2] Muraoka R, Nakano K, Kurihara S, Yamada K, Kawakami T. Immunohistochemical expression of heat shock proteins in the mouse periodontal tissues due to orthodontic mechanical stress. European Journal of Medical Research. 2010;**15**(11):475-482

[3] Kawakami T, Nakano K, Shimizu T, Kimura A, Okafuji N, Tsujigiwa H, Hasegawa H, Nagatsuka H. Histopathological and immunohistochemical background of orthodontic treatment. International Journal of Medical and Biological Frontiers. 2009;**15**(7/8):591-615

[4] Matsuda H, Muraoka R, Tomoda M, Nakano K, Okafuji N, Yamada K, Kawakami T. Immunohistochemical observation of BMP in the mouse orthodontic periodontal tension sides. Journal of Hard Tissue Biology. 2009;**18**(4):181-184

[5] Muraoka R, Nakano K, Matsuda H, Tomoda M, Okafuji N, Kurihara S, Yamada K, Kawakami T. Immunohistochemical observation of heat shock proteins expression in mouse periodontal tissues due to orthodontic mechanical stress. Journal of Hard Tissue Biology. 2009;**18**(4):193-197

[6] Muraoka R, Nakano K, Matsuda H, Tomoda M, Okafuji N, Yamada K, Kawakami T. A consideration on the role of HSP70 appearing in the periodontal tissues due to experimental orthodontic force. Journal of Hard Tissue Biology. 2011;**20**(4):275-282

[7] Muraoka R, Tsujigiwa H, Nakano K, Katase N, Tamamura R, Tomida M, Okafuji N, Nagatsuka H, Kawakami T. Transplanted bone marrow-derived cell migration into periodontal tissues and cell differentiation. Journal of Hard Tissue Biology. 2011;**20**(4):301-306

[8] Matsuda H, Harada T, Muraoka R, Tomoda M, Okafuji N. Immunohistochemical observation of osterix appearing in the mouse orthodontic periodontal tissues. Journal of Hard Tissue Biology. 2011;**20**(4):283-288

[9] Tomoda M, Nakano K, Muraoka R, Matsuda H, Yamada K, Kawakami T. Immunohistochemical changes of heat shock protein 27 expression in the mouse periodontal tissues exposed to orthodontic mechanical stress. Journal of Hard Tissue Biology. 2012; **21**(1):43-50

[10] Tomida M, Tsujigiwa H, Nakano K, Muraoka R, Nakamura T, Okafuji N, Nagatsuka H, Kawakami T. Promotion of transplanted bone marrow-derived cell migration into the periodontal tissues due to orthodontic mechanical stress. International Journal of Medical Sciences. 2013;**10**(10):1321-1326

[11] Watanabe T, Nakano K, Muraoka R, Shimizu T, Okafuji N, Kurihara S, Yamada K, Kawakami T. Role of Msx2 as a promoting factor for Runx2 at the periodontal tension sides elicited by mechanical stress. European Journal of Medical Research. 2008;**13**:425-431

[12] Watanabe T, Okafuji N, Nakano K, Shimizu T, Muraoka R, Kurihara S, Yamada K, Kawakami T. Periodontal tissue reaction to mechanical stress in mouse. Journal of Hard Tissue Biology. 2007;**16**:71-74

[13] Takaya T, Mimura H, Matsuda S, Nakano K, Tsujigiwa H, Tomita M, Okafuji N, Fujii T, Kawakami T. Cytological kinetics of periodontal ligament in an experimental occlusal trauma model. International Journal of Medical Sciences. 2015;**12**:544-551

[14] Mimura H, Takaya T, Matsuda S, Nakano K, Muraoka R, Tomida M, Okafuji N, Fujii T, Kawakami T. Functional role of HSP47 in the periodontal ligament subjected to occlusal overload in mice. International Journal of Medical Sciences. 2016;**13**:248-254. DOI: 10.7150/ijms.14129

[15] Ritossa F. A new puffing pattern induced by temperature shock and DNP in drosophila. Cellular and Molecular Life Sciences. 1962;**18**:571-573

[16] Milton JS. Heat shock proteins. The Journal of Biological Chemistry. 1990;**265**:12111-12114

[17] Lindquist S, Craig EA. The heat-shock proteins. Annual Review of Genetics. 1988;**22**: 631-677

[18] Arrigo AP, Landry J. Expression and function of the low molecular weight heat shock proteins. In: Morimoto RI, Tissières A, Georgopoulos C, editors. The Biology of Heat Shock Proteins and Molecular Chaperones. North America: Cold Spring Harbor Laboratory Press; 1994. pp. 335-373

[19] Pan H, Halper J. Regulation of heat shock protein 47 and type I procollagen expression in avian tendon cells. Cell and Tissue Research. 2003;**311**:373-382

[20] Merryman WD, Youn I, Lukoff HD, Krueger PM, Guilak F, Hopkins RA, Sacks MS. Correlation between heart valve interstitial cell stiffness and transvalvular pressure: Implications for collagen biosynthesis. American Journal of Physiology. Heart and Circulatory Physiology. 2006;**290**:H224-H231

[21] Oguro A1, Sakurai T, Okuno M, Nagata K, Atomi Y. The change of HSP47, collagen specific molecular chaperone, expression in rat skeletal muscle may regulate collagen production with gravitational conditions. Biological Sciences in Space. 2004;**18**:150-151

[22] Waldo CM. Method for the study of tissue response to tooth movement. Journal of Dental Research. 1953;**32**:690-691

[23] Keagle JN, Welch WJ, Young DM. Expression of heat shock proteins in a linear rodent wound. Wound Repair and Regeneration. 2001;**9**:378-385

[24] Svanberg G. Influence of trauma from occlusion on the periodontium of dog with normal or inflamed gingivae. Odontologisk Revy. 1976;**25**:165-178

[25] Stahl SS. Accommodation of the periodontium to occlusal trauma and inflammatory periodontal disease. Dental Clinics of North America. 1975;**19**:531-542

[26] Lindhe J, Ericsson I. The influence of trauma from occlusion o reduced but healthy periodontal tissues in dogs. Journal of Clinical Periodontology. 1976;**3**:110-122

[27] Biancu S, Ericsson I, Lindhe J. Periodontal ligament tissue reactions to trauma and gingival inflammation. An experimental study in the beagle dog. Journal of Clinical Periodontology. 1995;**22**:772-779

[28] Glickman I, Smulow JB. Effect of excessive occlusal forces upon the pathway of gingival inflammation in humans. Journal of Periodontology. 1965;**36**:141-147

[29] Kaku M, Uoshima K, Yamashita Y, Miura H. Investigation of periodontal ligament reaction upon excessive occlusal load-osteopontin induction among periodontalligament. Journal of Periodontal Research. 2005;**40**:59-66

[30] Hratl FU. Molecular chaperone in cellular protein folding. Nature. 1996;**381**:571-579

[31] Sakurai Y, Okuyama N, Tamamura K, Owawa R, Ito H, Yamasaki A. Expression of collagen-specific stress protein Hsp47 in rat epithelial tissue. Ohu University Dental Journal. 2007;**34**(4):131-136

[32] Nagata K, Saga S, Yamada KM. A major collagen-binding protein of chick embryo fibroblasts is a novel heat shock protein. The Journal of Cell Biology. 1986;**103**:223-229

[33] Nagata K, Saga S, Yamada KM. Characterization of a novel transformation-sensitive heat-shock protein (HSP47) that binds to collagen. Biochemical and Biophysical Research Communications. 1988;**153**:428-434

[34] Nagai N, Yorihuzi T, Hosokawa N, Nagata K. Human genome has a functional hsp47 gene (CBP2) and pseudogene (pshsp47). Gene. 1999;**227**(2):241-248

[35] Marutani T, Yamamoto A, Nagai N, Kubota H, Nagata K. Accumulation of type IV collagen in dilated ER leads to apoptosis in Hsp47-knockout mouse embryos via induction of CHOP. Journal of Cell Science. 2004;**117**(Pt 24):5913-5922

[36] Tsujimura K, Morishita M, Kawahara K, Fukunaga M, Tsuruda K, Iwamoto Y. A study on the expression of heat shock protein genes in the human periodontal ligament fibroblasts. Journal of the Japanese Society of Periodontology. 1995;**37**(2):287-293

[37] Yamashita S, Maeshima A, Nojima Y. Involvement of renal progenitor tubular cells in epithelial-mesenchymal transition in fibrotic rat kidneys. Journal of the American Society of Nephrology. 2005;**16**:2044-2051

12

Advanced Regenerative Techniques Based on Dental Pulp Stem Cells for the Treatment of Periodontal Disease

Ana-Maria Seciu, Oana Craciunescu and Otilia Zarnescu

Abstract

Recent progress in periodontology intended to reduce the risk represented by periodontal disease for systemic disorders and general human health condition. In this chapter, we overview the advantages and limitations of current techniques based on occlusive membranes for periodontal regeneration. Special emphasis is paid to advanced techniques using stem cells from dental pulp for the regeneration of bone defects caused by the chronic periodontal disease. Stem cells isolation, *in vitro* expansion and characterization techniques are presented. Therapeutic strategies of stem cells delivery using natural polymeric carriers are discussed. Stem cell-scaffold constructs application in bone tissue engineering is proposed, taking into account the marked decline of healing, and regenerative processes in elderly individuals. Future researchers envisage multiple effects of engineered constructs with antimicrobial, anti-inflammatory, and regenerative activity for periodontal treatment.

Keywords: cell carrier, collagen, dental pulp, periodontitis, regenerative medicine, scaffold, stem cells, tissue engineering

1. Introduction

Periodontium is a structural and functional tissue, which facilitates the anchoring of teeth in the maxillary and mandibular bones. It consists of two hard tissues, the cementum and the alveolar bone, and two soft tissues, the gingival connective tissue, and the periodontal ligament [1]. The periodontal tissues provide structural support at the tooth-jaw interface, a resilient attachment of the teeth during mastication and protection against the pathogenic microbial flora from the oral cavity [2]. Periodontal remodeling is a necessary process in response to occlusal changes and dental abrasion, while the gingiva can initiate an immune response against pathogenic bacterial flora [3]. At the molecular level, tissue remodeling is accomplished by resorption and deposition of extracellular matrix components [4].

Periodontitis is the second most common oral infectious disease after dental caries, which affects the periodontium. It is a result of the inflammatory response caused by the accumulation of bacterial plaque at the gingival edge of the tooth. In its first phase, gingivitis, an inflammatory process occurs in the gingival tissue causing oral discomfort, but the following phases of periodontal disease are characterized by progressive destruction of the supporting tissues of the tooth, increased dental mobility, impairment of dental function, and, finally, tooth loss [5]. Periodontitis involves a cascade of temporally and spatially coordinated molecular processes, which degrade the host tissues in a similar way to other tissue remodeling actions. Researchers indicated the involvement of main components of the periodontal ligament extracellular matrix in the initiation and progression of periodontitis [1, 2], but the molecular mechanisms have not been identified. The presence of chronic inflammation in association with bacterial plaque leaded to enzymatic degradation of the extracellular matrix components and an increase of soluble glycosaminoglycans fractions [6], carboxy-terminal telopeptides of type I collagen (COL) molecule [7], and the 40 kDa pro-apoptotic fragment of fibronectin (FN) [8]. In addition, increased levels of pro-inflammatory cytokines (tumor necrosis factor TNF-α, interleukin IL-1β), matrix metalloproteases (MMP-8, MMP-9) and apoptosis events called anoikis, which induce detachment of cells from the matrix, were observed [9]. The main mechanism of tissue damage encountered in periodontitis is extracellular matrix degradation, in particular, COL catabolism, by matrix metalloproteinases (MMP-1, MMP-3, MMP-8, MMP-9, and MMP-13). These enzymes are synthesized and activated by resident fibroblasts and macrophages during the inflammatory process, under the action of proinflammatory cytokines [10]. Their activity is regulated at the transcriptional level, post-translational level and through tissue inhibitors of metalloproteinases [11]. Other mechanisms coordinated by external bacterial virulence factors or proinflammatory cytokines secreted by host T-lymphocytes, at the inflammatory situs, induce the expression of receptor activator of nuclear factor kappa-B ligand (RANKL). RANKL is expressed by numerous cell types, including osteoblasts and lymphocytes, and is found in soluble form or associated with the cell membrane [12]. RANKL binds to its monocyte-expressed receptor RANK, inducing the formation of multinucleated osteoclasts. In the same time, osteoprotegerin (OPG) is a secreted receptor that acts as a competitive inhibitor of RANKL. Unlike healthy periodontal tissues, there are very high levels of RANKL and low OPG concentrations found in the gingival crevicular fluid of damaged periodontal tissues [13]. The balance within RANKL/RANK/OPG system controls the physiological processes involved in bone turnover and loss. Besides tissue damage, the cytokine network promotes fibroblast activation and proliferation, which can lead to fibrosis [5].

Periodontal disease presents a high risk for the general health, leading to systemic diseases, such as rheumatoid arthritis, chronic bronchitis, and pulmonary fibrosis [14]. Periodontal therapy targets the structural and functional regeneration of the complex structure of the periodontium, aiming the restoration of cementum lining the tooth root and the periodontal ligament attached to the cementum, together with the formation of new alveolar bone and gingiva. In the same time, the subgingival space needs protection against the pathogenic bacterial flora [2]. Stem cell biology has enabled the development of innovative cellular therapies that stimulate the endogenous regenerative process of the periodontal tissue [15]. Thus, two-dimensional (2D) cell sheets or three-dimensional (3D) cell aggregates served as grafting materials, but only for small periodontal defects due to their low stability [16]. There are numerous stem cell sources with potential application in periodontal regeneration involving both oral and extra-oral tissues. A major problem of stem cells clinical application in periodontal regeneration strategies is their low survival rate after transplantation [17]. In order to improve the therapeutic properties of stem cells, they are implanted in biomaterials that must meet the requirements of the biological environment. A detailed investigation of stem cells-biomaterial interaction, in correlation with the role of stem cells secretome represented by cytokines, growth factors and chemokines is needed. Tissue engineering is a strategic approach for periodontal regeneration in controlled conditions. Clinically meaningful results were obtained using complex biomaterials capable of spatial and temporal guiding of the periodontal regeneration [18]. The use of composite biomaterials can be complementary to existing clinical procedures, such as guided tissue regeneration (GTR) or combined with cellular therapies and/or bioactive molecules. These emerging technologies of regenerative medicine were tested *in vitro*, in preclinical studies, and clinical trials for periodontal tissue engineering [1, 19]. They facilitate the integration of stem cells into the surrounding milieu and functional reconstruction of the periodontal complex [16].

This chapter describes the advantages and limitations of current techniques and proposes advanced techniques based on stem cells and cell carriers for the treatment of periodontal disease. Special emphasis is paid to dental pulp stem cells (DPSCs) isolation, expansion conditions *in vitro,* and their use for the regeneration of bone defects caused by the chronic periodontal disease. Their delivery after injection within natural polymeric carriers is discussed as a new therapeutic strategy for periodontal lesions.

2. Current techniques of periodontal regeneration

2.1. Guided tissue regeneration

Many clinical and biological factors can impair the process of periodontal tissue regeneration. The tissue is in permanent contact with the external environment of the oral cavity and presents a risk of infection during the regeneration process. There are several types of mechanical stress, caused by occlusal forces or dental gum stretching, which affects the mucous membranes and reduces bone resorption. Surgical techniques of periodontal tissue regeneration include root surface modification, bone grafting, and GTR. The most common regenerative treatment GTR is based on the application of barrier membranes, in order to restrict epithelial and gingival connective cells in periodontal defects and to increase the number of cementoblasts and osteoblasts that synthesize extracellular matrix and, finally, new functional tissue [20]. On GTR market, several products are intended for the clinical treatment of intraosseous defects or class II fissure defects. They consist of non-resorbable membranes of synthetic materials (expanded polytetrafluoroethylene, nylon on silicone) or resorbable membranes made of organic materials, presenting different composition, and structure. In case of using non-resorbable membranes, bone regeneration is low, and a second surgery is needed to remove them. The resorbable membranes composed of COL types I or III extracted from bovine tendon or porcine skin are enzymatically degraded and their resorption time varies with the cross-linking degree. Polymeric membranes of polylactic acid or copolymeric materials of polylactic acid/polyglycolic acid are biocompatible, but their degradation depends on composition, pH, and presence of enzymes and bacterial infection [21]. Resorbable membranes, such as Avitene® are obtained from bovine pericardium crosslinked with diphenylphosphorylazide, Collistat® is a semi-occlusive membrane (pore size 0.004 μm) prepared from bovine dermis, BioMend® is made of type I COL from bovine tendon and exhibit variable efficacy, depending on the shape and size of the defect [22], Paroguide® from COL, and chondroitin sulfate (CS) helps to repair the periodontal ligament, cementum, and alveolar bone, without signs of inflammation [23]. Resorbable membranes have many beneficial properties as medical products, being hemostatic, chemotactic, and biocompatible, but they are not stable enough to allow the formation of new tissue. These membrane barriers are used during GTR to stimulate selective cell repopulation of the periodontal defects. Therefore, biocompatibility is the most important feature of a barrier membrane and any sign of cytotoxicity can lead to irreversible destruction of the periodontal tissue. In addition, the membranes must exhibit structural and mechanical properties, in order to maintain space and to resist against external forces. They should initiate tissue integration and be easily used in order to reduce intervention time and patients discomfort [24].

2.2. Limitations

Clinical trials have showed that periodontal treatment is effective in achieving the primary goal of preventing disease progression and loss of affected tooth. Long-term studies on periodontal disease noted that 95% of treated teeth were not lost for 10 years [25]. Although there are encouraging results, existing treatment methods have numerous limitations, and indicate the lack of complete periodontal tissue regeneration. Thus, most treatments of periodontal pocket lead to gingival retraction, which can progress over time in poor esthetics, increases tooth mobility, and affects dental functions [5]. In intraosseous defects, minor regeneration of periodontal tissue may occur in the apical region of the defect [26]. GTR can induce partial remodeling and restoration of the cortical bone, but total regeneration of bone or periodontal ligament does not occur [27]. It was noted that the biological process of epithelium growth and differentiation needed a layer of connective tissue to mediate the passage of signaling molecules [28]. Studies suggested that, in contrast to superficial connective tissue of the gingiva, deep connective tissue prevented epithelial migration and leaded to formation of a simple epithelium, phenotypically similar to the junctional epithelium [28]. Besides epithelium ingrowth, specific signaling pathway involved in the periodontal repair process is not known.

3. Stem cell therapy for periodontal regeneration

Stem cell research is one of the most promising areas of biology due to its therapeutic implications [29]. Stem cells are defined as immature, undifferentiated cells with self-renewal capacity, clonogenicity (the ability to form cell colonies), and cellular differentiation capacity [30]. The regenerative capacity of adult tissues depends on their own stem cell populations that have the ability to self-renew and form progenitor cells capable of differentiating into specialized cells. Mesenchymal stem cells (MSCs) are pluripotent cells that can differentiate into any cell type from all three embryonic layers, including periodontal tissue associated cells. Due to their differentiation capacity, widespread tissue distribution and promising results obtained in both preclinical and clinical models of tissue repair, MSC are increasingly used in tissue engineering. Ideal stem cells must be non-immunogenic, easy to obtain, highly proliferative, and have the ability to differentiate into desired cell type. Extraoral stem cells from adipose tissue and bone marrow, as well as intraoral stem cells from periodontal ligament, dental pulp, papilla, and follicle cells were used in periodontal tissue engineering, to repair damaged parodontium [24, 31, 32]. Dental tissues are easily accessible sources of stem cells, which can be used in cell therapy of periodontal disease and maxillofacial reconstruction due to their ability to form bone, dentin and pulp tissue [15, 33, 34].

3.1. Dental pulp stem cells (DPSC) role in periodontal regeneration

The dental pulp is the vital organ of the tooth, presenting very good repair and regenerative capacity. DPSC with high proliferative capacity and multipotency were used in orthopedics and maxillofacial reconstruction for regeneration of bone and dental tissues, respectively [35]. DPSC transplantation into the human alveolar bone initiated dental pulp regeneration [36]. In addition, a graft of DPSC from the child to the parent differentiated into osteoblasts and regenerated the mineralized tissue [37] or into odontoblasts responsible for reparative dentin secretion [38, 39]. Cultivation of a large number of DPSC in medium without xenogeneic serum granted these cells with major impact in regenerative medicine and clinic applications [40, 41]. Moreover, DPSC were reprogrammed into induced pluripotent stem cells at a higher rate than other cell types [42], confirming their periodontal tissue regenerative capacity [43, 44].

MSC was first isolated from the adult dental pulp by Gronthos et al. [45] and, then, from primary dentition extracted during periodontal and oral surgery [46]. DPSC from primary dentition presented higher proliferative capacity and differentiation potential, compared to DPSC from permanent teeth [47]. Still, scientific interest has lately turned to adult DPSC because the processing and storage of stem cells from primary dentition is not possible for the majority of the population [29]. DPSC were also isolated from inflamed pulp tissue and their markers profile was similar to that of cells from normal tissue [48]. DPSC is easily accessible and available in a larger amount than MSC from bone marrow due to their high proliferation rate [49, 50].

The regenerative quality of DPSC can be influenced by the isolation process and biological parameters, such as the age of the donor, its general health status and oral health, long-term storage conditions and post-freeze viability [29, 51, 52]. Dental pulp aging results in changes that are difficult to distinguish from physiological and pathological processes. An obvious change caused by aging is pulp size decrease due to continuous secretion of dentinal matrix (secondary dentinogenesis). As a result, the number of constituent cells (odontoblasts, fibroblasts, MSC) decreases, COL and crosslinked fibers increase, lipid infiltration and calcification take place [53]. These changes suggest a decline of DPSC characteristic functions with increasing age. In conclusion, isolation of DPSC is recommended from healthy young adult donors, in order to present clinical applicability in stem cell therapy.

3.2. DPSC isolation

Both explant culture and enzymatic digestion protocols are efficient for DPSC isolation from adult teeth, considering a pulp weight of at least 0.2 g for establishing a viable primary culture [54]. Third molars (wisdom tooth) are usually used after their extraction during mandatory surgical or orthodontic treatment of healthy adults (21–34 years), with patient's agreement, according to the bioethics rules in force. Immediately after extraction, the molars are placed in 10 mM sterile phosphate buffered saline (PBS) supplemented with a mixture of antibiotics (200 U/ml penicillin, 500 μg/ml streptomycin, 400 μg/ml neomycin, and 2.5 μg/ml amphotericin) and transported to the lab, on ice, for processing or storage at 4°C, for up to 24 h (**Figure 1**). Dental pulp is extracted from the pulp chamber of molars and subjected to enzymatic digestion in a solution of 3 mg/ml type I collagenase and 4 mg/ml dispase, at 37°C, for 1 h (**Figure 1**). The obtained cell suspension is filtered through 70 μm cell strainer and cultured in minimum essential medium eagle-alpha modification (α-MEM) supplemented with 20% fetal bovine serum, 100 μM L-ascorbic acid, 2 mM L-glutamine and 1% antibiotics mixture, in a humid atmosphere with 5% CO_2, and at 37°C. The culture medium is changed every 3 days.

3.3. DPSC properties

DPSC present typical characteristics of MSC isolated from other sources, like specific phenotype, *in vitro* renewal capacity, distinctive cell surface antigens, and clonogenicity [38]. Periodic observation of DPSC seeded in a culture plate is usually performed using an inverted microscope. At 24 h of *in vitro* cultivation, DPSC adhered to the plastic surface, and in the first week of cultivation, they started to form colonies, similar to mesenchymal-type stem cells. At 12 days of cultivation, the colonies reached confluence, and the first passage was performed. Hematoxylin-eosin staining of confluent DPSC revealed the fibroblast-like morphology, characteristic for the mesenchymal phenotype (**Figure 2A**). DPSC culture processed for transmission electron microscopy [55] exhibited typical ultrastructure of MSC with spherical or irregular shaped nucleus (N) containing a large amount of euchromatin and mitochondria-rich cytoplasm (**Figure 2B**). Some cells presented rough endoplasmic reticulum (ER) with dilated cisterns (**Figure 2B**).

DPSC cultures cultivated in standard conditions were investigated for self-renewal by colony-forming units (CFU-F) analysis. At 14 days of cultivation, cell clusters of different sizes and densities were observed (**Figure 2C**). This demonstrated that subpopulations of cells were able to generate new colonies from a single cell.

MSC immunophenotyping consists in cell surface antigens analysis using flow cytometry. DPSC at passage 3 (2×10^5 cells) were washed in PBS and incubated with primary antibodies directed to specific antigens, at 4°C, for 30 min. After centrifugation at 1200 rpm, for 10 min, cells were resuspended in PBS and analyzed at a flow cytometer. Unlabelled cells were used as a control. Data are processed as histograms using provided software and the results are expressed as percentages. Flow cytometry of DPSC cultures showed similar profile to that of mesenchymal-type stem cells. Specific markers, such as CD29, CD44, CD73, and CD90 were expressed at high levels, ranging between 96 and 100%. DPSC were negative for hematopoietic markers, CD34, CD45, and CD133, in accordance with previous studies [56]. STRO-1 is a specific marker present in stromal precursors from bone marrow with multiple differentiation

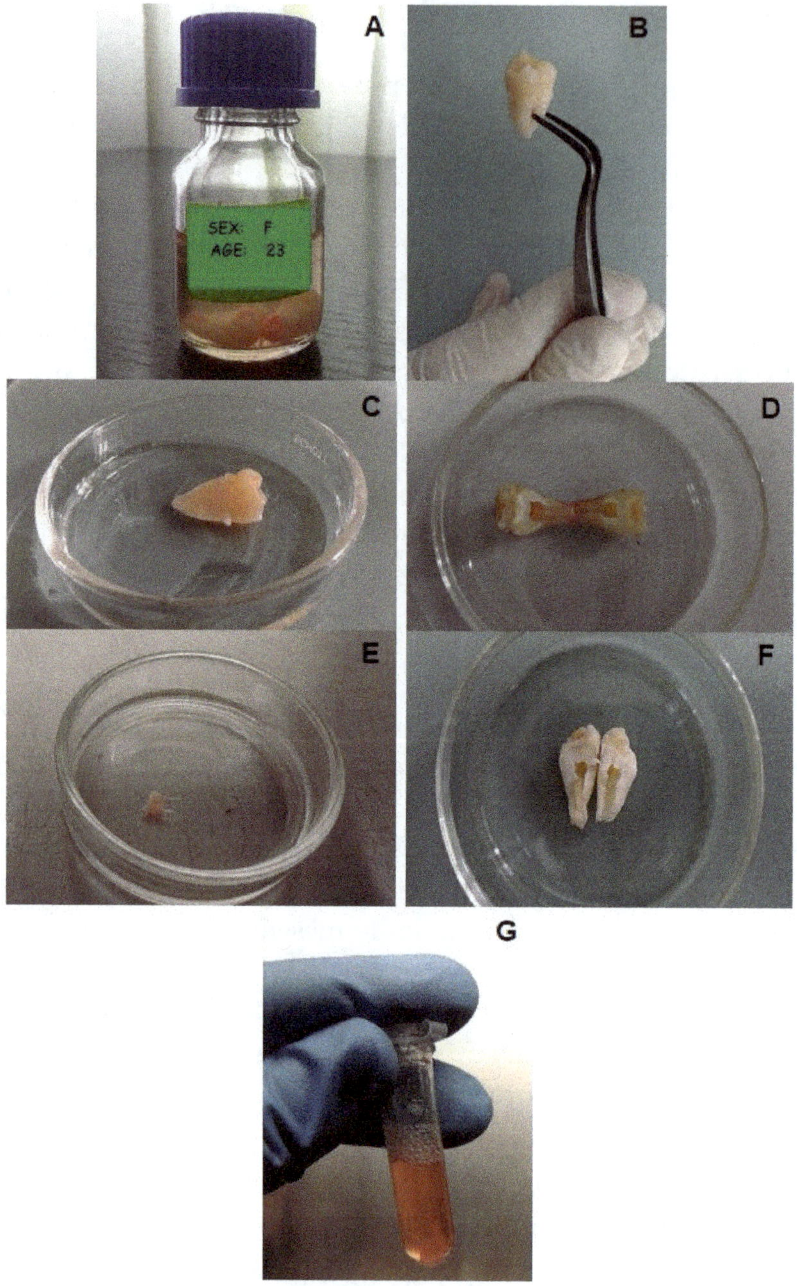

Figure 1. Isolation of stem cells from the third molar dental pulp by enzymatic digestion. The sample was transported to the lab on ice (A). Third molar (B) was thoroughly washed in 70% ethanol and PBS, pH 7.4 (C). The pulp chamber was mechanically exposed (D), the dental pulp was extracted (E) and the tooth remained empty (F). The dental pulp was digested in enzymatic solution (G).

potentials and, in particular, osteo/odontogenic. To date, DPSC populations expressing this marker [57, 58], as well as populations characterized by STRO-1 negative immunophenotype [56] were reported.

3.4. DPSC multidifferentiation capacity

DPSC exhibit plasticity and can be differentiated into osteoblasts, odontoblasts, osteocytes, chondrocytes, adipocytes, myocytes, cardiomyocytes, neural, and hepatocyte cells [29, 35, 59].

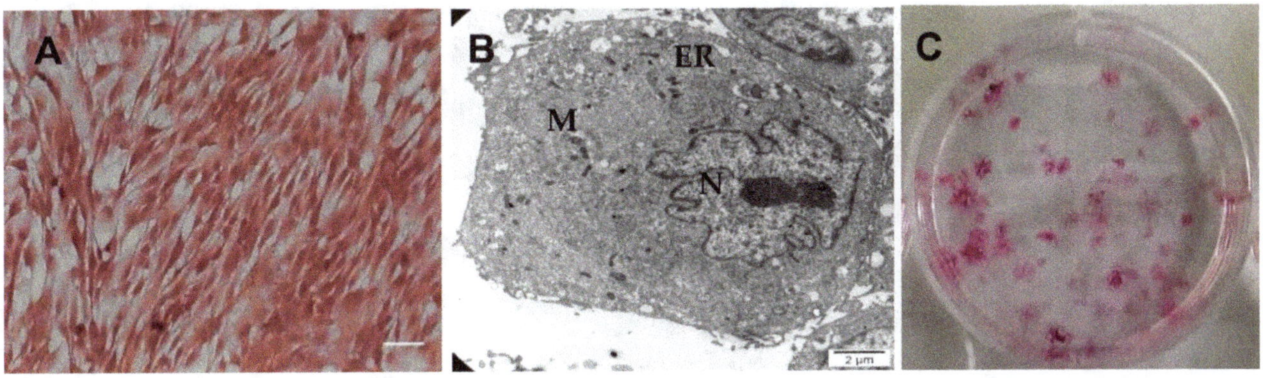

Figure 2. Light micrograph of DPSC at confluence showed characteristic spindle-shaped cell morphology (A, hematoxylin-eosin staining, bar = 10 µm). Transmission electron micrograph of DPSC revealed the N, mitochondria (M), and rough ER (B, bar = 2 µm). Colony-forming unit analysis of DPSC detected cell clusters after 14 days of *in vitro* cultivation (C, hematoxylin-eosin staining).

For DPSC differentiation, isolated cells are expanded *in vitro* by trypsinization and, at passage 5, 6, are seeded in 6-wells culture plates, at a density of 5×10^4 cells/ml in α-MEM until reaching confluence. Then, the culture medium is replaced with osteogenic differentiation medium based on 1 µM dexamethasone, 20 mM sodium β-glycerophosphate, and 45 mM L-ascorbic acid-2-phosphate [60]. The plates are incubated in a humid atmosphere with 5% CO_2, for 21 days and the medium is changed every 3 days. For adipogenic differentiation of DPSC, the monolayers are cultivated in specific induction media based on 5 µg/ml insulin, 10^{-6} M dexamethasone, 0.5 mM isobutylmethylxanthine, and 60 µM indomethacin [60]. Chondrogenic differentiation is performed in pellet mass culture (2×10^5 cells/pellet) placed in conical polypropylene tubes, centrifuged at 500 × *g*, for 5 min and cultivated in specific induction medium based on 5 µg/ml linoleic acid, 1× insulin-transferrin-selenium concentrate, 10 ng/ml transforming growth factor β1, 14 µg/ml ascorbic acid, and 10^{-7} M dexamethasone [60]. Specific staining protocols are used to analyze the morphology of differentiated stem cells.

Osteogenic differentiated cells fixed in 4% paraformaldehyde solution in PBS were stained with 2% alizarin red S, for 30 min [61], and images acquired at an inverted light microscope. DPSC cultivated in osteogenic differentiation medium, for 21 days presented characteristic calcium mineral deposits, visualized as strong red color (**Figure 3A**). Adipogenic differentiated cells stained with 0.5% Oil Red O solution in isopropanol, for 30 min [61] showed morphological changes, intracellular lipid droplets accumulation and reduced proliferation rate (**Figure 3B**). The spheroid of chondrogenic differentiated cells stained with 1% Alcian blue solution, pH 2.5, for 30 min [61] presented specific proteoglycans storage within the extracellular matrix (**Figure 3C**).

Morphological observations can be confirmed by immunofluorescence [55] or microarray investigations [62] that evidentiate specific markers expression at protein and gene level, respectively. In osteogenic differentiated DPSC, analysis of osteocalcin, osteopontin, and type I COL is performed. Adipogenic differentiation is marked by secretion of adiponectin and lipoprotein lipase, while DPSC differentiated toward chondrocytes express aggrecan, SOX-9 and type II COL [60, 62]. In each experimental model, control DPSC grown as undifferentiated cells in normal culture medium have no reaction for these specific markers.

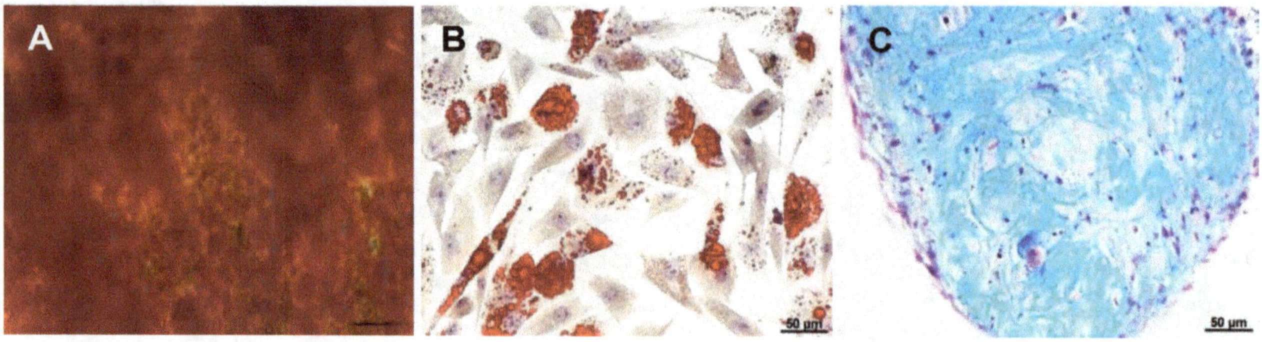

Figure 3. *In vitro* multilineage differentiation of DPSC after three weeks of cultivation in specific culture media. Osteogenesis was evidentiated by calcium deposits (A, Alizarin red S staining, bar = 100 μm). Adipogenesis was observed as intracellular lipid droplets accumulation (B, Oil Red O staining, bar = 50 μm). Chondrogenesis was showed by proteoglycans deposits in the extracellular matrix (C, Alcian blue staining, bar = 50 μm).

4. Advanced techniques for periodontal regeneration

Gene therapy and cell therapy are two advanced techniques that represent an effective solution to maximize the delivery of molecules involved in periodontal regeneration and to reduce limitations of currently used regenerative treatments. Gene therapy is a strategy for modulating host immune response triggered by dental microbiota. It consists of the direct insertion of certain genes into patient cells or indirect gene delivery using a carrier [24]. Their cellular transport is considered a more secure approach because it requires isolation of target cells and insertion of therapeutic genes under controlled conditions [32].

Cell therapy envisages induction of complete periodontal regeneration using triple complexes of cells injected in scaffolds containing bioactive molecules. The scaffold helps maintain the space of lost tissue and to protect the regenerated tissues of infection and mechanical stress. In addition, a tailored scaffold in terms of viscosity can promote high percentage of cells retention in injectable transplantation therapies [63]. Bioactive molecules, including bone morphogenetic proteins (BMP), enamel matrix protein derivatives and growth factors, such as platelet-derived growth factor, were also used to stimulate periodontal regeneration. BMP are multifunctional polypeptides that belong to the transforming growth factor-β superfamily, their main feature being the ability to induce ectopic bone formation. Bone regrowth in periodontal defects was achieved in various animal models by BMP application together with carrier systems [24]. Growth factors have regulatory effects on immune function, proliferation, and differentiation of periodontal tissue cells. Both *in vitro* and *in vivo* studies demonstrated the efficiency of platelet-derived growth factor in increasing osteoblast cells population for bone regeneration, endothelial cell multiplication for the capillary formation and fibroblasts proliferation for collagen synthesis and connective tissue regeneration [24].

4.1. Cell-scaffold constructs for periodontal regeneration

Solid biomaterials in which the cells of interest are seeded represent the most used cell transport method [64]. Their great advantages are the ease of application and the ability to encapsulate and concentrate cell suspensions at the target site. After implantation, these cells-biomaterial constructs stimulate cell proliferation and differentiation, resulting in tissue development [15]. The structure and porosity of biomaterials are important to allow nutrients absorption and to avoid cell apoptosis in the central region of the construct. Also, the structural integrity and mechanical properties of solid biomaterials should be adjusted for specific applications of bone and periodontal regeneration. Analysis of 1-year clinical trial on 7 adult patients (24–40 years old) demonstrated that a construct of autologous DPSC in 3D COL sponge could restore the mandible bone defects occurring after molar extraction, with final regeneration scores of 70–100% [40]. Other polymeric composites, hybrid materials or biomaterials incorporating biological active factors, such as platelet-rich plasma and fibrin-rich plasma, have been developed to transport DPSC for human periodontal tissue formation [65–68]. Implantation in animal models demonstrated repair of affected cementum, periodontal ligament, and alveolar bone. *In vitro* and *in vivo* studies demonstrated that DPSC in 3D systems have high osteogenic potential and increased the bone tissue production [38, 69]. Further tailoring is needed in order to be used as dental implants for bone tissue engineering.

4.2. DPSC-scaffold constructs fabrication

Natural proteic, polysaccharidic, and glycoproteic polymers having high molecular weight, such as COL types I, III, and V, CS contained by decorin and biglycan proteoglycans and FN were reviewed as main components of the oral extracellular matrix [4]. They were mixed in different weight ratios, at room temperature, for 2 h, to obtain biocompatible variants of composite material with regenerative properties. The mixtures were conditioned as 3D porous scaffolds by lyophilization [70]. Sterile scaffolds (~0.25 cm^3) were placed in 24-wells culture plate and 200 μl α-MEM culture medium supplemented with fetal bovine serum, containing 5×10^5 DPSC were injected into the scaffold. Cell suspension was absorbed during 30 min of incubation in a humid atmosphere with 5% CO_2, at 37°C. Cell-scaffold constructs were covered with 500 μl culture medium and incubation continued in standard conditions. The culture medium was changed every 48 h.

4.3. Biologic activity of DPSC-scaffold constructs

Assessment of cell viability, membrane integrity, cell adhesion, and proliferation are useful tools, in order to select optimal ratios between scaffold's polymers and to establish DPSC cultivation conditions.

A method for assessing DPSC viability within cell-scaffold constructs cultivated in standard conditions, for different periods of time is live/dead assay based on cellular esterase activity. Calcein AM penetrates living cells membrane and is transformed into fluorescent calcein under the action of esterases. Ethidium homodimer-1 penetrates only cells with the damaged membrane, intercalates DNA double helix, and emits red fluorescence. Live/dead assay allows simultaneous staining of live and apoptotic cells, measuring both cell viability and plasma membrane integrity. For the experiment, DPSC-scaffold constructs incubated in standard cultivation conditions, for 72 h are washed in PBS and, then, 20 μM calcein-AM and 5 μM ethidium homodimer-1 in PBS are added. The plates are incubated in the dark, at room temperature, for 20 min. The images of cell-scaffold constructs are acquired at 490 nm using an inverted fluorescence microscope equipped with a photo camera. A large population of viable cells colored in green was observed in COL-CS-FN composite material after 72 h of cultivation (**Figure 4A**). Adhered cells were distributed throughout the entire scaffold. Cells in different stages of apoptosis, colored in red, were present in very low number, indicating a very good biocompatibility of the natural composite scaffold toward stem cells from dental pulp tissue.

For observations on DPSC infiltration capacity and the degree of cell colonization within composite materials, scanning electron microscopy is a useful technique. Cross sections of cell-scaffold constructs cultivated in standard conditions, for 48 h are fixed in 2.5% glutaraldehyde in cacodylated buffer, at room temperature, for 20 min. Then, samples are visualized using an environmental scanning electron microscope, operated at 15 kV, in an inert nitrogen atmosphere. Scanning micrographs showed that DPSC infiltrated the 3D composite scaffold and adhered to pore walls as isolated cells (**Figure 4B**) or group of cells (**Figure 4C**).

For cell proliferation assessment in cell-scaffold constructs, MTS test is applicable after PBS washing to remove unattached cells. Cells are incubated with 3-(4,5-dimethylthiazol-2-yl)-5-(3-carboxymethoxyphenyl)-2-(4-sulfophenyl)-2H-tetrazolium (MTS) and phenazine methosulfate, at 37°C, for 3 h. The tetrazolium salt is reduced in the presence of mitochondrial dehydrogenases from the viable cells and generates a colored product. Thus, its quantity measured as optical density at 490 nm is directly proportional to the number of metabolically active cells. The degree of DPSC proliferation in COL-CS-FN composite scaffold was reported to a control of DPSC on the 2D plastic surface. The results showed that, at 48 h of cultivation, cell proliferation was 1.46 times higher than in control and, at 96 h of cultivation, DPSC proliferated 1.62 times more than in control. These data indicated that 3D composite scaffold stimulated DPSC proliferation.

The influence of FN on cell adhesion within DPSC-scaffold constructs can be analyzed using DNA fluorometric assay. The constructs are minced and mixed with a lysis solution of 30 mM saline sodium and 0.2 mg/ml sodium dodecyl sulfate, at 37°C, for 1 h. The mixture is then centrifuged at 13,000 × *g*, for 15 min and the supernatant used to determine the DNA content.

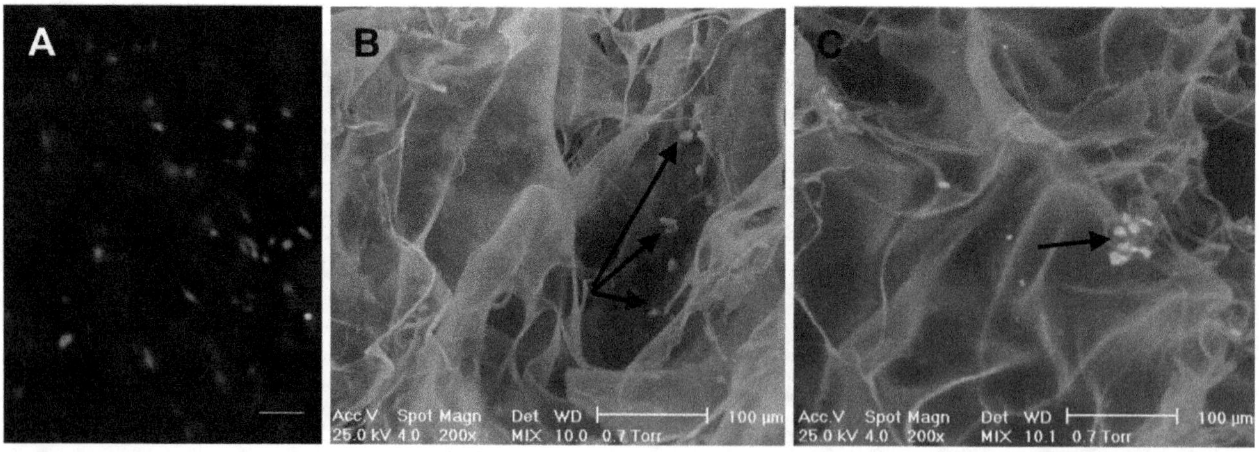

Figure 4. Constructs of DPSC in 3D porous composite scaffold based on collagen, CS and fibronectin in 10:1:10^{-8} (w/w/w) ratio. Fluorescence microscopy showed viable DPSC in biocompatible constructs after 72 h of cultivation in α-MEM (A, bar = 50 μm). Scanning electron micrographs revealed isolated DPSC (B, bar = 100 μm) or cell groups (C, bar = 100 μm) within the composite scaffold.

Briefly, over 10 μl of supernatant, 190 μl of working solution is added, followed by a vortexing step, incubation at room temperature, for 2 min, and the optical density is recorded at a fluorometer for nanoquantities. Taking into account a content of 8 μg DNA/cell [71], the results can be expressed as cell count/scaffold. Statistical analysis using Student's test on control-sample pairs of interest show differences considered significant at $p < 0.05$. The results obtained for DPSC cultivated in COL-CS-FN composite scaffold in standard conditions, for 96 h showed the significantly higher number of DPSC (786,675 ± 23,600 cells/scaffold) than in COL-CS scaffold (718,335 ± 25,100 cells/scaffold). This could be due to FN presence in materials composition and indicated its usefulness for improvement of cell adhesion. FN supports cell adhesion through synergistic action of both integrin-binging regions and N-glycans [72]. Variation of FN concentration and distribution is a topic of interest for cell-scaffold construct fabrication.

Further incubation of DPSC-scaffold constructs in standard conditions indicated that cell adhesion and proliferation decreased, probably as a result of cell migration outside the porous scaffold. Tailoring the pore size of 3D materials by polymer concentration, lyophilization temperature or cross-linking should adjust the adhesion and proliferation of DPSC for longer periods of cultivation.

4.4. Osteogenic properties of DPSC-scaffold construct

Osteogenic differentiation of DPSC is of interest in repairing bone defects, including in dentistry for elderly people with a deficit of stem cells. DPSC-scaffold constructs could serve as biomimetic experimental models, in order to improve the fabrication of dental materials with modified surfaces, and enhanced bioactivity. Individual components of ECM, like type I COL and FN, promote osteogenic differentiation of stem cells, but the process is influenced by environmental culture conditions [73]. COL-CS-FN composite scaffolds injected with DPSC were cultivated in specific osteogenic differentiation medium, for 21 days. Conditioned medium was harvested at 3, 6, 9, and 12 days of cultivation and analyzed for secretion of specific markers, such as alkaline phosphatase, calcium, and type I COL, using specific and sensitive techniques.

MSC are characterized by the low activity of alkaline phosphatase, while its increased activity is an index of cell differentiation into fully functioning osteoblasts. The analysis of alkaline phosphatase activity uses 50 μl supernatant incubated with 7.34 mM p-nitrophenyl phosphate in diethanolamine buffer, pH 9.8, containing 2.58 mM $MgCl_2$, at 37°C, and for 30 min. The reaction is stopped with 1 M NaOH solution and the optical density is recorded at 410 nm using a microplate reader. The alkaline phosphatase activity is calculated using a standard curve of p-nitrophenol and expressed as mM p-nitrophenol/min. For comparable results, the protein concentration of cell supernatants is determined using Bradford method. The results obtained for DPSC in COL-CS-FN scaffolds indicated that alkaline phosphatase activity increased by 4 times in the first 10 days of cultivation in osteogenic medium (**Figure 5**). After another 10 days of cultivation, the enzymatic activity reached 10 times higher values than at 3 days of cultivation. The steep slope of alkaline phosphatase activity profile demonstrated the differentiation of DPSC into osteoblasts within 3D composite scaffolds of COL-CS-FN cultivated in osteogenic differentiation medium.

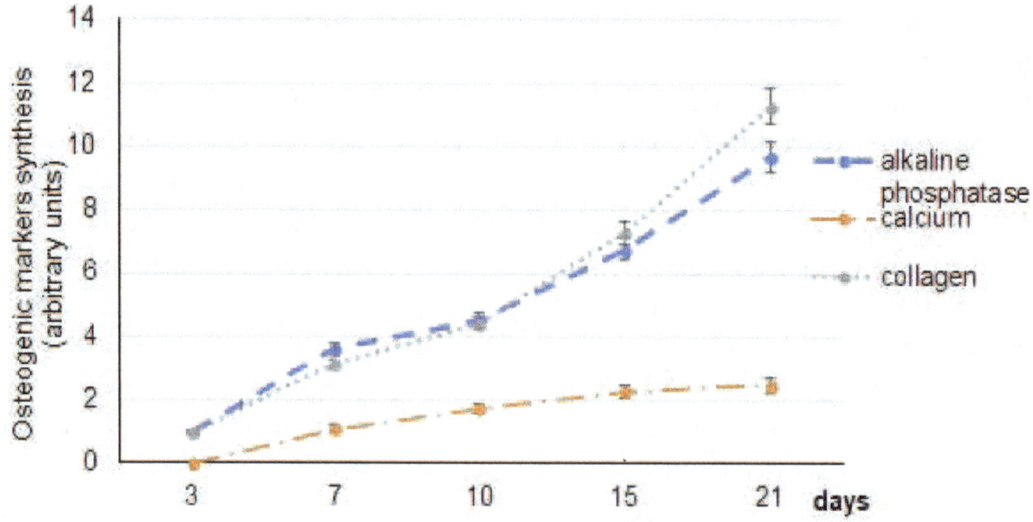

Figure 5. DPSC cultivated within 3D porous composite scaffold based on collagen, CS, and fibronectin in 10:1:10^{-8} (w/w/w) ratios, in the presence of osteogenic induction medium, for 21 days. Increasing quantities of alkaline phosphatase, calcium, and type I collagen showed DPSC differentiation into osteoblasts.

Determination of calcium amount deposited by cells can be performed using a quantification assay kit based on o-cresolphthalein dye reagent, which forms purple stable complexes with calcium ions. Supernatant of culture medium (50 μl) is incubated with 90 μl chromogenic reagent and 60 μl buffer, at room temperature, for 10 min. The optical density is recorded at 575 nm using a microplate reader and final results are expressed as nm calcium/μl. In case of DPSC in COL-CS-FN composite scaffold, the results indicated a rapid increase of calcium secretion in the first 10 days of osteogenic differentiation and, then, the values reached a plateau (**Figure 5**).

An important marker of stem cells differentiation into osteoblasts is type I COL synthesis. To avoid the interference of COL present in composite materials or degraded during incubation in the culture medium, it is recommended to use an antibody that specifically detects the propeptides from the C-terminal end of type I procollagen molecule. These are enzymatically cleaved and released into the medium only during the synthesis of triple helical COL molecule. The amount of type I procollagen secreted is quantified by incubation of 50 μl culture supernatant in 96-wells culture plate pre-coated with a specific monoclonal antibody, at 37°C, for 1 h. After subsequent washing steps, as provided by ELISA protocol, the incubation with peroxidase conjugate polyclonal antibody is performed, followed by substrate addition. Optical density is read at 450 nm using a microplate reader and the results are calculated as ng type I procollagen/ml. The results obtained for DPSC in COL-CS-FN scaffold presented similar variation to that of alkaline phosphatase activity (**Figure 5**). The curve profile of procollagen synthesis increased throughout the entire cultivation period, but higher concentrations of type I procollagen were registered after 10 days of cultivation in osteogenic medium (**Figure 5**).

In conclusion, specific markers of osteoblastic differentiation, alkaline phosphatase, calcium, and type I COL were secreted by DPSC cultivated in direct contact with COL-CS-FN composite materials. This indicates the possible use of these constructs not only as experimental models *in vitro* but as materials with osteogenic effect in periodontal tissue engineering. In addition, the values of all markers were significantly higher ($p < 0.05$) than those obtained in 2D DPSC cultures. The values demonstrated that 3D porous composite materials had a positive effect on calcium secretion and mineralization process useful in bone repair, as well as the capacity of cell-scaffold constructs to improve new extracellular matrix formation.

5. Conclusions

Periodontitis is a very common condition that poses a challenge to oral tissue engineering. Periodontal disease affects all four tissues of the periodontium, namely the gingival tis sue, periodontal ligament, cement and alveolar bone and can be partially treated by clas sic periodontal surgical methods. Specialized therapeutic methods, such as GTR, stem cell therapies, and innovative biomaterials including bioactive molecules, envisage the functional reconstruction of the periodontal complex, and reduction of periodontal disease risk for general health. Stem cells from numerous sources have potential application in periodontal regeneration because they are non-immunogenic, have high proliferation rate and ability to differentiate into the desired cell type. Stem cells from dental pulp are easy to obtain and currently studied in combination with 3D porous biomaterials of certain porosity, mechani_ cal and regenerative properties. Cell culture data demonstrated that COL-CS-FN composite material had the capacity to improve the secretion of osteogenic markers and the synthesis of bone matrix. These studies are important and can provide progress in periodontology, especially for elderly individuals presenting marked decline of healing and regenerative pro cesses. Future researchers envisage multifunctional engineered constructs with antimicrobial, anti-inflammatory, and regenerative activity for use in periodontitis treatment.

Acknowledgements

This work was supported by the Ministry of Research and Innovation, CNCS—UEFISCDI, project No PN-III-P4-ID-PCE-2016-0715 within PNCDI III and National Programme Nucleu No. 30N/18180.

Author details

Ana-Maria Seciu[1], Oana Craciunescu[2*] and Otilia Zarnescu[1]

*Address all correspondence to: oana_craciunescu2009@yahoo.com

1 Faculty of Biology, University of Bucharest, Romania

2 National Institute of Research and Development for Biological Sciences, Bucharest, Romania

References

[1] Han J, Menicanin D, Gronthos S, Bartold PM. Stem cells, tissue engineering and periodontal regeneration. Australian Dental Journal. 2014;**59**(Suppl 1):117-130

[2] Reed D, Diekwisch T. Biological aspects of periodontal repair. In: Vishwakarma A, Sharpe P, Songtao S, Ramalingam M, editors. Stem Cell Biology and Tissue Engineering in Dental Sciences. 1st ed. Academic Press: Elsevier Inc; 2015. pp. 445-458

[3] Dickinson BC, Moffatt CE, Hagerty D, Whitmore SE, Brown TA, Graves DT, Lamont RJ. Interaction of oral bacteria with gingival epithelial cell multilayers. Molecular Oral Microbiology. 2011;**26**:210-220

[4] Glim JE, Everts V, Niessen FB, Ulrich MM, Beelen RH. Extracellular matrix components of oral mucosa differ from skin and resemble that of foetal skin. Archives of Oral Biology. 2014;**59**:1048-1055

[5] Hughes F. Periodontium and periodontal disease. In: Vishwakarma A, Sharpe P, Songtao S, Ramalingam M, editors. Stem Cell Biology and Tissue Engineering in Dental Sciences. 1st ed. Academic Press: Elsevier Inc; 2015. pp. 433-444

[6] Giannobile WV, Riviere GR, Gorski JP, Tira DE, Cobb CM. Glycosaminoglycans and periodontal disease: Analysis of GCF by safranin O. Journal of Periodontology. 1993;**64**: 186-190

[7] Giannobile WV, Lynch SE, Denmark RG, Paquette DW, Fiorellini JP, Williams RC. Crevicular fluid osteocalcin and pyridinoline crosslinked carboxyterminal telopeptide of type I collagen (ICTP) as markers of rapid bone turnover in periodontitis. A pilot study in beagle dogs. Journal of Clinical Periodontology. 1995;**22**:903-910

[8] Jee SW, Wang S, Kapila YL. Specific pro-apoptotic fibronectin fragments modulate proteinase expression in periodontal ligament cells. Journal of Periodontology. 2004;**75**: 523-530

[9] Dai R, Iwama A, Wang S, Kapila YL. Disease-associated fibronectin matrix fragments trigger anoikis of human primary ligament cells: p53 and c-myc are suppressed. Apoptosis. 2005;**10**:503-512

[10] Sorsa T, Tjaderhane L, Konttinen YT, Lauhio A, Salo T, Lee HM, Golub LM, Brown DL, Mantyla P. Matrix metalloproteinases: Contribution to pathogenesis, diagnosis and treatment of periodontal inflammation. Annals of Medicine. 2006;**38**:306-321

[11] Aioub M, Lezot F, Molla M, Castaneda B, Robert B, Goubin G, Nefussi JR, Berdal A. Msx2−/− transgenic mice develop compound amelogenesis imperfecta, dentinogenesis imperfecta and periodental osteopetrosis. Bone. 2007;**41**:851-859

[12] Kawai T, Matsuyama T, Hosokawa Y, Makihira S, Seki M, Karimbux NY, Goncalves RB, Valverde P, Dibart S, Li YP, Miranda LA, Ernst CW, Izumi Y, Taubman MA. B and T lymphocytes are the primary sources of RANKL in the bone resorptive lesion of periodontal disease. American Journal of Pathology. 2006;**169**:987-998

[13] Bostanci N, Ilgenli T, Emingil G, Afacan B, Han B, Toz H, Atilla G, Hughes FJ, Belibasakis GN. Gingival crevicular fluid levels of RANKL and OPG in periodontal diseases: Implications of their relative ratio. Journal of Clinical Periodontology. 2007;**34**:370-376

[14] Kaur S, White S, Bartold PM. Periodontal disease and rheumatoid arthritis: A systematic review. Journal of Dental Research. 2013;**92**:399-408

[15] Chen FM, Sun HH, Lu H, Yu Q. Stem cell-delivery therapeutics for periodontal tissue regeneration. Biomaterials. 2012;**33**:6320-6344

[16] Liu A-Q, Hu C-H, Jin F, Zhang L-S, Xuan K. Contributions of bioactive molecules in stem cell-based periodontal regeneration. International Journal of Molecular Science. 2018;**19**:1016-1030

[17] Dan H, Vaquette C, Fisher AG, Hamlet SM, Xiao Y, Hutmacher DW, Ivanovski S. The influence of cellular source on periodontal regeneration using calcium phosphate coated polycaprolactone scaffold supported cell sheets. Biomaterials. 2014;**35**:113-122

[18] Ivanovski S, Vaquette C, Gronthos S, Hutmacher DW, Bartold PM. Multiphasic scaffolds for periodontal tissue engineering. Journal of Dental Research. 2014;**93**:1212-1221

[19] Shimauchi H, Nemoto E, Ishihata H, Shimomura M. Possible functional scaffolds for periodontal regeneration. Japanese Dental Science Review. 2013;**49**:118-130

[20] Ramseier CA, Rasperini G, Batia S, Giannobile WV. Advanced regenerative technologies for periodontal tissue repair. Periodontology. 2012;**2000, 59**:185-202

[21] Tatakis DN, Promsudthi A, Wikesjo UM. Devices for periodontal regeneration. Periodontology 2000. 1999;**19**:59-73

[22] Behfarnia P, Khorasani MM, Birang R, Abbas FM. Histological and histomorphometric analysis of animal experimental dehiscence defect treated with three bioabsorbable GTR collagen membrane. Dental Research Journal. 2012;**9**:574-581

[23] Parodi R, Carusi G, Santarelli G, Nanni F, Pingitore R, Brunel G. Guided tissue regeneration employing a collagen membrane in a human periodontal bone defect: A histologic evaluation. International Journal of Periodontics and Restorative Dentistry. 1997;**17**:282-291

[24] Shin SY, Rios H, Giannobile W, Oh TJ. Periodontal regeneration: Current therapies. In: Vishwakarma A, Sharpe P, Songtao S, Ramalingam M, editors. Stem Cell Biology and Tissue Engineering in Dental Sciences. 1st ed. Academic Press: Elsevier Inc; 2015. pp. 459-469

[25] Chambrone L, Chambrone D, Lima LA, Chambrone LA. Predictors of tooth loss during long-term periodontal maintenance: A systematic review of observational studies. Journal of Clinical Periodontology. 2010;**37**:675-684

[26] Cortellini P, Tonetti MS. Clinical and radiographic outcomes of the modified minimally invasive surgical technique with and without regenerative materials: A randomized-controlled trial in intra-bony defects. Journal of Clinical Periodontology. 2011;**38**:365-373

[27] Caton J, Bostanci N, Remboutsika E, De Bari C, Mitsiadis TA. Future dentistry: Cell therapy meets tooth and periodontal repair and regeneration. Journal of Cellular and Molecular Medicine. 2011;**15**:1054-1065

[28] Hill MW, Mackenzie IC. The influence of subepithelial connective tissues on epithelial proliferation in the adult mouse. Cell and Tissue Research. 1989;**255**:179-182

[29] Young A, Kingsley K. Dental pulp stem cell: A review of factors that influence the therapeutic potential of stem cell isolates. Biomaterials and Biomedical Engineering. 2015;**2**:61-69

[30] Dominici M, Le Blanc K, Mueller I, Slaper-Cortenbach I, Marini F, Krause D, Deans R, Keating A, Prockop DJ, Horwitz E. Minimal criteria for defining multipotent mesenchymal stromal cells. The International Society for Cellular Therapy position statement. Cytotherapy. 2006;**8**:315-317

[31] Lin NH, Gronthos S, Bartold PM. Stem cells and future periodontal regeneration. Periodontology 2000. 2009;**51**:239-251

[32] Rios HF, Lin Z, Oh B, Park CH, Giannobile WV. Cell- and gene-based therapeutic strategies for periodontal regenerative medicine. Journal of Periodontology. 2011;**82**:1223-1237

[33] Bluteau G, Luder HU, De Bari C, Mitsiadis TA. Stem cells for tooth engineering. European Cells and Materials. 2008;**16**:1-9

[34] Ledesma-Martinez E, Mendoza-Nunez VM, Santiago-Osorio E. Mesenchymal stem cells derived from dental pulp: A review. Stem Cells International. 2016;**2016**:4709572

[35] Verma K, Bains R, Bains VK, Rawtiya M, Loomba K, Srivastava SC. Therapeutic potential of dental pulp stem cells in regenerative medicine: An overview. Dental Research Journal. 2014;**11**:302-308

[36] Sun HH, Jin T, Yu Q, Chen FM. Biological approaches toward dental pulp regeneration by tissue engineering. Journal of Tissue Engineering and Regenerative Medicine. 2011;**5**:e1-e16

[37] Yamada Y, Ito K, Nakamura S, Ueda M, Nagasaka T. Promising cell-based therapy for bone regeneration using stem cells from deciduous teeth, dental pulp, and bone marrow. Cell Transplantation. 2011;**20**:1003-1013

[38] Tatullo M, Marrelli M, Shakesheff KM, White LJ. Dental pulp stem cells: Function, isolation and applications in regenerative medicine. Journal of Tissue Engineering and Regenerative Medicine. 2015;**9**:1205-1216

[39] Neves VCM, Babb R, Chandrasekaran D, Sharpe PT. Promotion of natural tooth repair by small molecule GSK3 antagonists. Scientific Reports. 2017;**7**:39654

[40] D'Aquino R, De Rosa A, Lanza V, Tirino V, Laino L, Graziano A, Desiderio V, Laino G, Papaccio G. Human mandible bone defect repair by the grafting of dental pulp stem/progenitor cells and collagen sponge biocomplexes. European Cells and Materials. 2009;**18**:75-83

[41] Govindasamy V, Ronald VS, Abdullah AN, Ganesan Nathan KR, Aziz ZA, Abdullah M, Zain RB, Kasim NH, Musa S, Bhonde RR. Human platelet lysate permits scale-up of dental pulp stromal cells for clinical applications. Cytotherapy. 2011;**13**:1221-1233

[42] Yan X, Qin H, Qu C, Tuan RS, Shi S, Huang GT. iPS cells reprogrammed from human mesenchymal-like stem/progenitor cells of dental tissue origin. Stem Cells and Development. 2010;**19**:469-480

[43] Duan X, Tu Q, Zhang J, Ye J, Sommer C, Mostoslavsky G, Kaplan D, Yang P, Chen J. Application of induced pluripotent stem (iPS) cells in periodontal tissue regeneration. Journal of Cellular Physiology. 2011;**226**:150-157

[44] Ye JH, Xu YJ, Gao J, Yan SG, Zhao J, Tu Q, Zhang J, Duan XJ, Sommer CA, Mostoslavski G, Kaplan DL, Wu YN, Zhang CP, Wang L, Chen J. Critical-size calvarial bone defects healing in a mouse model with silk scaffolds and SATB2-modified iPSCs. Biomaterials. 2011;**32**:5065-5076

[45] Gronthos S, Mankani M, Brahim J, Robey PG, Shi S. Postnatal human dental pulp stem cells *in vitro* and *in vivo*. Proceedings of the National Academy of Sciences of USA. 2000;**97**:13625-13630

[46] Miura M, Gronthos S, Zhao M, Lu B, Fisher LW, Robey PG, Shi S. SHED: Stem cells from human exfoliated deciduous teeth. Proceedings of the National Academy of Sciences of USA. 2003;**100**:5807-5812

[47] Daltoe FP, Mendonca PP, Mantesso A, Deboni MC. Can SHED or DPSCs be used to repair/regenerate non-dental tissues? A systematic review of *in vivo* studies. Brazilian Oral Research. 2014;**28**:1-7

[48] Alongi DJ, Yamaza T, Song Y, Fouad AF, Romberg EE, Shi S, Tuan RS, Huang R. Stem/progenitor cells from inflamed human dental pulp retain tissue regeneration potential. Regenerative Medicine. 2010;**5**:617-631

[49] Alge DL, Zhou D, Adams LL, Wyss BK, Shadday MD, Woods EJ, Gabriel Chu TM, Goebel WS. Donor-matched comparison of dental pulp stem cells and bone marrow-derived mesenchymal stem cells in a rat model. Journal of Tissue Engineering and Regenerative Medicine. 2010;**4**:73-81

[50] La Noce M, Paino F, Spina A, Naddeo P, Montella R, Desiderio V, De Rosa A, Papaccio G, Tirino V, Laino L. Dental pulp stem cells: State of the art and suggestions for a true translation of research into therapy. Journal of Dentistry. 2014;**42**:761-768

[51] Horibe H, Murakami M, Iohara K, Hayashi Y, Takeuchi N, Takei Y, Kurita K, Nakashima M. Isolation of a stable subpopulation of mobilized dental pulp stem cells with high proliferation, migration, and regeneration potential is independent of age. PLoS One. 2014;**9**:e98553

[52] Kellner M, Steindorff MM, Strempel JF, Winkel A, Kuhnel MP, Stiesch M. Differences of isolated dental stem cells dependent on donor age and consequences for autologous tooth replacement. Archives of Oral Biology. 2014;**59**:559-567

[53] Tranasi M, Sberna MT, Zizzari V, D'Apolito G, Mastrangelo F, Salini L, Stuppia L, Tete S. Microarray evaluation of age-related changes in human dental pulp. Journal of Endodontics. 2009;**35**:1211-1217

[54] Alsulaimani RS, Ajlan SA, Aldahmash AM, Alnabaheen MS, Ashri NY. Isolation of dental pulp stem cells from a single donor and characterization of their ability to differentiate after 2 years of cryopreservation. Saudi Medical Journal. 2016;**37**:551-560

[55] Dulugiac M, Moldovan L, Zarnescu O. Comparative studies of mesenchymal stem cells derived from different cord tissue compartments-the influence of cryopreservation and growth media. Placenta. 2015;**36**:1192-1203

[56] Bonnamain V, Thinard R, Sergent-Tanguy S, Huet P, Bienvenu G, Naveilhan P, Farges JC, Alliot-Licht B. Human dental pulp stem cells cultured in serum-free supplemented medium. Frontiers in Physiology. 2013;**4**:357-363

[57] Lei M, Li K, Li B, Gao LN, Chen FM, Jin Y. Mesenchymal stem cell characteristics of dental pulp and periodontal ligament stem cells after *in vivo* transplantation. Biomaterials. 2014;**35**:6332-6343

[58] Attar A, Eslaminejad M, Tavangar M, Karamzadeh R, Dehghani-Nazhvani A, Ghahramani Y, Malekmohammadi F, Hosseini SM. Dental pulp polyps contain stem cells comparable to the normal dental pulps. Journal of Clinical and Experimental Dentistry. 2014;**6**:e53-e59

[59] Akkouch A, Zhang Z, Rouabhia M. Engineering bone tissue using human dental pulp stem cells and an osteogenic collagen-hydroxyapatite-poly (L-lactide-co-ε-caprolactone) scaffold. Journal of Biomaterials Applications. 2014;**28**:922-936

[60] Graneli C, Thorfve A, Ruetschi U, Brisby H, Thomsen P, Lindahl A, Karlsson C. Novel markers of osteogenic and adipogenic differentiation of human bone marrow stromal cells identified using a quantitative proteomics approach. Stem Cell Research. 2014;**12**:153-165

[61] Kiernan J. Histological and Histochemical Methods: Theory and Practice. 4th ed. Oxfordshire: Cold Spring Harbor Laboratory Press; 2008. 606 p

[62] Yi Q, Liu O, Yan F, Lin X, Diao S, Wang L, Jin L, Wang S, Lu Y, Fan Z. Analysis of senescence-related differentiation potentials and gene expression profiles in human dental pulp stem cells. Cells, Tissues, Organs. 2017;**203**:1-11

[63] Amer MH, Rose FRAJ, Shakesheff KM, White LJ. A biomaterials approach to influence stem cell fate in injectable cell-based therapies. Stem Cell Research and Therapy. 2018;**9**:39-54

[64] Fisher OZ, Khademhosseini A, Langer R, Peppas NA. Bioinspired materials for controlling stem cell fate. Accounts of Chemical Research. 2010;**43**:419-428

[65] Scheller EL, Krebsbach PH, Kohn DH. Tissue engineering: State of the art in oral rehabilitation. Journal of Oral Rehabilitation. 2009;**36**:368-389

[66] Vaquette C, Fan W, Xiao Y, Hamlet S, Hutmacher DW, Ivanovski S. A biphasic scaffold design combined with cell sheet technology for simultaneous regeneration of alveolar bone/periodontal ligament complex. Biomaterials. 2012;**33**:5560-5573

[67] Costa PF, Vaquette C, Zhang Q, Reis RL, Ivanovski S, Hutmacher DW. Advanced tissue engineering scaffold design for regeneration of the complex hierarchical periodontal structure. Journal of Clinical Periodontology. 2014;**41**:283-294

[68] Kim JH, Park CH, Perez RA, Lee HY, Jang JH, Lee HH, Wall IB, Shi S, Kim HW. Advanced biomatrix designs for regenerative therapy of periodontal tissues. Journal of Dental Research. 2014;**93**:1203-1211

[69] Ito K, Yamada Y, Nakamura S, Ueda M. Osteogenic potential of effective bone engineering using dental pulp stem cells, bone marrow stem cells, and periosteal cells for osseointegration of dental implants. International Journal of Oral and Maxillofacial Implants. 2011;**26**:947-954

[70] Craciunescu O, Moldovan L. Designing bio-inspired composite materials for medical applications. In: Cuppoletti J, editor. Nanocomposites and Polymers with Analytical Methods. 1st ed. Rijeka: Intech; 2011. pp. 309-334

[71] Ahlfors JEW, Billiar KL. Biomechanical and biochemical characteristics of a human fibroblast-produced and remodeled matrix. Biomaterials. 2007;**28**:2183-2191

[72] Hsiao C-T, Cheng H-W, Huang C-M, Li H-R, Ou M-H, Huang J-R, Khoo K-H, Yu HW, Chen Y-Q, Wang Y-K, Chiou A, Kuo J-C. Fibronectin in cell adhesion and migration via N-glycosylation. Oncotarget. 2017;**8**:70653-70668

[73] Linsley C, Wu B, Tawil B. The effect of fibrinogen, collagen type I, and fibronectin on mesenchymal stem cell growth and differentiation into osteoblasts. Tissue Engineering Part A. 2013;**19**:1416-1423

Permissions

All chapters in this book were first published in PDI, by InTech Open; hereby published with permission under the Creative Commons Attribution License or equivalent. Every chapter published in this book has been scrutinized by our experts. Their significance has been extensively debated. The topics covered herein carry significant findings which will fuel the growth of the discipline. They may even be implemented as practical applications or may be referred to as a beginning point for another development.

The contributors of this book come from diverse backgrounds, making this book a truly international effort. This book will bring forth new frontiers with its revolutionizing research information and detailed analysis of the nascent developments around the world.

We would like to thank all the contributing authors for lending their expertise to make the book truly unique. They have played a crucial role in the development of this book. Without their invaluable contributions this book wouldn't have been possible. They have made vital efforts to compile up to date information on the varied aspects of this subject to make this book a valuable addition to the collection of many professionals and students.

This book was conceptualized with the vision of imparting up-to-date information and advanced data in this field. To ensure the same, a matchless editorial board was set up. Every individual on the board went through rigorous rounds of assessment to prove their worth. After which they invested a large part of their time researching and compiling the most relevant data for our readers.

The editorial board has been involved in producing this book since its inception. They have spent rigorous hours researching and exploring the diverse topics which have resulted in the successful publishing of this book. They have passed on their knowledge of decades through this book. To expedite this challenging task, the publisher supported the team at every step. A small team of assistant editors was also appointed to further simplify the editing procedure and attain best results for the readers.

Apart from the editorial board, the designing team has also invested a significant amount of their time in understanding the subject and creating the most relevant covers. They scrutinized every image to scout for the most suitable representation of the subject and create an appropriate cover for the book.

The publishing team has been an ardent support to the editorial, designing and production team. Their endless efforts to recruit the best for this project, has resulted in the accomplishment of this book. They are a veteran in the field of academics and their pool of knowledge is as vast as their experience in printing. Their expertise and guidance has proved useful at every step. Their uncompromising quality standards have made this book an exceptional effort. Their encouragement from time to time has been an inspiration for everyone.

The publisher and the editorial board hope that this book will prove to be a valuable piece of knowledge for researchers, students, practitioners and scholars across the globe.

List of Contributors

Apoorv Goel, Lester Jack Windsor and Steven Blanchard
Indiana University School of Dentistry, Indianapolis, USA

Aysan Lektemur Alpan
Faculty of Dentistry, Department of Periodontology, Pamukkale University, Denizli, Turkey

Kai Ling Siew, Esmonde Francis Corbet and Wai Keung Leung
Faculty of Dentistry, The University of Hong Kong, Hong Kong SAR, China

Chui Ling Goo
Faculty of Dentistry, The National University of Malaysia, Malaysia

Victor Goh
Faculty of Dentistry, The University of Hong Kong, Hong Kong SAR, China
Faculty of Dentistry, The National University of Malaysia, Malaysia

David G. Gillam
Centre for Oral Bioengineering, Institute of Dentistry, Barts and the London School of Medicine and Dentistry QMUL, London, UK

Dominiki Chatzopoulou
Oral Immunobiology and Regenerative Medicine, Institute of Dentistry, Barts and the London School of Medicine and Dentistry QMUL, London, UK

Oleh Andrukhov, Christian Behm, Alice Blufstein and Xiaohui Rausch-Fan
Division of Conservative Dentistry and Periodontology, University Clinic of Dentistry Medical University of Vienna, Austria

Mônica Fernandes Gomes, Andrea Carvalho De Marco, Lilian Chrystiane and Miguel Angel Castillo Salgado
Center of Biosciences Applied to Patients with Special Health Care Needs (CEBAPE)
Institute of Science and Technology, UNESP, São José dos Campos, São Paulo, Brazil

Lilian Chrystiane Giannasi
Center of Biosciences Applied to Patients with Special Health Care Needs (CEBAPE), Institute of Science and Technology, UNESP, São José dos Campos, São Paulo, Brazil
Metropolitan University of Santos, UNIMES, Santos, São Paulo, Brazi
Universitary Center of Anápolis, UniEVANGÉLICA, Anápolis, Goiás, Brazil

Hiroyasu Endo and Takanori Ito
Department of Oral Diagnosis, School of Dentistry at Matsudo, Nihon University, Japan

Terry D. Rees
Department of Periodontics, Texas A&M College of Dentistry, Dallas, TX, USA

Hideo Niwa
Department of Head and Neck Surgery, School of Dentistry at Matsudo, Nihon University,

Kayo Kuyama
Department of Oral Pathology, School of Dentistry at Matsudo, Nihon University, Japan

Maya Oshima, Tae Serizawa, Shigeo Tanaka and Masamichi Komiya
Department of Oral Surgery, School of Dentistry at Matsudo, Nihon University, Japan

Morio Iijima
Department of Removable Prosthodontics, School of Dentistry at Matsudo, Nihon University, Japan

Fardad Shakibaie and Laurence Walsh
School of Dentistry, The University of Queensland, Brisbane, Australia

Krishna Kripal
Rajarajeswari Dental College and Hospital, Bangalore, India

Kavita Chandrasekaran
Department of Periodontology, Rajarajeswari Dental College and Hospital, Bangalore, India

Rina Muraoka and Hirokazu Matsuda
Matsumoto Dental University School of Dentistry and Hospital, Shiojiri, Japan

Keisuke Nakano
Okayama University Graduate School of Medicine, Dentistry and Pharmaceutical Sciences

Hidetsugu Tsujigiwa
Faculty of Science, Okayama University of Science, Okayama, Japan

Ana-Maria Seciu and Otilia Zarnescu
Faculty of Biology, University of Bucharest, Romania

Mihoko Tomida, Norimasa Okafuji and Kazuhiro Yamada
Matsumoto Dental University School of Dentistry and Hospital, Shiojiri, Japan
Matsumoto Dental University Graduate School of Oral Medicine, Shiojiri, Japan

Toshiyuki Kawakami
Matsumoto Dental University Graduate School of Oral Medicine, Shiojiri, Japan

Oana Craciunescu
National Institute of Research and Development for Biological Sciences, Bucharest, Romania

Index

www.ingramcontent.com/pod-product-compliance
Lightning Source LLC
LaVergne TN
LVHW081020210926
848485LV00004B/907